THE CANCER BREAKTHROUGH YOU'VE NEVER HEARD OF

YOUR GUIDE TO LIMITED SURGERY
IN THE TREATMENT OF CANCER

THE CANCER BREAKTHROUGH YOU'VE NEVER HEARD OF

YOUR GUIDE TO LIMITED SURGERY
IN THE TREATMENT OF CANCER

Richard A. Evans, MD

Texas Cancer Center
Houston, Texas

Printer: Paragon Press, Honesdale, PA
Cover Photo: Alexanders/Houston
Charts on pages 103 and 104 from *CA: Cancer Journal for Clinicians*, January/February 2001, Vol. 51, No. 1, pp. 27-28. Reprinted by permission of J.B. Lippincott Co., Philadelphia, PA

Cataloging-in-Publication Data

Evans, Richard A.
    The cancer breakthrough you've never heard of/ Richard A. Evans

ISBN 0-9708664-0-2

Library of Congress Control Number: 2001090805

    1. Cancer----Surgery. I. Title

RD651.E93 2001   616.99'4
                            QBI01-200676

Copyright © 2000 by Richard A. Evans, M.D.

All right reserved. No part of this publication may be reproduced, stored in a retrieval system, or transmitted, in any form or by any means, electronic, mechanical, photocopying, recording or otherwise, without the prior written permission of the copyright owner.

Printed in the United States of America

10 9 8 7 6 5 4 3 2

For copyright permission or quantity discounts please contact the Texas Cancer Center, 1011 Augusta Dr. Suite 210, Houston, Texas 77057, 713-975-6270.

Contents

Preface to the Revised Addition, i
Acknowledgments, ix
Preface, xi
Introduction, 1

Part One   Understanding Cancer

1. The History of Cancer Surgery,   13
2. The Behavior of Cancer,   34
3. The Defense Against Cancer,   57
4. The Seed and the Soil,   71

Part Two   Treating Cancer

5. Principles of Treatment,   83
6. Bladder Cancer, 112
7. Breast Cancer, 123
8. Cancer of the Cervix,   139
9. Malignant Melanoma,   151
10. Cancer of the Penis,   161
11. Prostate Cancer,   168
12. Cancer of the Rectum,   187
13. Soft Tissue Sarcoma,   202
14. Cancer of the Vagina,   211
15. Cancer of the Vulva,   218
16. Barriers to Change,   227
17. Conclusion and Ten Questions to Ask Your Doctor,   237

Appendix I.   Selected Studies in Conservative Surgery,   245

Appendix II.   Selected Studies in Conservative Surgery (1995 - 2001),   285

Notes   310

Notes II,   329

Glossary,   337

Index,   355

The Last Word,   367

Order Form,   371

About the Author,   373

Suggested Reading,   375

I wish to dedicate this book with love to my parents
Betty Timmerman Evans
and
Samuel Rostron Evans

Preface to the Revised Addition

In 1995, this book was published under the title *Making the Right Choice: Treatment Options in Cancer Surgery*. I decided to change the name of the book to draw greater attention to a major change that has occurred in our understanding of cancer. Over the past ten to fifteen years academic surgeons and research scientists have made an important discovery. Following limited surgery, cancer which reappears locally does not spread! *This is the cancer breakthrough you've never heard of.* It is explained in different ways and repeated in almost every chapter throughout this book. This breakthrough is important, because it greatly diminishes the need for radical surgery in the treatment of early, curable cancer. But, this important breakthrough continues to be underrated, ignored or even disputed by many practicing cancer specialists. They remain intellectually and emotionally committed to the principles of radical surgery and aggressive cancer treatment. This results in unnecessary suffering - physical, emotional, and financial - for many patients with cancer.

For decades surgeons have relied upon radical surgery to remove every last cancer cell. (Sometimes radiation therapy has been added to complete the job.) They have believed that if one cell were left behind after surgery, that cell could become a deadly threat. It might grow into a new tumor - a local recurrence. Surgeons and radiation therapists have thought that this recurrence could spread to other parts of the body (metastasize) and eventually take the life of the patient. Scientific research has proven that this is incorrect. We now know that promptly-treated cancer which recurs locally following conservative surgery is not life threatening. *Again, this is the cancer breakthrough you've never heard of.*

But, many cancer specialists, especially surgeons and radiation therapists, continue to embrace the old ideas about cancer. They are caught in a paradigm shift, unable to accept the great change that is occurring in our understanding of cancer.

A SECOND MISTAKE

These same cancer specialists make a second mistake. They erect invisible barriers which prevent patients from learning about the success of conservative treatment. They give lip service to the benefits of a second opinion, but insure that most patients hear only a narrow range of treatment options. All patient who seek a second opinion, should obtain that opinion from an *advocate* of the competing point of view.

THE NEW ENGLAND JOURNAL OF MEDICINE

Even the prestigious *New England Journal of Medicine* has published guest editorials containing erroneous information on this subject. In 1995, Dr. I. Craig Henderson of the University of California, San Francisco, said,"Local failure is a particularly difficult consequence of therapy for most patients because it is readily apparent and is thus a constant reminder that the tumor is no longer curable."[1] I wrote a letter-to-the-editor stating, "This is incorrect."[2] Henderson acknowledged his error:"If the new cancer is of the same stage or a lower one than the original cancer the patient's prognosis remains largely unchanged."

In 1998, Dr. Samuel Hellman of the University of Chicago said, "... local recurrence often leads to distant metastases that are likely eventually to decrease overall survival."[3] In a letter-to-the-editor I said that I was surprised that Hellman would make an inaccurate statement on such an important subject.[4] I continued that I was even more surprised that the *New England Journal of Medicine* would again publish this erroneous idea. Hellman did not retract his assertion and tried to support it with studies of women with advanced cancer, who had been treated with radical surgery. He ignored the many studies of women with early cancer, treated with conservative surgery. (See page 250.) My letter in the *New England Journal of Medicine* continued, "At this rate, it is going to be many years indeed before American physicians have a clear understanding of the often-innocent behavior of locally recurrent breast cancer after limited surgery."

Radiation therapy may provide a minute survival advantage for a few patients with moderately advanced disease. But, this benefit is overshadowed by its failure to prolong the lives of patients with early breast cancer.

ADDITIONS TO THIS BOOK

Since 1995, additional medical research has been published about all of the cancers discussed in this book. All of the research evidence supports the principles outlined in this book. This new medical research is summarized in Appendix II. I have found no studies which conflict with the principles of conservative surgery described here.

The chapter on prostate cancer was completely revised. I devote more attention to several forms of conservative treatment which are challenging radical surgery and external beam radiation therapy (cobalt). Radiation seed implants, hormonal therapy and cryosurgery are among these effective treatment options. While aggressive treatment causes permanent impotence in most patients, conservative treatment is much less likely to do so. Less aggressive treatment has been practiced for many years, but, even now, relatively little has been published in the medical literature. Radical prostatectomy and external beam radiation continue to be the dominant forms of treatment in U.S. medical centers. Men may have difficulty finding physicians who can effectively champion these newer, less aggressive forms of treatment.

THE EVIDENCE

By late 1976, I had read over sixty articles on breast-sparing surgery for breast cancer. These studies came from dozens of institutions in North American and Europe. They all involved some type of lumpectomy with or without radiation therapy. The studies involved over a thousand patients treated over a span of many decades - beginning in the 1920's. Overall patient survival was a principle focus of these studies. Every article I read carried a single message: breast-sparing surgery is effective treatment for breast cancer. Conservatively treated patients seemed to live just as long as those treated with radical surgery. Yet in the United States a woman with breast cancer could have obtained two opinions or two dozen opinions. Unless she went to Houston to see surgeon John Stehlin or radiation therapist Eleanor Montague, or unless she went to Cleveland to see surgeon George Chile, she was going to have a mastectomy, in spite of the enormous body of evidence to the contrary.

American surgeons were ignoring the scientific evidence supporting limited surgery. They were loathe to break from the tradition of radical surgery which dominated the thinking and practice of 20th century surgeons.

MY CONTRIBUTIONS

In the late 1970's I found several studies which suggested that locally recurrent breast cancer which followed limited surgery was not a threat to survival. In 1980, I published an explanation for the innocent behavior of locally recurrent cancer.[5] This explanation is explained in chapters 3 and 4 of this book. It remains as sound today as it was in 1980.

Since 1980, I have published over 50 letters-to-the-editor and original articles. (See my curriculum vitae on our web site: www.texascancercenter.com) I have frequently suggested that the lessons we have already learned from breast cancer apply to most, if not all, other malignancies. No one has successfully refuted this suggestion. Many surgeons have written favorably about my work. These comments are summarized in my curriculum vitae on our web site.

Leading cancer surgeons are still baffled by the results of some of their own research. In 1996, Intergroup Melanoma Trial published the results of a randomized trial of 740 patients with localized melanoma, 1.0 to 4.0 mm thick.[6] Half of the patients received an elective lymph node dissection (ELND), when the melanoma was removed. The other patients had their lymph nodes left intact. If the lymph nodes later became enlarged with cancer cells, they were removed. The primary patients to benefit from an ELND were those with thin lesions, 1.0 - 2.0 mm. This was surprising, because these patients were the *least* likely to have positive regional lymph nodes. Why did ELND benefit those patients least likely to have positive lymph nodes? The authors of this study offered no explanation for their surprising results. My explanation can be found on page 258. My explanation has been repeatedly published in the medical literature.[7,8,9,10,11,12,13] It remains the only explanation of this surprising observation. It has never been refuted. (It is also published on our web site, www.texascancercenter.com, under the section: Treatment Options/Melanoma/Medical Mysteries. In this book see Appendix II, malignant melanoma.).

OTHER CANCERS

The success of limited surgery has now been well documented, using the most accurate form of clinical research - randomized, prospective trials. This is true for malignant melanoma, the soft tissue sarcomas, and cancer of the bladder, breast, and rectum. Many physicians have found conservative treatment to be successful for other malignancies, as well. Dr. Daniel Dargent of Lyons, France, has now treated over 50 patients with cancer of the cervix using local excision. Doctors in California are treating prostate cancer with treatment which preserves potency in many patients. Dr. Israel Barken of San Diego has controlled prostate cancer in patients using cryosurgery which usually spares the nerves which control erection. Drs. Stephen Strum and Bob Leibowitz of Los Angeles have successfully treated hundreds of men with hormonal therapy. In the U.S. how many patients with cancer of the cervix or prostate are aware of these conservative forms of treatment?

THE TEXAS CANCER CENTER

In 1998, I helped establish the Texas Cancer Center, a 501 (c) (3) nonprofit organization, dedicated to educating cancer patients about their full range of prudent treatment options. All proceeds from the sale of this book benefit the Texas Cancer Center. We established a web site, www.texascancercenter.com. Much of the information in this book has been published on the site, including the names of our board members: Bob Camp, CPA, Peter D. de Ipolyi, M.D., Samuel R. Evans, Robert Farrell, Henry Groppe, Jr., G. Riley Hetherington, Alberto A. J. Maillard, M.D., Joe Reynolds, and Gray Wakefield.

We intend to update our site as additional medical research is published. These additions can be found under the sections called "New Medical Research." We also intend to offer this book on the Internet as an e-book at www.cancerebook.com. We also offer a consultation service through our web site. Our mission is to ensure that all patients facing treatment for cancer have access to the information they need in order to choose the treatment that is right for them. We hope that this book helps patients, their families and loved ones to achieve this goal.

Joe Reynolds is a lawyer, who has studied cancer as if he were preparing for trial. For a few months he became a "world authority" on DCIS (ductal carcinoma in situ) when he needed to help a family member make important decisions about treatment. For years Henry Groppe has supported Dr. Dean Ornish and his belief that low fat diets can reverse coronary artery disease. Henry has promoted the use of biofeedback to treat drug and alcohol addiction. He has recognized the importance of ideas that were once dismissed by recognized medical "authorities." Henry has learned that established "belief systems" can hold great power within any profession - power that can interfere with real progress.

Riley Hetherington is a lawyer and a master behind the podium. Riley understands what Ogden Nash had in mind when he said: "We're making great progress, but we're going in the wrong direction." Robert Farrell has been a friend since childhood. Cancer has touched his life and inspired him to help others to learn and to conquer.

Dr. Al Maillard is a head and neck surgeon. We have been friends for over 25 years. We have spent countless hours discussing the ideas in this book. Gray Wakefield has a passion for service to others. His accounting skills and experience with non-profit organizations have been of great help to the Texas Cancer Center. Bob Camp has been my accountant and friend for twenty years.

I am, of course, indebted to Sam Evans, my father. He has been a life long source of encouragement; a man who looks for the good in both people and the challenges of life. He is a man of great integrity, an inspiration to his family, a model for all who know him, and a man who walks humbly with his Lord..

Since 1985, Karl Virtue has been my friend through First United Methodist - Houston. He has helped me with fund raising activities in many organizations.

I am grateful for the support and friendship of Dr. Ralph Moss. His book, *The Cancer Industry,* inspired my first call to him over ten years ago. That call lasted over an hour and it's been that way ever since. Ralph has spent his entire professional career studying alternative medicine and is an independent and objective source of information. He provides a consultation service on his web site www.cancerdecisions.com. Ralph was a house guest when he came to Houston and helped us launch the Texas Cancer Center in 1998.

I appreciate the wise counsel and friendship of Dr. Israel Barken. He was also a house guest when he came to speak before the Rotary Club of Houston. I am also grateful to the countless family members and friends who have been of support throughout this long mission - to tell cancer patients what the best cancer doctors know about their disease.

> Richard A. Evans, M.D.
> Houston, Texas
> February 14, 2001

1. Henderson IC. Paradigmatic shifts in the management of breast cancer. N Engl J Med 332:951-952, 1995.
2. Evans RA. Adjuvant chemotherapy in breast cancer. N Engl J Med 333;596-597, 1995. (letter)
3. Hellman S. Stopping metastases at their source. N Engl J Med 337:996-997, 1997.
4. Evans RA. Radiation therapy and chemotherapy in high-risk beast cancer. N Engl J Med 338:331, 1998. (letter)
5. Evans RA. Host resistance to carcinoma of the breast. South Med J 73:1261-1263, 1980.
6. Balch CM, Soong S-J, Bartolucci AA, and others. Efficacy of an elective regional lymph node dissection of 1 to 4 mm thick melanomas for patients 60 years of age and younger. Ann Surg 224:255-266, 1996.
7. Evans RA. Elective lymph node dissection for clinical stage I malignant melanoma. J Surg Oncol 57:31-2, 1994. (letter)
8. Evans RA. Review and current perspectives of cutaneous malignant melanoma. J Am Coll Surg 179:764-767, 1994. (letter)
9. Evans RA. Elective lymph node dissection for malignant melanoma: the tumor burden of nodal disease. Anticancer Res 15:575-80, 1995.
10. Evans RA. Elective lymph node dissection (ELND) for malignant melanoma. Ann Surg 221:435-6, 1995. (letter)
11. Evans RA. Malignant melanoma: primary surgical management (excision and node dissection) based upon pathology and staging. Cancer 76:2384-5, 1995.(letter)
12. Evans RA. Melanoma recurrence surveillance: Patient or physician based? Ann Surg 223:445-6, 1996. (letter)
13. Evans RA. Recent advances in the care of the patient with malignant melanoma. Ann Surg 227:607-8, 1998. (letter)

Acknowledgments

I am indebted to the members of the Department of Physiology at Tulane Medical School, who kindled my interest in immunology and encouraged me to pursue graduate work in that field: the late Drs. Nicholas DiLuzio and W. Cliff Newman, and Drs. Joseph Pisano and Cliff Crafton. Cliff and I spent hundreds of hours talking about immunology's puzzles. Dr. DiLuzio would tell his students, "As a physician you can only treat one patient at a time. As a scientist you can benefit the whole world with what you discover." Dr. John McDonald, now Chairman of the Department of Surgery at Louisiana State University—Shreveport, introduced me to the exciting field of organ transplantation.

I thank Dr. Halsted Holman of the Department of Medicine, Stanford Medical School, for giving me an opportunity to do research in his lab. At that time I met Dr. Randy Morris, then a medical student and now Director of the Transplantation Immunology Laboratory at Stanford. I taught Randy everything I knew about immunology in a few hours. He is still teaching me.

I also wish to thank Dr. John Stehlin, Jr., and Dr. Peter de Ipolyi, who introduced me to the field of surgical oncology. My interest in conservative surgery for cancer was sparked by John Stehlin's pioneering work in breast cancer. Dr. Stehlin began performing breast-sparing surgery in 1970. I also thank the late Dr. George Crile, Jr. I visited Dr. Crile and his wife, Helga Sandburg Crile, twice in their home in Cleveland. In 1979, I sat in his living room reading a manuscript he was about to publish. I was excited to see his excellent results with breast-sparing surgery. (Most of his patients had no radiation therapy.) Dr. Crile read my paper, which was about to be published in the *Southern Medical Journal*. He pointed to one sentence: "For instance, a patient who survives a carcinoma of 2 to 3 cm in diameter without developing distant metastases may be expected to survive a similar volume of tumor in adjacent breast or lymphatic tissue." He said, "This is the way I have felt about breast cancer all of my life." His son-in-law and daughter, Dr. Caldwell and Mrs. Ann Esselstyn, were also gracious hosts. Dr. Esselstyn practices surgery at the Cleveland Clinic.

I thank the supporters and staff of the Houston Academy of Medicine/Texas Medical Center Library. This invaluable resource made this work possible.

There are countless physicians, surgeons, immunologists, and scientists who have been supportive of this work. I particularly wish to thank those gynecologists and urologists who reviewed chapters pertaining to tumors outside of my field. They helped greatly to improve the accuracy of these chapters. The treatment recommendations presented here are my own. Review of these chapters does not constitute an endorsement of the recommendations presented here.

The gynecologists were: Dr. Neville F. Hacker, Royal Hospital for Women, Paddington, Australia; Dr. Joseph L. Kelly, University of Pittsburgh School of Medicine, Pittsburgh, Pennsylvania; Dr. Peter E. Schwartz, Yale University School of Medicine, New Haven, Connecticut; and Dr. Erich Burghardt, University of Graz, Graz, Austria. The urologists were: Dr. Edward M. Blight, Jr., Loma Linda University School of Medicine, Loma Linda, California; Dr. Jan-Erik Johansson, Örebro Medical Center Hospital, Örebro, Sweden; Dr. Joseph N. Macaluso, Jr., Urologic Institute of New Orleans, New Orleans, Louisiana; Dr. Thomas A. Stamey, Stanford University School of Medicine, Stanford, California; and Dr. W. Bedford Waters, Loyola University School of Medicine, Chicago, Illinois.

I wish to thank my agent, Mike Doran of the Southern Literary Agency. Mike struggled with lengthy manuscripts more suited for a medical audience and converted them into plain English. He came to understand and believe in my message. I wish to thank Rudy Shur, the Managing Editor of the Avery Publishing Group, who refined the message and agreed to put up with another doctor learning how to write. He provided the professional experience needed to bring this book to you. I also thank Lisa James for her excellent editorial assistance.

Preface

If a man will begin with certainties, he shall end in doubts; but, if he will be content to begin with doubts he shall end in certainties.

Francis Bacon, 1605

This book has been written for people who have been diagnosed with cancer, and for the people who care for them. In it, I explain why I believe that conservative surgery—surgery that tries to preserve bodily form and function by removing as little tissue as possible—is a good option for some cancer patients. But before I can explain how to use this book, I have to explain how I came to believe in conservative surgery, because I want you to understand the principles on which my beliefs are based.

MY EXPERIENCE WITH IMMUNOLOGY AND CANCER TREATMENT

I became interested in immunology when I was a sophomore at the Tulane University School of Medicine in the late 1960s. While working in the Department of Physiology, under the late Dr. Nicholas DiLuzio, I was captured by the potential of this emerging field of science. The control of transplantation rejection and the cure of cancer were two of immunology's powerful lures. I learned that laboratory research was a slow process. Each productive experiment was preceded by a dozen that failed. Failures were due to mistakes in technique, to errors in the experimental design, and to errors in our most recent scientific ideas. Scientists had to be adaptable: ready to correct mistakes, ready to design new experiments, ready to change their ideas.

My own laboratory work in the medical schools at Tulane

and Stanford led to no great discoveries, though I was surrounded by them much of the time. I did learn that immunologists, like most scientists, walk on marbles long before their feet touch solid ground. I learned that progress was made as scientists exchanged ideas, argued, and changed their theories, always steering toward a clearer view of the truth. Science was fun, like solving a puzzle.

In 1971, I received an M.S. degree in physiology and immunology and an M.D. from Tulane, and by the late 1970s, I was completing my training in general surgery in Houston. Surgeons seemed to work by a rigid set of rules meant to be heeded, but seldom questioned. Cancer surgeons relied upon ideas that had been passed down for almost a century. The number one rule of cancer surgery was to remove every single cancer cell, and every cell that may become cancerous. This was called radical surgery. (This book uses the phrase conservative surgery to mean the opposite of radical surgery. This somewhat confusing terminology is discussed in the Introduction.) Radical surgery was considered necessary in order to control the disease and ultimately cure the patient. Though this sounded reasonable, its functional and cosmetic consequences were sometimes devastating.

Radical surgery included the following operations: radical mastectomy (removal of the breast, nearby lymph nodes, and chest muscles), cystectomy (removal of the bladder), hysterectomy, and amputation of an extremity. The complications of radical surgery depended upon the location of the cancer, but they included permanent colostomy, impotence, and infertility. In spite of the overwhelming consequences of their treatment, cancer surgeons had resisted change for decades. Their ideas about cancer surgery were untouchable.

This seemed to be in sharp contrast with the scientists I knew, who lived in a world that thrived upon change. Progress was measured by change—an increase in knowledge. Among scientists, ideas were exchanged and challenged in the quest for understanding. Without change, progress was impossible. Among cancer surgeons, the challenge of sacred ideas often led to personal antagonism. Surgeons and scientists seemed to view change from opposing points of view.

I have since learned that surgeons and scientists are not fundamentally different. The two fields were simply in different phases of development. Immunology was a new field, and scientists were collecting information. General principles were just forming. The field of cancer surgery had been established a hundred years earlier. Its principles were well established—as I came to learn, too well established.

MY INTRODUCTION TO CONSERVATIVE SURGERY

Fortunately, I met two physicians who were challenging the prevailing ideas: Dr. John Stehlin, Jr., a cancer surgeon at St. Joseph Hospital in Houston, and Dr. Eleanor Montague, a radiation therapist at M. D. Anderson Hospital, also in Houston. They were both treating breast cancer with techniques that saved a woman's breast through removal of the tumor followed by radiation therapy. They had studied the experience of dozens of doctors, primarily in Europe, who had treated hundreds of patients using breast-sparing techniques. They didn't know the answers to all the questions about breast-sparing surgery, but they knew the questions that needed to be asked. They understood the limits of their own knowledge and had a clear idea of how to learn more. Dr. Stehlin had started a cancer research lab in which human tumors could be grown and studied in mice. He was also a pioneer in the treatment of malignant melanoma and was one of the first to successfully use heat in the treatment of advanced cancer. Dr. Montague had a clear idea of what surgery and radiation treatment could and could not accomplish. She struggled to explain the baffling results of breast cancer research. (She could also pepper her colleagues with facts and insight, which left many of us begging for mercy.) It seemed clear to me that Dr. Stehlin and Dr. Montague were on the leading edge of a great change in cancer treatment.

Dr. George Crile, Jr., of the Cleveland Clinic was the other strong advocate of breast-sparing procedures in this country. His campaign had begun in the 1950s, and his great contributions are discussed in Chapter 1 and elsewhere.

In the late 1950s, a group called the National Surgical Adjuvant Breast Project (NSABP) began to coordinate the work of dozens of medical schools in the United States and Canada. These investigators studied many aspects of breast cancer treatment and helped make breast cancer one of the most thoroughly studied of all cancers, perhaps the most thoroughly studied. By the late 1970s, the NSABP was beginning to challenge traditional ideas about cancer surgery. The results of one of its studies were just being released, and the conclusions were intriguing.

In some patients with breast cancer, a few tumor cells spread to the lymph nodes in the armpit (the axillary lymph nodes). This NSABP study concluded that these patients could wait until these nodes became enlarged with tumor cells before the nodes had to be removed. Patients with breast cancer could be followed for several months with tumor cells growing in their lymph nodes. Delayed treatment did not impair survival. (The details of this study are presented in Chapter 1.)

This surprising observation seemed to contradict the number one principle of cancer surgery, namely, the prompt removal of every cancer cell. Could cancer surgeons prudently perform an incomplete cancer operation? Could they really remove the cancerous mass in the breast, but leave microscopic cancer cells behind in the lymph nodes? This was the first scientific study to reach this startling conclusion. (Dr. Crile had reached a similar conclusion in the 1960s based upon his own clinical experience.)

When I asked my teachers in surgery about this puzzling study, I received this answer: "We remove the lymph nodes to see if they have cancer in them, which helps us decide if chemotherapy is needed." Chemotherapy is often prescribed for patients whose cancer has spread to their lymph nodes. Yes, that was a good reason to remove the nodes. But it did not explain why patients did so well if cancer-containing nodes were allowed to remain in the patient. "Why?" I asked. There was no reply. This study never attracted much attention among practicing surgeons, because it did not alter their surgical practice. Axillary lymph nodes continued to be removed regardless of the reason.

As I wrestled with this dilemma, I came up with some ideas that were eventually published in 1980, in the *Southern Medical Journal*.[1] I felt that the presence of cancer in a patient's breast resulted in a war between the tumor and the patient, previously described by scientists as the tumor-host conflict. The patient may have lost the battle in the breast, but I came to believe that most patients were still able to defend themselves against the spread of cancer to distant organs. They did this by killing cancer cells circulating within the blood stream. Animal studies at that time demonstrated that cancer cells begin to circulate within the blood stream from the time a tumor is very small, the size of a mustard seed. These cells had to be killed in some manner to prevent the appearance of distant metastases.

I concluded that a patient who could kill cancer cells circulating from a breast cancer could also kill cells circulating from a cancer in the lymph nodes. Thus, the cancer cells left behind in a lymph node were of no risk to the patient, if they were removed in a timely fashion. If a patient survived her primary breast cancer without developing distant metastases, she could be expected to survive the appearance of a similar amount of cancer in the treated breast or an axillary lymph node. I also believed that cancers which grew too large might broadcast many cancer cells into the blood stream, enough to overwhelm the patient's defense system.

I discussed these ideas with many colleagues, who were generally supportive. By 1989, the NSABP lumpectomy trial (discussed in Chapter 1) proved that lumpectomy was as effective as mastectomy in the treatment of breast cancer. (Lumpectomy is the removal of the tumor itself, along with a narrow margin of healthy tissue.) The study also proved that the surgeon did not have to remove every last cancer cell. A few remaining cancer cells did not decrease survival, as long as the resulting tumor was removed promptly. This is perhaps the most important finding of the lumpectomy trial. Unfortunately, it received very little publicity. These results were identical to the earlier study of axillary lymph nodes, and they supported my ideas.

In the fifteen years that I have struggled with these ideas, I have studied the findings of surgeons in the United States, Canada, Europe, and Japan. The papers I have read in my extensive research now fill a four-drawer file cabinet. All of the information conforms to a simple idea, a basic principle of tumor-patient interaction.

THE TUMOR-PATIENT CONFLICT

For many years, scientists have talked about the conflict between the tumor and the patient. If a tumor grows within a breast or other organ, it has won this local battle against the immune defenses of the patient, but the war is not over. A patient can still survive by preventing the cancer's spread to distant organs through the actions of the immune system. To be sure, the presence of cancer cells anywhere in the body is frightening. The diagnosis of cancer is frightening. But the pivotal event is the spread to distant organs. If the tumor can be removed before it has spread, the patient is cured of the disease.

Patients who can kill cancer cells circulating from a primary breast cancer can also kill cancer cells circulating from a recurrent cancer. Surgeons who perform conservative surgery have a second chance to cure the patient, as long as the recurrent tumor is removed before it sheds a large number of tumor cells into the blood stream. I also believe that many of the lessons learned from the study of breast cancer apply equally well to other cancers.

CHALLENGING ACCEPTED CANCER SURGERY IDEAS

By the 1990s, I found myself explaining the main idea of this book—that patients who can fight the spread of cancer from one tumor can fight its spread from a recurring tumor—to doctors and friends. Everyone understood this simple principle. There was one obvious question: If it's this simple, why don't the leaders in cancer surgery agree with you?

My friend, Dr. Dan Jernigan, had the answer. He explained to me the ideas of Thomas Kuhn, who said that great changes in science do not occur in an orderly process, one experiment after another. Rather, scientists form theories about the world that are difficult to change. Each generation becomes passionately committed to established ideas. The earth rotates around the sun. Germs cause infection. These are now commonly accepted concepts, but in their time, these theories challenged contrary, but well-established, ideas. Chapter 1 discusses the changing ideas in cancer surgery. Chapter 16 elaborates on Kuhn's ideas.

George Crile, Jr., was criticized throughout his professional career for speaking out against radical surgery. In 1955, he wrote a book, *Cancer and Common Sense*.[2] The leaders of the American Medical Association and other prestigious organizations wrote, "Dr. Crile offers a dangerous, fatalistic philosophy of cancer. His thesis is contrary to the teachings of the country's 81 medical schools and to the experience of Physicians and Surgeons."[3] Crile later speculated that the sentence which precipitated this reaction was: "But there is no clear evidence that immediate treatment is any more effective than treatment given a little later." Crile was not referring to a delay of weeks or months, but of a few days between a breast biopsy and the operation, to give the patient time to consider her treatment options. Today, the delay Crile advocated thirty years ago is an accepted part of medical practice.

I am sure this book contains sentences that will cause debate. I have tried to make this book as accurate as possible, and welcome the comments and criticisms of those who can make it even better. I have sent manuscripts to dozens of authorities in various fields, requesting their suggestions. (Any errors, of course, are my own.) Regardless, writing that challenges prevailing convictions always generates controversy. Also, I am trying to simplify some fairly complex scientific information. Similarly, some statements made here may need to be modified for special situations. Beware of the type of criticism Crile experienced, criticism of a sentence or small section, lifted out of the context of the book. This book is not the final answer on any cancer treatment. I hope that it is a beginning toward greater acceptance of conservative surgery for many solid tumors. I look forward to discussions that will help clarify the points I am trying to make. I hope such dicussion will lead to better surgical treatment for patients with cancer. After all, that was the purpose for writing this book in the first place.

THE PURPOSE OF THIS BOOK

The purpose of this book is to present to you the information supporting conservative surgery. I summarize the experience of those who have practiced conservative treatment for many types of cancer. This book is written for the lay public. Some general knowledge of biology is helpful, but I've tried to make this book as easy to read and understand as possible—to explain everything in understandable terms. (The Glossary defines some of the medical terms used in this book.) However, some of the issues considered in this book are complicated. They cannot be discussed simply. If you are dealing with a decision that will affect the rest of your life, you should be willing to work toward the correct decision. Patients who face a mastectomy or a permanent colostomy do not need a book written for junior high school students. These issues are not that simple.

As I prepared this book, I read many popular books and articles from consumer magazines about the treatment of cancer. I wanted to see what information was already available. Magazine titles often sounded promising—"What a Woman Must Know about Breast Cancer," "Straight Talk about Cancer Treatment." While many of these articles informed women about breast-sparing surgery, most of them were shallow. Writers usually presented the prevailing philosophy of more treatment is better treatment.

For each cancer, I have tried to find all the relevant published studies. Writings from proponents of radical surgery, modified radical surgery, conservative surgery, radiation therapy, chemotherapy, and watchful waiting have all been reviewed. I have never deliberately excluded information contrary to the conservative viewpoint of this book. I have not selected only those articles that support conservative surgery.

This book is designed to help you make the right choice about your treatment—the choice that you think is right for you. The first requirement is that you have a choice. I am not attempting to talk you into any particular operation. I merely wish to gather into one place most of the information that supports conservative surgery for cancer. I want you to have access to information that is not readily available outside a medical school library. I want you to have as accurate an understanding as possible about your treatment options: the risks, the complications, the expected results.

Some may consider the surgical options presented here to be inadequate. In some cases, that may be true. Conservative treatment is not suited for all patients. My focus on conservative treatment should be balanced by that of those who support aggressive treatment. The supporters of aggressive treatment are easy to find. They have presented their views in countless books and magazine articles, some of which are listed in the Suggested Reading.

There was another important reason for writing this book. It may be years—perhaps decades—before the issues discussed

Preface   xix

here are ultimately resolved. Few of the cancers here have been studied in scientific trials, and none as thoroughly as breast cancer. For many cancers, these trials have not even begun. Several years are usually needed to plan and execute each study. Several hundred patients are often treated with the procedures under investigation. The patients must then be observed for an additional five to ten years. (Even today, some surgeons believe that ten years of follow-up is not enough.) Until the issues discussed in this book are ultimately resolved, patients and their doctors must rely upon the knowledge gained from those doctors and patients who have experience with conservative treatment methods.

I have not included detailed descriptions of treatment or of preoperative and postoperative care. I have tried not to repeat information that is widely available elsewhere.

WHAT CANCERS ARE COVERED IN THIS BOOK AND WHY

During the early 1990s I spent many hours investigating other cancers besides breast cancer, which is covered in Chapter 7. Initially, I looked at malignant melanoma (Chapter 9), the soft tissue sarcomas (Chapter 13), and rectal cancer (Chapter 12). These malignancies are within my specialty of general surgery. There was a large amount of information about those malignancies, enough to see their strong correlation with breast cancer.

Later, I read about those malignancies outside of my own specialty, in the fields of urology and gynecology. Urologists treat cancer of the bladder (Chapter 6), penis (Chapter 10), and prostate (Chapter 11). Gynecologists treat cancer of the cervix (Chapter 8), vagina (Chapter 14), and vulva (Chapter 15). Many of the lessons we have learned from breast cancer seem to be valid for these cancers as well. However, I have had little formal training in urology and gynecology and have had little, if any, experience treating patients with these cancers.

In deciding what cancers to write about, I considered whether aggressive treatment of a specific cancer would significantly affect bodily function or appearance. For example, cancer of the large intestine can be treated with an operation that usually has no lasting consequences. However, cancer of the rectum is sometimes treated with surgery that requires a permanent colostomy. Thus, I discuss the treatment of only rectal cancer.

In addition to this factor, I have not included cancers of the head and neck, because most head and neck surgeons already practice the types of conservative surgical techniques recommended in this book. Because of the mutilating effects of radical surgery, these surgeons excise just enough tissue to remove the cancerous cells. There is some debate about the extent of surgery needed to treat cancer of the thyroid gland, as patients who have had their entire gland removed must take thyroid hormone daily for the rest of their lives. Since the benefit of conservative surgery is so small, I decided to not cover this complex and controversial subject.

HOW TO USE THIS BOOK

This book does not need to be read from front to back. You may wish to turn first to a chapter about a particular cancer in Part Two and return later to Part One, which explains what we currently understand about cancer. The important themes of this book are repeated several times.

Part One of this book focuses on the history of cancer surgery and biological behavior of cancer. In Chapter 1 you will study the history of cancer treatment and learn what led the practicioners of modern medicine to favor aggressive therapy. You will see how doctors have changed their ideas about cancer over the past hundred years. Chapter 2 covers the basic science of cancer—how cancer cells grow and spread. This chapter includes a section on the things we don't know about cancer, the things that cause the great debates about treatment. Chapter 3 covers the patient's defenses against spreading tumor cells. In Chapter 4 I discuss the ongoing battle between the patient and the cancer, and explain why I believe surgeons have a second chance to cure cancer following a conservative operation.

Part Two focuses on the treatment of cancers in different parts of the body. Chapter 5 summarizes the role of surgery, radiation, chemotherapy, and other therapies in the treatment of cancer. It is divided into the same sections as the remaining chapters on treatment, and thus serves as a model for each of the other chapters. (The only exception is that each of the other

Part Two chapters begins with a section on anatomy and physiology, which provides some basic information about the specific part of the body being discussed.)

Each of the chapters in Part Two covers the following topics: types of tumors affecting a certain organ, how specific tumors are graded for severity, routes of tumor spread, available screening tests, signs and symptoms, how a specific tumor is diagnosed, staging systems designed to determine how extensive the cancer is, the types of treatment available, analysis of how effective conservative surgery is in dealing with a specific cancer, and what sort of follow-up is required.

Many of the supporting clinical studies are presented in Appendix I. I have tried to review all the clinical information currently available and summarize the most important studies here. I have not hand-picked selected studies that agree with the conservative orientation of this book.

GETTING YOUR DOCTOR'S ADVICE

If you find parts of this book too technical, seek the help of your family doctor. Your doctor should certainly be willing to discuss your concerns with you. You will be charged for an office visit; in such a critical matter, his advice is well worth its cost. I believe that family physicians should play and will play a greater role in advising their patients about controversial treatment. Physicians do not need to perform surgery to understand the results of surgery. They do not need to administer radiation therapy or chemotherapy to become familiar with their benefits and complications. I hope you will include your family doctor in this important decision.

Introduction

Lay me on an Anvil, O God.
Beat me and hammer me into a crowbar.
Let me pry loose old walls,
Let me lift and loosen old foundations.

Carl Sandburg, 1920

Over one million Americans are diagnosed with cancer each year, and each year almost half of them are cured. In 1971, the United States government initiated a War on Cancer. About $25 billion has been spent on cancer research since then, but cancer deaths in the United States have increased 7 percent during this war.

Most patients who are cured of cancer are cured with surgery and surgery alone. Patients often ask, "How much surgery is really necessary? Must I endure a disfiguring operation to survive this dread disease?" Patients may see their options as aggressive treatment on one hand, or death on the other. Fortunately, this is not so.

Recent medical research suggests that many patients can be successfully treated with conservative surgery—surgery that preserves the patient's bodily form and function. This book has been written to help you understand how much surgery is needed to successfully treat cancer. If you fear that traditional treatment may cause harm to you or a loved one, read and consider the information presented here. I think you will find it reassuring.

This book presents the advantages of conservative surgery for many patients with curable cancer. The treatment recommendations in this book are not greatly different from current surgical practice. Every treatment recommended here is currently offered in one or more medical centers in the United States or Europe. For example, the Cleveland Clinic has been treating breast cancer with partial mastectomy without radiation therapy since the 1950s. They report on their excellent results in journals and at professional meetings. So this is not a book about "unconventional therapy." Many of these recommendations are controversial simply because they are not accepted by the majority of surgeons.

This book deals with early cancer, cancer that can be completely removed and usually cured with surgery alone. Some tumors may have already spread to distant organs. Conservative surgery is also suitable in these circumstances, because aggressive or radical surgery cannot cure disease that has already spread.

Radical surgical procedures have cured many people of breast cancer and other malignancies. In some cases, radical surgery is still suitable and successful. This is true for patients whose large tumors have responded somewhat to radiation or chemotherapy. Radical surgery may also be appropriate for some malignancies deep inside the body that cannot be easily observed for signs of recurrence. In these cases, removal of an extra margin of tissue may be justified. The benefits of radical surgery have been widely discussed and are well known to all surgeons. This book emphasizes conservative surgery because its benefits are not as widely accepted. My negative comments about radical surgery should be read in this light. I am not criticizing all radical procedures and the surgeons who have performed them. I simply wish to present other treatment options.

A WORD ABOUT WORDS

It is important to have a clear idea about the meaning of the words and phrases used here. While I have included a Glossary at the end of the book to help you with medical terminology, there are several terms you will need to understand from the beginning. Cancer is a general term for the uncontrolled growth and multiplication of cells. It includes three principal characteristics: a locally expanding mass, invasion into nearby tissues, and spread to distant organs. A "tumor" is an abnormal mass of tissue with no function that arises from preexisting tissue. A tumor does not have to be malignant, but for many years this word has been used as a polite word for cancer. In this book, "tumor" or "solid tumor" means malignant tumor.

Unfortunately, there are some phrases that even physicians and surgeons have yet to agree upon. For instance, many new terms have been used to describe limited breast surgery: "breast-sparing surgery," "lumpectomy," "wide excision," "partial mastectomy," "quadrantectomy." "Breast-sparing surgery," of course, includes all types of operations that preserve the breast. The other terms in the above list are arranged approximately in order from least aggressive to most aggressive surgery. They are all defined in Chapter 7. I prefer both the operation and the term "partial mastectomy."

There is still no accepted term that means the opposite of radical surgery. Some surgeons have used the term "conservative" surgery to fill this void in our vocabulary. But this has caused some confusion, because conservative also means traditional, and "conservative" surgery is certainly not traditional. Conservative also means cautious, and "conservative" surgery may not be the most cautious.

The phrases "conservation surgery," "preservation surgery," and "so-called conservative surgery" have also been tried. I use "conservative" surgery to mean removal of the entire tumor plus an adequate margin or rim of apparently normal tissue. This extra margin of tissue should be wide enough to produce results that are equivalent to the results of radical surgery. Conservative surgery is not a specific operation or list of operations. It is an attitude that attempts to preserve bodily form and function without compromising patient survival.

Doctors seldom use the word cure when talking about cancer. There is no test sensitive enough to detect small numbers of cancer cells. The five-year survival rate is the percentage of patients who are alive five years after treatment. This is still a widely used method for reporting treatment results. Patients who are alive and also free of disease after five years are unlikely to have trouble with the cancer again.

A LOOK AT THE METRIC SYSTEM

Discussions of limited surgery must eventually involve numbers. How big is the tumor? How much tissue should be removed? Most doctors use the metric system to answer these questions. If you are not comfortable with the metric system, it is not likely that you care to learn about it now. Instead of trying to teach you all about the metric system, let me ask you to first learn one number—2 centimeters. Two centimeters, abbreviated 2 cm, is about the diameter of a nickel, or about three quarters of an inch. This number appears repeatedly throughout this book. For many cancers, such as cancer of the breast, 2 cm is the dividing line between small tumors and those of intermediate size. Also, when removing a tumor, surgeons often measure about 2 cm away from the edge of the tumor. They remove the tumor along with about 2 cm of visibly healthy tissue. This is called a 2-cm margin.

What are the benefits and complications of removing more than 2 cm? What are the benefits and complications of removing less? What is a prudent margin of excision? This issue is the primary focus of this book. Your understanding of this discussion will be easier if you have a clear understanding of this measurement.

You should know a couple of other terms. Millimeters (mm) are occasionally used to describe, for example, how far a malignant melanoma may have penetrated into the skin. One millimeter is one tenth of a centimeter (about 1/32 of an inch).

Measurements of volume are occasionally used. One metric liter is a little larger than a quart. A thousandth of a liter is called a milliliter (ml). A milliliter can also be defined by forming a cube that is 1 cm on all sides—a cubic centimeter (cc). A milliliter and a cubic centimeter are identical. Five cc equals one teaspoon. About 30 cc go into one ounce.

DEALING WITH FEAR

The diagnosis of cancer always causes fear—fear that cancer may recur. No amount of surgery or radiation will eliminate the risk that cancer may recur at a distant site. Once cancer cells have started to grow in a distant organ, aggressive local treatment seldom controls the continued spread of disease. The risk of distant spread can be reduced by early detection, not by aggressive treatment. Cancer in distant organs may be treated in some cases by chemotherapy. But no patient should choose a radical operation or precautionary radiation therapy just because of fear. Patients, their families, and their doctors usually want to do everything possible to achieve a cure. But the spread of cancer to distant organs cannot be reduced by radical local treatment. Fortunately, it is uncommon today in the treatment of breast cancer for a surgeon to take the attitude that radical surgery is a patient's only hope, although that feeling may still exist when dealing with other cancers.

One of the best ways to reduce your fear is to join with others who share your concerns. Support groups have formed all over the country. The benefits of these groups is enormous. Often, you can find up-to-date medical information through them. (Some AIDS groups have disseminated information so quickly that patients learned about new discoveries before their doctors did.) You receive the reassurance of seeing others live through the struggles you are facing. There is even some evidence that participation in a support group actually prolongs the lives of its members. See Appendix II for a list of support groups and related resources.

FACTORS INFLUENCING YOUR TREATMENT OPTIONS

As you consider your treatment options, you should focus on two results of treatment: local recurrence and survival. Consider a patient with a 2-cm breast cancer. This patient's outcome is typical of many different types of cancer treated at a relatively early stage. Following the most aggressive surgery, radical mastectomy, her chances for local recurrence—recurrent disease near the site of the surgery—are 5 to 10 percent. Following the most conservative surgery, lumpectomy, her chances for local recurrence are as high as 40 percent. Regardless of the surgery, her chances for surviving five years are about 85 percent. This puzzling outcome is explained in Chapter 4.

Advocates of aggressive treatment may claim they can improve these survival figures to 87 or 88 percent. There are several problems with this claim. First, survival differences of 2 to 3 percent are very difficult to verify scientifically. Differences this small are often not differences at all. Second, even this survival advantage does not mean that aggressive treatment cures 2 to 3 percent more patients. In truth, these few patients may merely live a few months longer, yet still live past the five-year mark. In this example, 85 percent of patients will survive regardless of treatment, 12 to 15 percent will not survive regardless of the extent of treatment. Aggressive treatment may affect only 2 to 3 percent of patients, allowing them to live a few months longer, or it may affect none at all.

Precise figures of this sort are difficult to obtain. They require studies involving hundreds of patients, who are carefully observed for many years. For most cancers, precise figures are not available. As you will see in Part Two of this book, there is no reliable evidence that aggressive treatment (in surgery, removal of a wide margin of apparently healthy tissue) provides even this small survival advantage for patients with early-stage disease although some patients with more advanced cancer may benefit from other types of aggressive treatment, such as preoperative chemotherapy.

Only you can decide if a decrease in local recurrence or a possible small increase in survival is worth the consequences of aggressive treatment. For most cancers, there may not be a clear right or wrong choice. We all deal with risk in a different manner, from the way we handle our money to the way we drive. The right choice is the choice that is right for you after weighing all the evidence.

You must ultimately decide for yourself. Is there sufficient evidence that a particular cancer will behave according to the rules presented here? Do the benefits of a limited operation outweigh the possible risks? My purpose is not to suggest that all readers should pursue conservative treatment. I merely wish to provide readers with a clear understanding of their options. Americans are questioning many aspects of their health care, including their own treatment. Many want to participate in these important decisions. I primarily wish to provide the information patients need to make sound decisions. I support conservative treatment but I am primarily pro-choice. I should add, though, that conservative surgery requires careful follow-up evaluation by both the patient and the physician. It is only suitable for patients who can participate in a regular program of follow-up care.

All physicians are under great professional pressure to conform to established treatment practices. Furthermore, in these litigious times, physicians may be held responsible for poor results, especially if more treatment could have been given. (Chapter 16 summarizes many of the reasons why change is so difficult in medicine.)

But your own treatment does not have to be governed by these obstacles to progress. As patients and doctors enter an age of enhanced communication, sophisticated information is becoming easily available. Patients will be able to obtain information from computer networks and cable television. Eventually, you should be able to retrieve information on most cancers and view it in your own home. The issues this book deals with should be thoroughly discussed and debated in terms you can understand. Thus, many patients will be able to assume greater responsibility for decisions about their treatment.

This book was also written so that you might benefit from the remarkable changes that are occurring in our understanding and treatment of cancer. With the help of this book, you can make decisions based upon reason and common sense, not fear or tradition. You can gain the assurance that conservative surgery is safe surgery. Surgeons can prudently avoid damaging functional and cosmetic consequences of their treatment without compromising patient survival.

THE SIGNIFICANCE OF LOCAL RECURRENCE

For over a hundred years, surgeons have believed that they had to remove every cancer cell in order to cure their patients. Many cancers have been treated by some type of radical operation that removed the affected organ and a large amount of surrounding tissue. Nearly all cancer surgery was called "radical," because it *was* radical. Radical mastectomy for breast cancer is the best-known example. This operation included removal of the entire breast, the lymph glands in the armpit, and the muscles beneath the breast. Surgeons developed radical operations for many organs of the body. These operations were very disfiguring. The object was to remove all visible cancer and even those invisible cancer cells that were near the tumor.

Local recurrence was considered a very grave sign, almost a death sentence. Surgeons considered themselves responsible for recurrent cancer in the region of their operation. For most of the twentieth century, surgeons struggled to control malignant disease by greater application of their craft in trying to remove every last cancer cell. Larger and larger operations were devised to reduce the dreaded aftermath of local recurrence. But the larger operations were seldom effective. At the time, it was reasonable to remove as much cancer as technically possible. During the past forty years we have learned much about the successes and failures of radical surgery. We now realize that ever more radical surgery is seldom effective in controlling cancer. This does not discredit the many surgeons who have tried valiantly to conquer this disease with the knife.

Recently, precise scientific studies have dramatically changed our opinion about local recurrence. The multi-institutional National Surgical Adjuvant Breast Project (NSABP) conducted a lumpectomy trial for breast cancer. In 1989, this study proved that patients treated by tumor removal alone, in an operation called a lumpectomy, lived as long as those treated by total removal of the breast. This finding has greatly increased the practice of lumpectomy in this country.

This study also discovered something else, a finding that has received little publicity among physicians or the public. Patients who develop locally recurrent breast cancer following a lumpectomy have a second chance to be cured. A recurrent tumor can be promptly removed without any added risk to the patient's continued survival. This observation went against decades of experience with radical surgery. The nonthreatening behavior, or innocence, of locally recurrent cancer after conservative surgery is a surprising contradiction, an unexpected blessing for many cancer patients. Most surgeons now agree that local recurrence following breast-sparing surgery is not a grave sign. It is certainly not an ominous event, as it is when local recurrence follows radical mastectomy.

THE PATIENT'S DEFENSES AGAINST CANCER

For many years, scientists have talked about the conflict between the tumor and the patient, known as the tumor-patient conflict. There is evidence from both laboratory and clinical experience to suggest that patients fight cancer in many ways. For example, the presence of white blood cells within a tumor suggests that these cancer-fighting cells often attempt to kill the cancer. Just because a tumor grows within a breast or other organ doesn't mean that it can't be stopped. Patients can still survive by preventing cancer's spread to distant organs. (Lymph nodes are not considered distant organs.) As tumor cells circulate within the blood stream, they are attacked by cancer-fighting cells and chemicals. The patient whose tumor is removed before it spreads, or metastasizes, can be cured. The patient whose tumor is removed after the spread of disease is seldom cured. The tumor-host battle against spreading tumor cells is literally a life-and-death struggle.

In addition to this powerful battle between the cancer and the patient, many scientists and surgeons have also believed that random chance plays a major role. Cancer behaves unpredictably. An apparently healthy patient can die with a small tumor, while a fragile patient may survive a tumor that seems far worse. It has been reasonable to conclude that random chance is at work. But it is not entirely the work of chance.

I first published my ideas on this subject in 1980,[1] and they are ideas I continue to believe today. Cancer in a patient's body provokes the tumor-host conflict. The patient can still defend himself or herself against the distant spread of this disease via the immune system and other defense mechanisms. If the tumor is removed before it has spread, the patient can be cured of the cancer. Patients who prevail over their original tumor without developing distant metastases can even be expected to survive a recurrent tumor, for example, within the breast, or within the lymph nodes. The tumor-host conflict is not an ephemeral contest, subject to random chance. It is a reproducible battle between two adversaries. While the outcome of the first encounter may not be predictable, the outcome of future battles certainly is. The defense system of the patient, if it prevented the spread of cancer from the first tumor, can be relied upon to prevent the spread of cancer from a recurrence.

This helps to explain the findings of the NSABP lumpectomy trial mentioned earlier. Some women did have breast cancer cells growing within their lymph nodes. But these cancer cells did not spread, because the same defense mechanisms that prevented the distant spread of tumor cells from the first breast cancer could also prevent the spread of tumor cells from the enlarging lymph node. However, a patient's defense mechanisms are limited. Therefore, any locally recurrent cancer, whether within the breast or the lymph nodes, must be removed in a timely fashion.

Recent information suggests that other solid tumors may behave in a similar fashion. Local recurrence after limited surgery can be promptly removed without jeopardizing patient survival. Of course, there are differences among cancers, and only limited information about most cancers. But I have found no tumor that violates this simple principle. Sometimes, though, doctors can lose sight of the basic principles of cancer behavior because they are focused on the technical aspects of treatment. (See Chapter 2 for a fuller discussion of this topic.)

An accurate description of the tumor-patient conflict is obviously more complicated than this simple summary. It is presented in greater detail in Chapter 4 and is woven throughout the book. Chapter 1 focuses on local recurrence following cancer surgery and the steps that surgeons have taken to reduce this once dreaded complication. You will see that increasingly radical surgery did little to improve local recurrence results. Chapters 2 and 3 introduce you to the behavior of tumor cells and to the body's attempt to destroy them. These chapters may seem complicated, but they only scratch the surface of what scientists have learned about cancer in the last few decades. By the time you read Chapter 4, I hope you will share my confidence in our bodies' complex system of immune protection. I hope you will agree that the immune system is a reliable defense against the spread of residual tumor cells. This is the principle message of this book.

Part One

Understanding Cancer

1.
The History of Cancer Surgery

> *Pain, hemorrhage, infection, the three great evils which had always embittered the practice of surgery and checked its progress, were, in a moment, in a quarter of a century (1846–1873) robbed of their terrors.*
>
> William S. Halsted, 1904

Any cancer surgeon of a hundred years ago would have little difficulty working beside his modern-day colleagues, because the surgeon's scalpel remains the basic tool of cancer treatment. Over 90 percent of those patients who are cured of cancer today are still cured by surgery alone. While modern medicine has benefited greatly from this century's technological advances, the treatment of cancer has advanced due to changing ideas about the growth and spread of malignant disease. Technological marvels such as CAT scanners and laser beams have contributed little to the overall survival of patients with cancer. The greatest part of this improvement came about during the last two decades, the fruit of much careful research.

The central controversy among cancer surgeons has always been: how much normal tissue must a surgeon remove to be confident he "got it all"? In my view, attitudes established a hundred years ago have held back needed progress toward more conservative treatment. There has been a tendency to favor tradition over innovation. Reviewing this story is important, because all cancer patients are participants in a debate that is far from resolved.

Because breast cancer is so common, most of our knowledge about cancer surgery has been learned from the study of this type of cancer. Physicians have had an opportunity to treat breast cancer in many different ways. The history presented here focuses almost entirely upon this disease. The treatment histories of other malignancies are covered in the appropriate sections of Appendix I.

THE BEGINNING OF MODERN SURGERY

Surgery was practiced on the battlefield for centuries by barbers, who were often derided as little more than butchers. In the mid-1880s, a surgeon's skill was measured by his speed, which is understandable since he performed amputations and cared for wounds without anesthesia or antibiotics. "Respectable" physicians refused to be associated with such a brutal craft. Sir James Simpson, a discoverer of anesthesia, said, "A man laid on the operating table in one of our surgical hospitals is exposed to more chances of death than was the English soldier on the field of Waterloo."[1]

Things began to change in the last quarter of the nineteenth century. Ether anesthesia was becoming available in many hospitals. Joseph Lister had discovered that postoperative infection could be reduced by eliminating bacteria from the field of surgery, and surgeons washed their hands and instruments with greater frequency. Antiseptics (not antibiotics) were introduced. Surgeons in Germany developed instruments and techniques that improved the craft of surgery and helped control blood loss. Microscopes became widely available, and more pathologists could diagnose cancer. These major advances set the stage for the beginning of modern cancer surgery as we know it.

Into this setting stepped William S. Halsted, today called the "Father of American surgery." Halsted entered Columbia University's College of Physicians and Surgeons in 1874, at the age of 22. Four years later, he had completed medical school, internship, and surgical training. He went on to study in the great clinics of Germany and Austria for two years, a practice that was very common at the time. There he learned more about careful surgical technique and the importance of laboratory investigation. He was also introduced to the students of Rudolf

Virchow, the "Pope of German medicine." Virchow had discovered that all growth, tissue repair, wound healing, and even cancer formation depend on a process of continually dividing cells—"omnis cellula e cellula" (all cells come from cells). Old ideas, such as the notion that "evil humors" caused illness, were discarded. Pathologists began the analytic study of disease. Since most illnesses are caused by sick cells, Virchow helped to elevate medicine from witchcraft to science.

In 1880, Halsted returned to New York City, where he became a respected young surgeon. It is important to realize that in Halsted's day, most patients with cancer waited until their disease was far advanced before seeking the advice of a physician. The results of last-minute treatment were discouraging. As Halsted said, "Most of us have heard our teachers in surgery admit that they have never cured a case of cancer of the breast. . . . There are undoubtedly many surgeons in active practice who have never cured a cancer of the breast."[2]

At that time, breast cancer was treated with either removal of the tumor or complete removal of the breast. Halsted expanded upon the techniques he had learned in Germany and began to develop the radical mastectomy, an operation that removed the entire breast and much of the surrounding tissue.

THE THEORY BEHIND RADICAL SURGERY

To understand Halsted's surgical strategy, it is necessary to understand his theory of cancer spread. The word "cancer" is derived from the Greek word for crab, *karkinoma*. Indeed, the disease was considered analogous to a crab in its behavior: reaching out to destroy healthy tissue, withdrawing and becoming dormant, and then becoming destructively active again. While in Germany, Halsted had been told by the students of Virchow that cancer cells did not spread through the blood stream. All tumors, they said, spread by direct extension. Cancer spread to the liver and lungs directly through the layers of the body into these organs; cancer cells reached the brain by traveling up the lymphatic network in the neck.

This theory of "centrifugal spread" became the foundation of surgical oncology. We now know that Virchow was wrong. Cancer does spread to distant organs primarily through the blood stream. But at that time, Virchow's great reputation led to the acceptance of his ideas as holy writ. The views of those doctors who did believe that cancer spread via the blood stream did not prevail. This flawed perception of tumor spread supported aggressive surgical treatment.

Surgeons believed that if the tumor could be surrounded and removed, the patient could be cured. The centrifugal spread theory meant that cure was totally in the hands of the surgeon, who cut out the farthest tentacles of the tumor. Halsted's study of anatomy and physiology allowed him to design a breast cancer operation based upon accurate anatomical dissection. His radical mastectomy procedure removed the entire tumor, the entire breast, the underlying chest muscles, and the axillary (armpit) lymph nodes. His surgical technique was careful, gentle, meticulous, and lengthy, a superior replacement for the hasty, flamboyant style of his predecessors. The tumor was handled minimally and never cut in two. Lymph ducts between the tumor and the axillary lymph nodes were left intact. The surgeon removed the surgical specimen in one piece to avoid spilling tumor cells into the operative field. Halsted summarized a common notion of the time: "The division of one lymphatic vessel and the liberation of one cell may be enough to start a new cancer."[3] Certainly, no one wanted that.

In July 1885, former President Ulysses S. Grant died of cancer of the tongue, caused by many years of smoking and drinking. The extensive newspaper coverage of this event greatly elevated the public discussion of this previously "shameful" disease.[4] In the Victorian era, cancer was a private matter, seldom discussed. Grant's illness helped to bring cancer out in the open.

In 1892, Halsted started a thirty-year tenure as Professor of Surgery and Surgeon-in-Chief at the newly opened Johns Hopkins Hospital and Medical School in Baltimore. Two years later, Halsted wrote about the first fifty patients he had treated with his new operation—the radical mastectomy. Many of these patients had come to him with tumors the size of a hen's egg; others, the size of an orange. All the patients had axillary lymph nodes filled with cancer. In spite of this, Halsted's results were astonishingly good for his time. He reported that only three patients had developed local recurrence among the fifty he had treated. This was considered an overwhelming achievement. Halsted's radical mastectomy for breast cancer soon gained wide acceptance in the United States and Europe. For the first time, an American surgical procedure had been adopted abroad. This further contributed to the status of Halsted's procedure and to the pride of American surgeons.

It is difficult to overestimate Halsted's influence on the surgical treatment of cancer and the training of surgeons. The radical mastectomy became the "gold standard" against which all breast cancer treatment would be measured. His detailed surgical training program became a model for all surgical training in the United States.

Altogether, 17 surgical residents and 55 assistant residents finished Halsted's program, and 42 became teachers of surgery in similar programs across the United States and Canada.[5] From these programs, 166 chief residents in surgery graduated, all disciples of Halsted's ideas about cancer and surgical training. Many surgeons today are proud to trace their own academic lineage directly back to Halsted. Surgeon Sherwin Nuland, in his book, *Doctors: The Biography of Medicine*, said, "Even after almost thirty years of being a surgeon, my own occasional flutterings of self-doubt in the operating room can always be stilled by reminding myself that my professor was Gustaf Lindskog, whose professor was Samuel Harvey, whose professor was Harvey Cushing, whose professor was William Halsted . . . the quiverings are gone in the wink of an eye."[6]

The training of surgeons was different from that of other specialists. The eight-year program that Halsted developed was a great improvement over the old apprenticeship system. Surgeons-in-training spent many hours in the operating room learning from those who were two or three years older. Surgeons learned to make decisions quickly in the operating room. They teased their colleagues in internal medicine for spending endless hours discussing the diagnosis and treatment of patients with exotic diseases. A surgeon was expected to be decisive. The training program was shaped like a pyramid, with dozens of medical students at the bottom and one or two chief residents at the top. The structure has been compared to that of the military, and surgeons-in-training were expected to follow orders. At each medical school, the person in charge was the chairman of the department of surgery. He appointed residents and hired surgeons to the faculty who shared his views about surgery. It is not surprising that ideas about radical surgery became accepted very quickly.

THE GROWTH OF RADICAL SURGERY

The philosophy and techniques of radical surgery for breast cancer were soon applied to other types of malignancies. Ernst Wertheim of Vienna, Austria, popularized the radical hysterectomy for carcinoma of the cervix. Hugh Young performed the first radical prostatectomy for prostate cancer at Johns Hopkins in 1904. Halsted assisted him during this operation.

In 1908, Sampson Handley proposed that malignant melanoma should be removed with a two-inch margin of normal skin in all directions around the cancer. Surprisingly, this recommendation, which continues to be quoted in modern surgical literature, was based upon a single autopsy of a single patient who died of melanoma that had spread throughout her body. Handley was also a proponent of the theory of centrifugal spread.

Ernest Miles proposed a radical procedure for cancer of the rectum; it removed the entire rectum and surrounding tissue, resulting in a permanent colostomy. George Crile, Sr., developed the radical neck dissection for tumors of the head and neck, a procedure that removed the tumor along with the muscles, jugular vein, and lymph nodes of the affected side of the neck. Head and neck surgeons developed the *commando* operation, which removed part of the jawbone. (Its popularity has been attributed to its name, derived from the commandos of World War I.[7]) Some surgeons even removed the pelvis and both legs—the entire lower half of the body—in an operation called a hemicorpectomy.

In the 1910s, cancer caused 4.4 percent of the deaths in the United States, making it the eighth leading cause of death behind tuberculosis, heart disease, diarrhea, violence, pneumonia, kidney failure, and apoplexy (now known as stroke).[8] By and large, the medical profession was making some progress. Sociologist Lawrence Henderson put this period into perspective when he said, "Sometime between 1910 and 1912 in this country, a random patient, with a random disease, consulting a doctor chosen at random, had, for the first time in the history of mankind, a better than fifty-fifty chance of profiting from that encounter."[9] In 1913, the American Society for the Control of Cancer, which later became the American Cancer Society, was formed to distribute information about cancer and to compile statistics.

By the 1920s, surgeons were beginning to win their fight

against cancer. This was primarily because patients started seeking medical attention earlier, with smaller tumors. Some were actually cured of their disease. Radical surgery was saving some lives. Cancer, unmentionable during the Victorian era, was gaining public attention as a curable disease.

Now comes a paradox. At the time of radical surgery's apparent triumph, the premise behind it evaporated. The famous pathologist James Ewing, of Memorial Hospital in New York, published evidence that cancer cells did indeed spread to distant sites by circulating in the blood stream, not by growing tentacles out into adjacent organs. Surgeons decided that tumor cells broke off from the primary tumor and progressed in an orderly fashion to the lymph nodes and then into the blood stream. Lymph nodes were considered a partial barrier to the spread of tumor cells.

The fall of the centrifugal spread theory in the 1920s did not dampen the enthusiasm of American and European surgeons for radical surgery, and it's important to realize why this occurred. As patients lived longer, more of them returned with recurrent disease in the area of the surgical scar. This was called local recurrence, and it was often the first evidence of failure. Most patients with local recurrence were soon found to have cancer in distant organs—distant metastases. Local recurrence became the equivalent of a death sentence, since few patients lived more than an additional two years.[10-12] Surgeons mistakenly criticized themselves, believing that they were responsible for the recurrence, the spread of disease, and ultimately the death of the patient. Why? Because they had failed to remove enough tissue, or because tumor cells had spilled into the wound. Cushman Haagensen, the famous breast surgeon from Columbia-Presbyterian Hospital in New York, said, "The surgeon certainly is accountable . . for local recurrence in the field of operation."[13]

Most surgeons witnessed this pattern of recurrence repeatedly in their practices and suffered great anguish. Time after time, they returned to the operating room ever more determined to perform surgery that would eliminate every cancer cell. Surgeons continuously reiterated the importance of radical surgery to their colleagues and the surgical residents they trained. Another paradox was emerging: surgeons were seeing smaller and smaller tumors, yet performing more radical operations and removing more tissue.

EARLY CHALLENGES TO RADICAL SURGERY

In the first decades of the twentieth century, few doctors questioned the doctrine of radical surgery. Rudolf Matas of Tulane was one of the few. Ironically, Matas and Halsted were close friends—a relationship that endured in spite of their professional disagreement. In the United States, no one else dared to confront Halsted's radical mastectomy until more than a generation after his death in 1922. Instead, early challenges to Halsted came from abroad.

Radiation had first been introduced into cancer treatment in 1898 by Pierre and Marie Curie, who worked in Paris. By the 1920s, this treatment had gained wide clinical acceptance. In 1922, Geoffrey Keynes, an English surgeon (the brother of economist John Maynard Keynes), began using local excision and radiation therapy to treat breast cancer. He treated many patients with stage I breast cancer (no evidence of tumor cells in the lymph nodes). Over 70 percent of his patients survived five years, a respectable figure for the time. As the sole practitioner of local excision and radiation, he was criticized, and his results were unfairly compared with the best results of his colleagues. Eventually, he reverted to total removal of the breast, because 8 percent of his patients developed local recurrence. But this rate of recurrence was actually no higher than that following radical surgery, and even today would be considered a good result. In his autobiography, *The Gates of Memory*, Keynes wrote, "A built-in dogma of thirty years' standing dies hard, and I was regarded with grave disapproval and shaking of heads by the older surgeons of my own hospital."[14]

During this period, Duncan Fitzwilliams, working at St. Mary's Hospital in England, treated 93 patients with early breast cancer using excision alone. He claimed to have results equivalent to those of radical surgery. He said, "Those who have been brought up in the atmosphere of the radical operation with no experience of anything less extensive must remember that they are repeating dogma and not speaking from formed judgement. Medicine is never advanced by such action."[15] Sakari Mustakallio of the University Central Hospital in Helsinki, Finland, began treating patients with tumor excision and low-dose radiation therapy.[16] So did Vera Peters at the Princess Margaret Hospital in Toronto, Ontario, using a higher dosage of radiation.[17] Both obtained survival results comparable to those of the radical mastectomy. Robert McWhirter, a radiotherapist in Scotland, began removing the entire breast, but only the breast, an operation called a simple mastectomy. After surgery, he administered radiation to the lymph glands in the armpit. All those investigators achieved excellent survival results, although the low radiation doses used in Finland led to higher rates of local recurrence. In 1943, Frank Adair reported that 63 patients treated at Memorial Sloan-Kettering Hospital in New York with conservative surgery had survived as long as those treated with radical surgery. Nevertheless, Adair concluded, "But it would be disastrous if we were to take a step backward."[18]

Throughout this period, interest in finding better ways to treat cancer was growing. In 1937, the Congress established the National Cancer Institute to conduct cancer research. Cancer replaced tuberculosis as America's most dread disease. By the 1940s, cancer had become the second leading cause of death behind cardiovascular disease (heart attacks and stroke).

EVIDENCE AGAINST RADICAL SURGERY INCREASES

During the 1950s, a new generation of surgeons and radiation therapists continued the challenge to Halsted's ideas by practicing breast-sparing treatment of breast cancer. It came about in this way.

In England, surgeon Reginald Murley and radiotherapist I. G. Williams tracked down the records of patients who had been treated by Keynes twenty to thirty years earlier.[19] Murley supported radical surgery and expected to find that Keynes' conservative treatment had failed. He was surprised to find solid evidence that patients treated with simple excision and radiation therapy survived as long as those treated at the same hospital by radical surgery. This discovery led surgeons and radiotherapists in several hospitals throughout England to begin offering breast-sparing treatment.[20-22] (One study reported a high local recurrence rate if radiation was not used.[23,24]) What is more important, they began to challenge the notion that local recurrence was the cause of distant metastases. Williams and Murley said, "It is, however, possible that local recurrence per se is an infrequent source of distant metastases and that the appearance of the latter has been determined quite independent of the former."[25]

In 1954, Keynes wrote about his experience twenty to thirty years earlier in challenging the radical mastectomy: "Orthodoxy in surgery is like orthodoxy in other departments of the mind—it starts as a tentative belief in some particular course of action, but later begins to almost challenge a comparison with religion. It comes to be held as a passionate belief in the absolute rightness of that particular view. A dissentient view is regarded as a criminal subversion of the truth, and the holder is sometimes exposed to slander and abuse. . . . In speaking today of the unorthodox view of carcinoma of the breast, I do not mean to suggest the orthodoxy has been manifested in its more violent forms. None of us has been burnt at the stake, but feelings have run pretty high."[26]

In the United States, Murley told George Crile, Jr. (son of the doctor who had developed the radical neck dissection) of the Cleveland Clinic about the excellent results achieved by Keynes prior to World War II. Crile, like Murley, was a young surgeon who supported radical surgery. But he was intrigued by Murley's evidence. He persuaded his colleagues at the Cleveland Clinic to allow him to try this more conservative approach. Crile thus became the first American surgeon to practice conservative surgery for breast cancer. Most of his patients were treated with a partial mastectomy alone, that is, excision of the tumor plus a wide margin of healthy tissue. Radiation therapy was only used on those few patients with more advanced tumors.

Although his results were always comparable to those achieved through radical surgery, Crile was nevertheless criticized as an extremist. He said in his book, *Cancer and Common Sense*, "Those responsible for telling the public about cancer have chosen to use the weapon of fear. They have created a new disease, cancer phobia, a contagious disease that spreads from mouth to ear."[27]

THE EXTENSION OF RADICAL SURGERY TECHNIQUE

The gulf between the advocates of radical surgery and supporters of conservative surgery kept widening. Supporters of radical surgery developed elaborate mechanical techniques to reduce local recurrence. They excised so much tissue that skin grafts were often required to cover the surgical defect. The remaining skin was shaved very thin, to remove any possible tumor cells close to the skin. Surgical wounds were sometimes irrigated with a toxic solution to kill tumor cells that might have spilled into the wound. It was thought that cancer could spread prior to and during surgery, and surgeons handled tumors as if they were land mines. Residents in training were told not to touch the patient's breast to avoid shedding tumor cells into the blood. (Never mind that the patient may have been sleeping on her breast tumor for months.)

Rituals developed around the operation. Radical surgery specified the location of the biopsy incision (within the area of a mastectomy incision), the interval between diagnostic biopsy and surgery (only minutes), the location of the mastectomy incision (low, if possible), and so on. Surgeons were trained to remove the biopsy incision as part of the radical operation. Surgeons who failed to follow these procedures were subject to severe disciplinary measures. Many surgeons changed gowns, gloves, and instruments after the biopsy and again before closing the skin. The goal of surgery was to remove every cancer cell and to be certain that no malignant cell returned to the surgical incision. Surgeons focused almost completely upon the details of the operation. They believed that the precise execution of this intricate procedure was the patient's only chance for cure. This was, and in many cases still is, a reasonable conclusion. Surgeons were trying to maximize their only effective weapon against cancer. This commentary should not be interpreted as criticism of these heroic efforts.

The proponents of radical surgery moved ahead with more aggressive procedures. In the late 1940s, surgeons in Europe began performing an *extended* radical mastectomy. Besides removing the entire breast, the chest muscles, and the axillary lymph nodes, this procedure also excised lymph nodes located beneath the breastbone. Dr. Jerome Urban at Memorial Sloan-Kettering Hospital became a leading advocate of this procedure. Some patients whose cancers were located near the breastbone appeared to benefit from this procedure, but it never gained wide acceptance and was eventually abandoned. Leading surgeons at Columbia University and the Mayo Clinic pressed for even more extensive surgery. They divided the collarbone and removed the first rib to remove additional tissue! Fortunately, this procedure also was quickly abandoned. Even following radical surgery, radiation therapy was occasionally administered to eradicate residual tumor cells. While some of these procedures reduced local recurrence, unfortunately, none consistently improved patient survival. Radiation therapy was used primarily for advanced cancer.

The surgeon was very much in charge of the patient's care. He performed surgery hoping for a cure. If the patient developed local recurrence, he knew that cure was no longer possible. He could send the patient for radiation therapy, which could kill the tumor on the chest wall. This prevented the cancer from causing an offensive wound on the chest. The next form of treatment, introduced in the middle of the 1950s, was chemotherapy, which was used on patients with recurrent or advanced disease. Naturally, there was some competition between specialists. Each specialist wanted to maximize his own role.

By the 1950s, major cancer centers, beginning with the Mayo Clinic in Rochester, Minnesota, began to plan treatment early in the disease's course. According to an approach called multidisciplinary treatment, patients with advanced or complicated malignancies would be seen by a surgeon, radiation therapist, and oncologist simultaneously. These committees would plan the most effective treatment strategy. For example, chemotherapy or radiation treatment might be given prior to surgery to shrink the tumor. Thus, patients were no longer moved from one doctor to another as each exhausted his ability to control the patient's illness. The new approach improved the care of cancer and has been widely praised throughout the medical community.

BREAST-SPARING TREATMENT GAINS MOMENTUM

During the 1960s, perhaps because radiation therapy had been pioneered in Paris by the Curies, enthusiasm for breast-sparing surgery arose in France.[28-35] The leading French radiotherapist, F. Baclesse, reviewed his experience with 100 patients treated with local excision and radiation from 1937 to 1953. He concluded that his results were every bit as good as those of radical surgery. After that, physicians in Paris, Marseille, Creteil, and Villejuif began reporting excellent survival statistics following treatment that spared the breast.

But many patients were treated with inadequate tumor excision or no tumor excision at all. All too often they developed a local recurrence, and the breast was then totally removed. Under this circumstance, the operation was called a *salvage mastectomy*. The French then made a surprising observation. Investigators at the Curie Foundation concluded, "It appears that local recurrences following lumpectomy and radiotherapy or radical radiotherapy alone do not alter the prognosis."[36] Patients treated with a salvage mastectomy did surprisingly well, and over half lived another five years. This was far better than the one- or two-year survival rate seen among patients who developed recurrence following radical surgery.

In 1964, the first scientific study of breast-sparing surgery was begun at the Guy's Hospital in London. The study compared tumor excision plus low-dose radiation therapy with radical mastectomy. This trial initially concluded that the overall survival rate of patients treated with a partial mastectomy was equal to that following radical mastectomy. Unfortunately, many patients had disease that had spread to the axillary lymph nodes. The low dose of radiation used was not effective in killing this disease. Many of these patients developed extensive local recurrences and died because of this flaw in the study. The poor results among these patients were widely publicized by critics of conservative surgery, and the conservative movement was set back.

In the midst of this rancorous debate, George Crile, Jr., returned to the battle. In 1965, he published his experience with local excision, maintaining strongly, as before, that conservative treatment was safe and effective. At Harvard, Oliver Cope was also practicing breast-sparing surgery, with favorable results. In 1967, he presented his experience to a meeting of the New England Surgical Society, but the society refused to publish his report in its journal.

The excellent results of conservative treatment were subtly beginning to influence some advocates of radical surgery, who began reducing the scope of their procedures. Radical mastectomy left the patient only a thin layer of skin to cover the rib cage, giving the chest a washboard appearance. As early as 1963, American surgeon Hugh Auchincloss had suggested that most patients could be treated with a *modified* radical mastectomy. This operation did not remove the large pectoral muscle overlying the ribs of the chest wall. The modified procedure eliminated the washboard appearance because of the presence of a muscle between the skin and the ribs. The patient still lost the entire breast and the lymph nodes under the arm. Earlier studies in Europe had shown that the modified procedure did not compromise patient survival, and many English surgeons had already adopted this procedure. The modified procedure was gaining acceptance in the United States. Patients seeking conservative surgery were frequently told by their surgeons, "I do the modified procedure." These surgeons believed that they were modernizing the treatment of breast cancer. Even Halsted reported back in 1894 that he had done seven incomplete operations "due to the small size or recent appearance of the tumor."[37]

By the 1970s, the treatment of breast cancer was clearly one of the most argued subjects in medicine. In 1972, an editorial in the prestigious *British Medical Journal* said, "There is more controversy about the management of breast cancer than almost any other topic in tumor therapy, and more so now than ever before."[38] In 1970, John Stehlin of St. Joseph Hospital in Houston began to treat patients with partial mastectomy and radiation therapy. He, too, was severely criticized by his colleagues. In 1979, he published his experience with 79 patients, providing additional evidence that conservative surgery was as effective as more radical treatment. Those following the medical uproar were not surprised when he began his paper by saying, "The treatment of no other form of cancer has evoked such a degree of controversy and emotionalism as has that of carcinoma of the breast."[39] Samuel Hellman, an oncologist from the University of Chicago, has compared the persecution of those surgeons who opposed radical surgery to that of the accused heretics in the Spanish Inquisition.[40] I would only add that the dogma of radical surgery has applied to most cancers, not just cancer of the breast. Normally sedate medical meetings erupted in fierce debate. While some surgeons mentioned lumpectomy to their patients as an option, most of them continued to practice mastectomy.

THE TIDE BEGINS TO TURN

By 1975, over 150,000 American women were developing breast cancer annually. Crile had treated 291 patients with

surgery that saved the breast, but most American women were still treated with mastectomy. Over twenty medical centers in Finland, Canada, England, France, Italy, and the United States were treating patients with breast-conserving surgery and radiation. Over sixty articles on breast-sparing surgery has been published in prominent medical journals in the United States and abroad, and they all carried a single message: *patients treated with breast-conserving surgery and radiation live as long as those treated by mastectomy.* Except for Keynes, the first modern physician to practice breast-sparing surgery, no surgeon, no radiation therapist, and no institution has returned to total removal of the breast after starting to use breast-sparing therapy.
apy.

Nevertheless, American patients with breast cancer had a difficult time learning about alternative forms of treatment, much less finding a surgeon who advocated breast-sparing treatment. The vast majority of surgeons, intellectual descendants of William Halsted and his doctrine, were steadfastly committed to mastectomy. They pointed to the poor results of partial mastectomy in the past. They seldom mentioned that this procedure had not been seriously used since the nineteenth century, when it was used for the treatment of large tumors. Advocates of radical surgery said they were waiting for additional results from scientific trials of breast-sparing surgery.

In fairness, there were problems associated with some reports favorable to conservative surgery. In some studies, many patients returned with local recurrence. In others, the conservative treatment was restricted only to patients with early disease. Thus, the good results might have been due to patient selection and not to treatment. Still, the preponderance of circumstantial evidence suggested that partial mastectomy was a safe and effective procedure for patients with early breast cancer.

In 1973, Umberto Veronesi of Milan, Italy, began a scientific study comparing partial mastectomy plus radiation with radical mastectomy. Veronesi removed one-fourth of the breast and called the operation a *quadrantectomy*. This was the first such study since the Guy's Hospital trial. By 1980, 701 patients had been studied. Veronesi showed statistically that survival and local recurrence results were equal for the two forms of treatment.

A CONCERTED RESEARCH EFFORT BEGINS

Bernard Fisher of the University of Pittsburgh had begun to question some of Halsted's principles back in 1957, when he organized the multi-institutional National Surgical Adjuvant Breast Project (NSABP) to study various aspects of breast cancer treatment. Through a series of trials, this group has done far more than improve the surgical, radiation, and chemotherapeutic treatment of breast cancer.[41]

Working in the laboratory and in clinical trials, Fisher and the NSABP reversed many of Halsted's hypotheses. As already discussed, Halsted had concluded that tumor cells spread in an orderly manner and by direct extension to neighboring lymph nodes. The NSABP concluded that tumor cells do not progress in an orderly pattern, and that they break away from the tumor and travel to lymph nodes in clusters. Halsted believed that lymph nodes were barriers to the passage of tumor cells. The NSABP concluded that lymph nodes are not effective barriers to tumor spread. Halsted believed that positive lymph nodes could themselves become the cause of additional tumor spread. The NSABP concluded that positive lymph nodes are an indicator of a poor prognosis, and not its cause. If cancer cells are living within a patient's lymph nodes, her immune resistance is probably weak. Halsted believed that the tumor grew and spread on its own, independent of the patient. The NSABP concluded that a complex interaction between the tumor and the patient affects all aspects of the cancer. Halsted believed that the blood stream was unimportant in the spread of tumor cells. The NSABP concluded that the blood stream is very important in the spread of tumor cells. Halsted believed that cancer cells remained localized for a long time. The NSABP concluded that tumor cells begin to circulate early; they called breast cancer a systemic disease. Halsted believed that the type of surgical treatment was very important to a patient's outcome. The NSABP concluded that local treatment had little effect on survival.

The NSABP successfully challenged many of the ideas about breast cancer that had dominated the twentieth century. The Halstedian model was replaced by an alternative view of tumor spread. No individual, no institution has contributed more to our understanding of cancer than Bernard Fisher and the

NSABP. (There are still many questions about cancer that remain unanswered. These will be discussed more thoroughly in Chapters 2 and 3.)

In one very important study (trial B-04), the NSABP focused attention on the treatment of axillary lymph nodes. Surgeons treated over 1,000 women with breast cancer. None of the women had enlarged lymph nodes in the armpit. The lymph nodes were said to be clinically negative, that is, there was no evidence of cancer on clinical (physical) examination. Surgeons know that physical examination of these nodes is unreliable; 30 to 40 percent of patients with no palpable nodes are found to have microscopic tumor spread by the pathologist (pathologically positive) after the nodes have been removed.

In this study, all patients had a mastectomy, but the axillary lymph nodes were treated in three different ways: the nodes were surgically removed (40 percent of this group had positive nodes), the nodes were irradiated, or the nodes were not treated and only observed. About 18 percent of the patients in the last group developed lymph nodes enlarged with cancer and required an operation to remove them. (It was not explained why only 18 percent of patients developed enlarged lymph nodes, and not the full 40 percent found to have positive nodes in the group treated with surgery.)

The overall survival rates in all three groups were identical. In other words, there was no survival *advantage* to eliminating those cancer cells by either surgery or radiation therapy, and no *disadvantage* to leaving tumor cells alone and simply observing the patient. The NSABP concluded that the surgeons could prudently leave cancer cells behind in a patient's lymph nodes without hurting her chances for survival, an idea contrary to all previous notions about cancer surgery.

The innocence, or nonthreatening nature, of recurrence in the lymph nodes had first been reported by Crile in 1960. He believed that intact regional nodes offered a degree of immune protection.[42] He stated, "The survival rate of the patients treated with delayed treatment of the axilla [armpit] was similar to that of the patients treated by radical mastectomy."[43] This was a remarkable observation for its time. It was contrary to all established principles and practice of surgery.

This observation by Crile and its verification by the NSABP never attracted much attention among surgeons. They continued to remove lymph nodes to learn how far the disease had spread. Patients with positive lymph nodes were often treated with chemotherapy, while those with negative nodes were not. Thus, lymph node removal was performed to find out whether or not to administer chemotherapy. It was not performed to remove cancer. For some, this distinction was unimportant. The biological mystery was largely ignored.

A confounding issue now entered the discussion—*multicentricity*, or the observation that many patients with breast cancer had small areas throughout the breast that resembled early cancer. Surgeons argued that it was foolhardy to leave behind breast tissue that might become malignant. No surgeon wanted to say, "I think we got it all," or "We got most of the cancer." Radical surgeons argued that radiation therapy was a poor treatment for malignant tissue that could be surgically eliminated. It soon became clear that patients did not develop recurrent cancer nearly as often as the pathologists found these "multicentric" changes. Even today, radiation therapy is used to kill these cells.

EVIDENCE FOR CONSERVATIVE BREAST SURGERY GROWS

By the 1970s, the pioneers in breast-sparing surgery had concluded that local recurrence was not an ominous event. Sakari Mustakallio reviewed his thirty years of experience in Helsinki and concluded, "Thus, provided they are treated, regional metastases by no means impair the patient's prognosis."[44] Vera Peters in Toronto considered her thirty years of practice and observed, "Surgery alone is followed by a significantly higher recurrence rate, but an effect on survival could not be demonstrated."[45] J. M. Spitalier of Marseille, France, concluded, "Late recurrences were all operable and did not appear to be associated with decreased survival."[46] These surprising observations could be confirmed only with a scientifically sound study.

In 1976, the NSABP began its much-awaited lumpectomy trial and in 1985, it published the first results.[47] *Lumpectomy* was the removal of the tumor, along with a very narrow margin of normal tissue. All patients had their axillary (armpit) lymph nodes removed. This trial compared three different forms of treatment to the breast: modified radical mastectomy, lumpectomy alone, or lumpectomy plus postoperative radiation therapy. Pathologists were asked to verify that the edges of the removed tissue were free of tumor cells. However, everyone acknowledged that some microscopic tumor might have already spread into surrounding breast tissue, far from the eye of the pathologist.

The results were as follows. Patients treated with a modified radical mastectomy developed local recurrence about 8 percent of the time, patients treated with lumpectomy alone developed local recurrence 43 percent of the time, and patients treated with lumpectomy plus radiation therapy developed local recurrence 12 percent of the time.[48]

Those who developed local reccurence were treated with a second operation, either a salvage mastectomy or another lumpectomy. According to traditional surgical beliefs, patients who developed local recurrence should have fared poorly. But the survival results were surprising. Patients initially treated by lumpectomy alone *survived every bit as long* as those treated with aggressive treatment (mastectomy or lumpectomy plus radiation). The 43-percent recurrence rate among lumpectomy patients did not decrease overall survival. These results confirmed and extended earlier findings from Sweden, Canada, and France.

After conservative treatment, promptly treated recurrent cancer in the breast or neighboring lymph nodes can be removed with little, if any, risk to patient survival. This remarkable observation was the antithesis of one hundred years of surgical belief and practice. It suggested two important questions. One, does this observation apply to other malignancies? Two, why does local recurrence following conservative surgery appear to behave in such an innocent, or nonthreatening, fashion?

RESEARCH RAISES QUESTIONS

No cancer has been studied as thoroughly as breast cancer. For other malignancies, there has been much less experience with conservative surgery. It is uncertain whether the general lessons learned from breast cancer can be applied to other malignancies. But, as you will see in the last half of this book, there is increasing evidence that many cancers seem to behave like breast cancer. That is, local recurrence following limited surgery is not an ominous event.

Soft tissue sarcomas are tumors that arise from muscle, fat, or other body tissues. Before 1960, these cancers were often treated with amputation. Since then, surgeons have treated sarcomas with wide excision and postoperative radiation therapy. After reviewing the experience of many institutions, it is clear that radiation reduces local recurrence, but does not enhance overall survival. Murray Brennan of Memorial Sloan-Kettering Cancer Center conducted a scientific trial comparing patients using wide excision with or without radiation therapy. Brennan concluded, "[A] decrease in local recurrence is not accompanied by an improvement in the long-term survival rate." [49]

The same results have been found in the treatment of malignant melanoma. The World Health Organization (WHO) Collaborating Centres for Evaluation and Treatment of Melanoma collected 593 cases.[50] Patients treated with narrow margins of excision had an increased rate of local recurrence, but their overall survival was not decreased. The WHO trial showed no correlation between the width of excision and eventual mortality. (Studies of other kinds of cancers are summarized in Appendix I.)

The innocent behavior of local recurrence is still a mystery—a mystery that has been largely ignored. Explanations have been suggested, but none has received general acceptance. Some surgeons believe that a few microscopic cancer cells left behind at surgery may spread and ultimately prove fatal. Others believe that the those few cells may grow into a detectable tumor, but that the recurrence can be removed without jeopardy to the patient's life. This distinction is very important for patients who wish to preserve their bodily form and function. Every stroke of the surgeon's knife *depends on his or her perception of local recurrence.*

I believe that the dilemma of local recurrence has a logical explanation. Just as small primary cancers are usually harmless, so also small recurrent cancers may be innocent. I will present my explanation in Chapter 4. Some knowledge of the interaction between a cancer and the patient is helpful to understand this dilemma. This interaction is discussed next in Chapters 2 and 3.

As the twentieth century draws to a close, so ends the first hundred years in the modern treatment of cancer. Radical surgery is being modified, and conservative surgery is finding greater acceptance. Many leaders in the field of surgical oncology believe that additional trials of conservative surgery are necessary before traditional treatment is altered. The eradication of every possible cancer cell is still the primary objective. Fear of local recurrence continues to be the basis of cancer treatment.

In 1992, George Crile, Jr., America's pioneer in partial mastectomy and conservative surgery for cancer, died of lung cancer. He had devoted his professional life to protecting women from disfiguring surgery. In his autobiography, *The Way It Was*, Crile says: "In retrospect most of what I said has been proved to be correct. However, to my knowledge none of my critics has ever retracted their statements."[51]

Over a period of thirty years, Crile had become immune to the criticism of his fellow surgeons. He was not honored for his pioneering work in breast cancer because the leaders in American surgery were still defending their outmoded surgical principles.

But this has not stopped the accumulation of evidence supporting conservative surgery.

It is a sad commentary on American surgery that surgeons like George Crile and John Stehlin have not been widely honored for their pioneering work. The leaders in American surgery have seen their cherished ideas and their radical operations replaced by new ideas and conservative operations. They have been too proud to recognize the pioneers who brought about this great change. In the fields of gynecology and urology, these new ideas are only beginning to gain acceptance. It will be many years indeed before conservative surgery is widely practiced.

The twentieth century saw tumultuous change in the principles and practice of cancer surgery. It may take the persistence of informed patients to bring this process to completion.

2.

The Behavior of Cancer

Anybody who has been seriously engaged in scientific work of any kind realizes that over the entrance to the gates of the temple of science are written the words: Ye must have faith. It is a quality which the scientist cannot dispense with.

Max Planck, 1932

Scientists have learned much about the behavior of cancer in the past twenty years. Changes in surgical treatment are only a small part of the great progress being made in all areas of cancer research. Environmental hazards have been identified and reduced. Individuals are understanding and improving their personal habits. Early detection programs are gaining acceptance for breast, cervical, and rectal cancer. Scientists are learning much at the genetic, biochemical, and molecular levels. They have put into place hundreds of pieces of a very intricate puzzle, and a picture is beginning to emerge. The picture is that of a struggle between cancer cells on one side, and the patient's defense system on the other.

It is well known that advances in treatment have been disappointing. In 1971, President Richard Nixon declared a "War on Cancer." Many authors have reviewed the string of optimistic predictions and disappointments that followed.[1] The principal focus of cancer research has been upon finding a "cure" or a more effective therapy. But it is very difficult to treat a disease that one barely understands. NASA required an understanding of aviation and jet propulsion to send a man to the moon. Likewise, cancer researchers require an understanding of tumor growth and spread in order to design effective therapy. This chapter reviews much of the progress made in this area. Most of this knowledge has been gained in the past twenty-five years. (Chapter 3 deals with the mechanisms used by the body to prevent the spread of tumor cells.)

There are two sides in a great battle: the cancer and the patient. This is called the tumor-patient conflict. For many years, physicians have seen evidence that patients fight their cancer. (Scientists have been studying this battle in animals for decades. They have called it the tumor-host conflict.) Because of cancer's unpredictable behavior, doctors have assumed that random chance plays an important role in this battle; the random growth and spread of cancer cells fights the beleaguered defenses of the patient. As we learn about the biology of cancer, we realize that the growth and spread of tumor cells is governed by more than random chance.

THE UNANSWERED QUESTIONS

Before I begin to explain what has been discovered in recent years, it is important for you to consider the questions about cancer that remain unanswered. Conflicts over treatment are based upon conflicting answers to these questions.

When do cancer cells from a growing tumor begin to circulate in the blood stream?

Doctors used to believe that most tumors must reach about the size of a grape before tumor cells could be shed into the blood stream, because few patients with smaller tumors developed distant metastases. As recently as the 1970s, scientists believed that some tumor cells simply were pushed mechanically into nearby blood vessels by the pressure of a growing tumor.

Physicians have trouble studying the circulation of cancer because it is almost impossible to find cancer cells within a patient's blood stream. Within each drop of blood there are 250,000 to 500,000 white blood cells and hundreds of millions of red blood cells. No instrument can automatically identify cancer cells in a blood sample, and it is difficult using a microscope to find cancer cells among so many normal blood cells.

However, some progress has been made. In animals, scientists have found tumor cells in the blood flowing out of a tumor. In humans, scientists have identified tumor cells in blood vessels flowing away from large tumors. Most scientists agree that tumor cell circulation begins to occur early, well before a tumor can be clinically detected. Lance Liotta, an authority on tumor cell metastasis (spread) at the National Cancer Institute, states in a prominent cancer textbook, "For many common epithelial tumors [such as the carcinomas included in this book], the onset of tumor cell dissemination [spread] occurs soon after primary tumor vascularization [blood vessel formation]. It has been calculated that most metastases from breast cancer are initiated when the primary tumor is less than 0.125 cm."[2] (This is slightly larger than two drops of water.)

Most of this research was done in the 1970s. But not all physicians, especially surgeons, have accepted Liotta's conclusion. Today, scientists are trying to learn how tumor cells spread and create metastases, information presented later in this chapter. Scientists are now trying to identify the size at which each type of cancer begins to shed tumor cells.

It is important to distinguish here between the circulation of tumor cells in the blood stream and the development of distant metastases. The latter are established colonies of growing tumor cells that are able to sustain themselves from the nutrients in their environment.

Why do some tumors form distant metastases while others do not?

As the tumor grows, the probability of distant spread increases. Cancer cells have extraordinary capabilities that allow them to grow, invade, and spread. Tumors can spread in three different ways: locally by direct extension, via lymph vessels, and via the blood stream. In a single tumor, only about one in every million cells can metastasize. Cancer cells vary widely in their ability to spread. Tests are now available that can identify which tumors have the greatest chance of spreading. But even with elaborate tests, tumors can behave unpredictably. Some consider the unpredictability to be due to random chance. Others believe that the immune system plays a role in regulating the spread of tumor cells.

Are some patients better able to fight spreading cancer cells than others?

Patients fight cancer cells with a variety of defense mechanisms in much the same way they fight infection. Some doctors argue that the development of distant metastases depends almost completely on the tumor. They believe that the appearance of a cancer is evidence that the immune system has failed to do its job. The patient's defenses are defunct. However, the immune system is very complex. Most doctors believe that, even after a cancer has developed, the immune system can continue to function. Working within the blood stream and in distant organs, it can destroy tumor cells before they establish distant tumor colonies. Today, there are no tests that can accurately measure a patient's ability to fight circulating tumor cells. But researchers are beginning to discover clues about the ways in which patients differ in this important struggle. Because of the many factors involved in immune protection, it may be years before clinically useful tests are available.

So is the spread of cancer primarily a random process?

Like seeds spread by the wind, some aspects of tumor spread are subject to random chance. The park in my neighborhood is surrounded by large, old oak trees. Every autumn, acorns fall on the surrounding soil. They are spread and destroyed by humans, animals, wind, and other forces of nature. There are no saplings growing in this park or in nearby yards. Much of what occurs to these acorns may be considered random chance. But the soil in the park and the urban environment are not conducive to the growth of new trees. I do not expect this situation to change in the future. Like the soil surrounding these oak trees, patients resist the growth of tumor "seeds" in distant organs. It is logical to expect that the relationship between a patient and any residual cancer is stable over a period of many years.

If a few cancer cells are left inside the patient after surgery, can those remaining cells cause distant metastases?

The spread of cancer is subject to forces both random and unknown. No one can predict what will occur in an individual patient the first time cancer appears. But once a patient has been exposed to a cancer for several months, it is possible to reach some conclusions. If no metastases have developed, removal of the tumor will cure the patient. (Of course, it is important that the tumor is removed before the cancer becomes too large and overwhelms the patient's defenses with the sheer volume of cells being produced.) If the tumor recurs from a few unseen cells in the area of surgery, these cells are unlikely to spread. Like the acorns that fall every year, these tumor cells are restrained by the forces of the environment. This idea is very important to the issues considered in the book. It is discussed in Chapter 4.

If a patient develops, for example, a breast cancer, then a local recurrence, and then a distant metastasis, which cancer caused the distant metastasis?

In looking at a single patient, it is usually impossible to determine if a distant metastasis arose from the primary tumor or a local recurrence. Occasionally, a patient develops two separate types of tumors, and the source of the distant metastasis is clear. Answers to this difficult question have come from carefully planned scientific studies. The NSABP lumpectomy trial, discussed in Chapter 1, demonstrated that recurrent (or persistent) breast cancer does not cause distant metastasis. Therefore, distant metastases must almost always be caused by the original (or primary) breast cancer. Many surgeons have reached similar conclusions for the soft tissue sarcomas, malignant melanoma, and other tumors. I consider this to be an unanswered question because the answer I have given is not universally accepted.

Why do people die of cancer?

Death from cancer can occur in many different ways. The function of the kidneys or the intestinal tract can be shut down by a localized tumor growth that obstructs either system. Clearly, tumor growth in the brain or other vital organ could have a fatal outcome. More commonly, however, patients are overwhelmed by the growth of large tumors in several parts of the body. By robbing normal tissues of nutrients, cancer causes the healthy areas of the body to become emaciated. Eventually, even the cancer cells begin to die at a rapid rate. This releases a great deal of cellular waste into the blood stream, disturbing the body's delicate internal environment. This includes such things as acid-base balance, blood oxygen, and levels of sodium, potassium, and other elements. Ultimately, the kidneys and liver are unable to eliminate this enormous burden of toxic waste.

These questions may seem simple. Perhaps you thought that scientists who can decode DNA should have answered them by now. But the information needed to answer them is complex. In order for you to wrestle with these questions, you will first need a general idea about the participants in the tumor-patient conflict. The rest of this chapter takes a detailed look at the spread of tumor cells. However, you do not have to learn all of the information presented here to understand the primary message of this book and how it can help you deal with your cancer. At any time during this chapter, you may skip ahead to Chapters 3 or 4, or to Part Two, without losing the continuity of the book.

If you want to keep going, you should first have a general feeling for the way in which doctors learn about cancer and how they reach conclusions. I believe you will then see why there are so many unanswered questions about cancer.

HOW WE LEARN ABOUT SCIENCE

Cancer research can be divided into two broad categories, basic science and clinical science. This distinction applies, of course, to all medical research. Medical schools across the country are organized along departmental lines that recognize this distinction.

Basic Science

Basic science is usually conducted in a laboratory, in test tubes and experimental animals. The complex maze of interactions between cancer cells and their hosts (the patients or animals with cancer) can be unraveled one step at a time in very controlled situations. Scientists have learned much about tumor growth and spread at the genetic and biochemical level, atom by atom. Each of these studies focuses on a very narrow facet of a complex puzzle. Most of the information discussed in this chapter is the result of basic research.

Some of this detailed information is beginning to play a role in treating patients. Much of it, though, does not yet figure in treatment. Studies in test tubes cannot determine how cancer cells behave when they must interact with all the cells and organs of a living being. Studies in animals cannot always determine how cancer cells behave in humans. To do this, doctors must conduct clinical studies.

Clinical Science

Clinical science involves the study of patients and is usually conducted in hospitals. There are two basic types of clinical studies: retrospective and prospective trials.

Most studies published today are *retrospective*—studies that look back. Physicians often report their experience with a particular cancer by reviewing patient charts from their practice or their hospital. These studies have many shortcomings. For example, patients with one type of cancer may have been treated with operation A or operation B. Let us assume that patients lived longer after operation A. The following questions have to be answered:

- Did these patients have less advanced cancers?
- Did the doctor who performed operation A see his or her patients more often during the months following surgery?
- Was surgeon A better than surgeon B?
- How did the study count patients who moved away or otherwise became lost?
- How did the study count patients who died of causes other than cancer?

A real-life example of the flaws found in retrospective studies is presented in Chapter 9 on malignant melanoma. Many surgeons have reported that patients with this disease live longer if their lymph nodes are also removed during the operation in which the melanoma is removed. I believe that retrospective studies have exaggerated the benefit of this operation. Many patients who had only their melanomas removed returned to their surgeons with nodes massively enlarged with cancer. They died as a result of the large recurrence. Many of them could have been cured if they had returned earlier. These retrospective studies focused on whether a certain operation was performed or deferred. They failed to adequately measure the quantity of tumor in the lymph nodes. The problem was not failure to remove the lymph nodes at the first operation, but failure to carefully watch for enlarging lymph nodes after the first operation.

Another example is the debate on breast-sparing surgery. By 1975, over sixty articles on breast-sparing surgery had been published in medical journals. These studies all reported that breast-sparing surgery was as successful as was more radical surgery in curing breast cancer. However, because of the kinds of problems mentioned above, doctors required more scientific studies before they adopted breast-sparing treatment.

Prospective studies are much better. These are studies which are planned and then carried out into the future. Physicians are not simply reviewing patient charts to find information. The trials are also usually *randomized*; patients are randomly assigned to one form of treatment or another. (Of course, patients must understand the nature of the study and agree to participate.) Here the sickest patients are evenly divided among the various treatments, and all physicians deliver each of the treatments under investigation. These studies follow a rigid set of rules and require years to complete. For example, the NSABP lumpectomy trial, discussed in Chapter 1, only accepted patients who met certain criteria: tumors that were 4 cm or less in diameter, tumors that were not attached to surrounding tissue, enlarged lymph nodes (if present) not attached to surrounding tissue, and so forth. In total, there were twenty-two criteria.

Prospective trials can find out if one operation is better than another, if one combination of chemotherapy drugs is better than another, and so forth. But these studies do not provide the detailed look at tumor growth and spread provided by laboratory studies.

Applying Basic Principles to Clinical Situations

Scientists and doctors are studying cancer from two directions. Basic scientists are unraveling cancer at the molecular level, and doctors are trying to improve treatment results at the clinical level. Much of what we will learn about cancer in this chapter, such as the role of DNA in cell mutation, is basic science. Basic science helps us formulate principles that apply to all cancers regardless of where in the body they originate. Studies of breast cancer, prostate cancer, and malignant melanoma have all contributed to our basic understanding of this disease.

However, I believe that these unifying principles can become lost in clinical situations, which involve treatments used on actual patients with specific cancers. Clinical science is divided into specialties based on anatomy (the different parts of the body). Surgeons in each speciality are often concerned primarily with the technical aspects of the operations they perform, and not with overall principles of cancer. Also, in trying to keep up with the flood of information within their own specialties, doctors often find it difficult to step back and view cancer from a basic science perspective. Thus, they often cannot see how information from urology, for example, may apply to gynecology or to general surgery. It is easy to become lost in the details of scientific research and lose sight of its general aims, in this case, learning about how cancer—any cancer—grows and spreads. But, just like basic scientists, I believe that surgeons of all specialties should be familiar with knowledge gained from all types of cancer.

Between basic science and clinical science lie the many unanswered questions mentioned above. But we have learned a great deal about how cells work and how they go wrong. We will begin by looking at a normal cell.

THE NORMAL CELL

Cancer is a complicated disease, but no more complicated than the growth and development of a single cell, an event we take for granted. A human cell is divided into two sections, the nucleus and the cytoplasm. The nucleus is the headquarters of the cell. It gives orders to the cytoplasm, which contains machinery needed to manufacture proteins and other chemicals that carry out the cell's function. The nucleus is also where cell division starts.

Both protein formation and cell division are controlled by twenty-three pairs of chromosomes made up of deoxyribonucleic acid (DNA). Twisting through the nucleus of the cell, DNA is made up of two strands that together resemble a spiral staircase, or a double helix. (Note that there are two different kinds of pairs: the chromosomes are paired, and then each chromosome is made up of paired DNA strands.) The chromosomes contain genes; each gene consists of segments of DNA. Within the DNA of *each* cell is the information needed to make *every* cell. The DNA contains all of the 100,000 genes required to form a complete person, information that is also known as the human genome. Surprisingly, these 100,000 genes represent only 3 percent of the entire human genome. The remaining DNA does not carry the codes to manufacture protein molecules. This so-called "junk DNA" may be responsible for gene repair and other functions.

HOW DNA CONTROLS CELL FUNCTION

To understand how DNA controls cell function, you must first understand how it is structured. We can then look at how DNA directs both cell division and protein formation.

The Structure of DNA

The structure of DNA can be compared to a simple ladder. To visualize the way DNA duplicates itself, you must saw the ladder in half, cutting each step in the middle. Now glue the ladder back together with weak glue. The upright boards represent long chains of sugar molecules alternating with phosphate compounds.

Attached to each sugar molecule is a nitrogen-containing compound, called a base. These bases stick out from the upright sugar-phosphate chain like the steps on the ladder. One base from each side of the ladder is paired with a base from the opposite side. Together, they form a step. The bases are loosely attached to each other, like the ladder steps that are weakly glued together. There are only four bases: adenine, thymine, guanine, and cytosine. Adenine is always paired with thymine, and guanine is always paired with cytosine. To visualize the shape of DNA, it is necessary to twist the ladder along its long axis, down the middle of the glued steps. The result is a double helix. It also helps to think of the simple children's toy called a Slinky, which is a long piece of metal tightly wound into a short length. In a similar fashion, the shape of the DNA molecule allows a lot of information to be stored in a short space.

DNA and Cell Division

Acting like the dots and dashes of Morse code, or the holes in an old-fashioned Wall Street ticker tape, the order of the bases is the genetic code. Before a cell divides, the spiral staircase unwinds and then separates down the middle, the steps of the ladder dividing in two. Each side of the ladder serves as a mold to create a complementary opposite strand of DNA from base molecules floating free within the nucleus. The sugar-phosphate upright chain is also reproduced from sugar and phosphate molecules floating about in the nucleus. This process is called *DNA synthesis*. After the DNA in the nucleus duplicates itself, the rest of the cell then divides. This process is called *mitosis*. Each daughter cell contains a complete set of twenty-three chromosome pairs. The time required for a cell to go through a complete reproductive cycle is called the *doubling time*.

Naturally, cell division is at its most active during fetal development. It is during this period that cells commit themselves to becoming one type of cell or another. As they become different, they are said to *differentiate*. Some cells become skin, others muscles, nerves, or even cancer-fighting white blood cells.

DNA and Protein Formation

DNA controls the cell by sending information to the cytoplasm. The double helix unwinds, exposing its bases (the ladder rungs): cystine, adenine, guanine, and thymine. The exposed DNA serves as a template to form a nearly identical compound called ribonucleic acid (RNA). This process is called *transcription*, because the RNA is practically a copy of the DNA. RNA differs from DNA in that it contains a different sugar, and that of the four bases, uracil replaces thymine. It is practically a complementary mirror image of the DNA.

The RNA travels out of the nucleus into the cytoplasm. It attaches to a ribosome, which manufactures proteins based upon the chemical code in the RNA. This process is called *translation*, because information is changed from one language to another. For example, the base sequence ACC (adenine-cystine-cystine) in DNA transcribes into UGG (uracil-guanine-guanine) in RNA, which then translates into the amino acid tryptophan. Tryptophan is one of twenty amino acids, chemicals that are the building blocks of protein molecules. These proteins make up cell products such as digestive enzymes, insulin, or blood clotting factors. Some cancer-causing chemicals interfere with this coding process. For example, aflatoxin, a fungal product, causes the substitution of thymine for guanine.

Manufactured proteins or other compounds are packaged and carried to the cell's surface. Here they can be released, or become part of a receptor on the surface. Receptors receive information from the environment. The receptors send signals into the cell, instructing it to manufacture products or to begin the process of cell division.

WHAT CAUSES CANCER?

Cancer gets started in many different ways. Genetic abnormalities, which can be inherited, make members of some families more susceptible to certain kinds of malignancies, such as breast, ovarian, and colon cancer. Chromosomes also can be injured by environmental toxins, such as smoke, asbestos, and radiation. Viruses inject abnormal DNA into the nucleus of a cell and alter the normal chromosomes. Alcohol, as well as certain drugs and chemicals, can also facilitate the development of cancer.

When a normal gene is transformed into a cancer-causing gene, it is called an *oncogene*. Oncogenes play a role in over 25 percent of human cancers. These genes are normally involved in the regulation of cell growth; for example, the normal *myc* gene is required for blood-forming cells to start making DNA.

About 100 different oncogenes have been identified so far. Of these, about 50 play a role in human tumors. (The rest affect laboratory animals.) For example, the first gene found to be responsible for hereditary breast cancer, BRCA1, was discovered in September 1994. However, it does not play a major role in most breast cancers because most breast cancers are not hereditary. Furthermore, scientists have discovered twenty-two different defects that can occur in this gene. This adds to the difficulty of developing a single blood test to identify patients who have inherited a BRCA1 gene.

Mistakes in Cell Division

Each time a cell divides, it must accurately duplicate its 3 billion pairs of bases. Sometimes mistakes are made, a mutation occurs, and an abnormal cell is created. When errors appear in a cell's DNA code, genes can recognize these mistakes. Within the nucleus of the cell, enzymes go to work cutting out the faulty DNA and replacing it with normal DNA. Damage to one strand of the DNA double helix is easy to repair, because the opposite strand contains the information needed to correct the mistake. Damage to both strands of DNA is much more serious, and can result in the production of an abnormal cell product, cancer, or cell death.

During this repair process, cell division is shut down by a gene called p53. This gene was originally identified as a gene that suppressed tumor growth (a *tumor-suppressor gene*). It was later discovered that this gene serves a function in the repair of damaged DNA in otherwise normal cells. (This is typical of cancer research. A substance is discovered that helps or hinders tumor growth. Later, someone discovers the normal function of this substance in healthy cells. For example, many cancer genes have a normal function during fetal development.)

Three-dimensional models of the p53 protein have been constructed. Scientists understand the various ways in which this protein can twist itself into the DNA double helix and hinder DNA duplication. It can hinder the growth and spread of tumor cells, when that process is driven by the action of overactive oncogenes. It can also become an oncogene itself if its DNA is damaged, and can thus contribute to tumor development. The abnormal p53 tumor-suppressor gene plays a role in about half of all human cancers.

About twelve different tumor-suppressor genes have been identified. These genes are able to slow the growth and spread of cells that have been turned ON by cancer-causing oncogenes or by other cancer-causing cell damage. One example is multiple tumor suppressor gene 1 (MTS1). MTS1 directs the cell to make p16, another protein that interferes with cell division. Researchers hope to retard tumor growth with medicines that act like normal p53 or p16 proteins. It has recently been shown that common antitumor agents are effective only in tumors with a normal p53 gene. Thus, tumor cells lacking a normal p53 resist the effects of radiation therapy and of various chemotherapy agents.[3] For many tumors, an abnormal p53 gene makes the prognosis worse.

How Cell Division Mistakes Become Cancerous

Scientists believe that cancer is seldom caused by a single event or cellular abnormality. They think that a regulatory gene (such as p53) must receive two or more attacks, or hits, from one of the cancer-causing agents mentioned earlier before it malfunctions. Sometimes, abnormal cell growth occurs that is premalignant, such as polyps of the colon or some forms of actively growing breast tissue. Over a period of several years, these cells can gradually become malignant due to additional attacks on the DNA. Even genes with inherited abnormalities require additional chromosome damage to initiate cancer. Chromosomal damage can increase the rate of cell division. A rapidly dividing cell is more likely to make errors as the DNA is duplicated. Each new error increases the chance for the cell to become malignant.

Cell growth is also regulated by other chains of DNA known as *telomeres*. A young cell has thousands of telomeres attached to the end of the chromosomal DNA, like the tip of a shoelace. Each time a cell divides, one or two dozen telomeres are lost. When all the telomeres have been lost, the chromosome breaks down and the cell dies. This is part of the normal aging process. Most cancer cells produce an enzyme called telomerase, which prevents the loss of telomeres. The biological clock of these cells is stopped. They become immortal, that is, malignant. (Agents have been found that block the action of this enzyme, allowing cancer cells to age and die normally. Perhaps one of them will become the "magic bullet"—a drug that kills cancer cells without harming normal cells.)

A cancer cell has been compared to an automobile with many accelerators, called oncogenes, and many brakes, called tumor-suppressor genes. Cells go through several phases as various accelerators are activated and various brakes cease to function. A cancer cell is able to invade and spread when all the accelerators are pressed to the floor and all the brakes have ceased to function.

HOW TUMORS GROW

Our bodies grow to a certain size and then stop growing. Our organs do the same. If we lose blood, we manufacture enough blood to replace what was lost and then stop. Cancer cells lack the signal to stop growing; they grow and grow. Cancer is initially a cell's failure to control its own division and growth, a failure that is continuously passed on to each new generation of cancerous cells. The ON-OFF switch for cell division is locked in the ON position.

Cancer is thought to begin from a single cell. It divides repeatedly. Some tumors double in size every few days, while others require several months. After a tumor has divided twenty times, it contains about one million cells. It is still so small that it cannot be felt or seen on an X-ray or scan. A cancer must double about thirty times to reach the diameter of 1 cm (3/8 of an inch). At this size it contains about one billion cells and can often be felt.

After a tumor has been removed, it is studied by a pathologist. He examines it with the naked eye and under the microscope. He can usually figure out if the tumor is malignant and where it arose, since most cancer cells resemble the normal tissue from which they grew. None of the tests for any of the following factors has an absolute influence on treatment decisions. But many doctors consider them when deciding whether to be more or less aggressive with chemotherapy and other treatment.

Tumor Grade

The pathologist can also see how many cells were dividing. The more dividing cells he sees, the faster the tumor was growing.

Slower-growing cancers are called *low grade* or differentiated. Again, the cancer cells are distinctive in that they closely resemble the normal tissue from which they were derived. They retain the unique characteristics of breast or lung tissue, for example. Patients with slow-growing tumors are usually less likely to develop distant metastases. If metastases do develop, they grow slowly too.

Some cancer cells often appear very abnormal, even "wild" to the trained eye. These fast-growing tumors are called *high grade* or undifferentiated. Undifferentiated tumors all appear similar. (They are "undifferent.") There are many rapidly dividing cells with little distinguishing form or architectural pattern. These tumors are more likely to spread, and have a poorer prognosis than low-grade tumors. These differences can be seen in Figure 2.1.

Chromosome Number

Besides a tumor's grade, or rate of growth, oncologists—doctors who specialize in the study and treatment of cancer—often consider the number of chromosomes present. Cancer cells frequently gain or lose chromosomes as they divide. (High-grade tumors with an abnormal number of chromosomes are associated with a very poor prognosis.)

Recently, pathologists have been able to measure cell growth more accurately by measuring the amount of DNA within the tumor cells. One test that measures DNA is called *flow cytometry*. Cells with a normal twenty-three pairs of chromosomes are called diploid. (In Greek, *diplous* means double and *-ploid* mean fold, the folds of the DNA.) Cells with an abnormal number of chromosomes are called aneuploid (*aneu-* means abnormal). Aneuploid cells often divide rapidly, causing a worse prognosis. Flow cytometry can measure the percentage of cells that have normal DNA. Flow cytometry can also measure the fraction of cells that are in the DNA synthesis phase, or S phase, of cell division. A tumor with a high fraction of cells in the S phase is growing rapidly and often behaves aggressively. Aggressive tumors double their size in a short period of time. For example, some lymphomas double in 40 hours, compared with a doubling time of 600 days for some adenocarcinomas.

Hormone Receptors

Another factor that decides the aggressiveness of a cancer is the presence or absence of hormone receptors. In the body, there are dozens of hormones, which are constantly acting on various cells. Hormones stimulate cells to carry out their normal function. Insulin helps cells burn sugar for energy. Thyroid

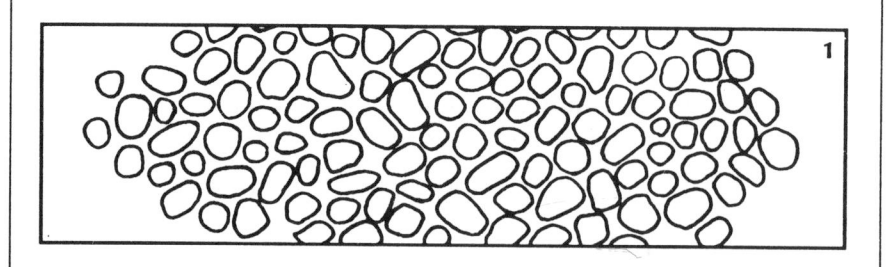

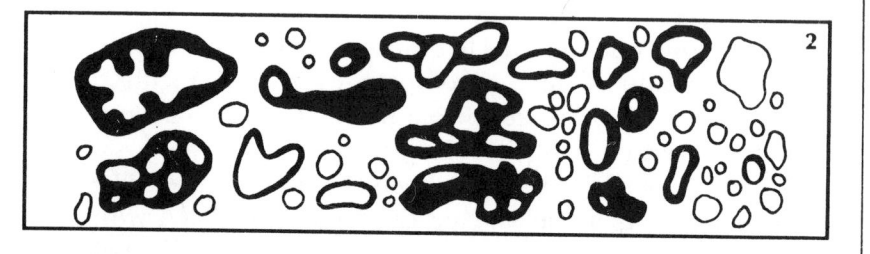

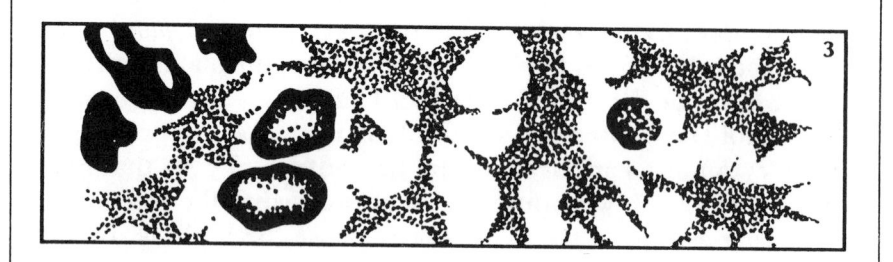

Figure 2.1 Tumor Grade as Seen in Prostate Cancer. As shown in this figure, the higher a cancer's grade, the more abnormal it appears under a microscope. Panel 1 shows a low-grade or well-differentiated cancer. The glands within the prostate are separate and of uniform size, and they form a nearly normal pattern. Panel 2 shows moderately differentiated cancer, in which the glands are still separate, but vary in size and shape. They form a more obviously abnormal pattern. Panel 3 shows a high-grade or poorly differentiated cancer, in which the glands are fused together in clumps. They show almost no pattern at all.

hormone helps us maintain our normal body temperature. Growth hormone stimulates cell growth. Estrogen, a female hormone, stimulates breast growth.

In order for a cell to respond to a hormone, it must have on its surface a hormone receptor. Each hormone and each receptor must fit perfectly, like a key in a lock. The hormone attaches to this receptor and triggers a series of events inside the cell. The cell ultimately responds to the stimulus of the hormone by either dividing or producing milk, stomach acid, or another product.

Cancer cells may have hormone receptors on their surfaces. For example, breast cancer cells that have estrogen receptors (estrogen-receptor positive) are more nearly like normal cells, and therefore less aggressive. Breast cancer cells that do not have estrogen receptors on their surface are less like normal cells, and therefore more aggressive. Because cancers that are estrogen-receptor positive are more like normal cells, patients with such cancers have a better prognosis than do those whose cancers are estrogen-receptor negative. Estrogen-receptor status also influences whether a tumor will respond to hormonal therapy. Tumors that are estrogen receptor-positive are more likely to respond to therapy that changes the patient's hormonal environment.

Hormone Production

Cancer cells can also manufacture a variety of hormones called growth factors that can stimulate the growth of cells. Some cells stimulate their own growth; these growth factors are called autocrines. Growth factors that stimulate nearby cells are called paracrines. Growth factors that stimulate the growth of distant cells are the classic endocrine hormones. A cell must have a specific growth factor receptor on its surface to be stimulated by that growth factor. For example, breast cancer patients whose tumors contain these receptors are more likely to develop recurrence after surgery. The ability to detect growth factors may help doctors to distinguish between patients with localized cancer and those whose disease has spread.

Some tumors produce a hormone called tumor angiogenesis factor, which stimulates the growth of capillaries into the tumor. These blood vessels are needed to bring oxygen and nutrients to the growing tumor. Without these new blood vessels, the tumor might outgrow its supply of vital nourishment and die. Growing endothelial cells (blood vessel cells) may also stimulate the spread of tumor cells.[4] Some researchers have shown that distant metastases and patient survival are significantly affected by the density of capillaries in early breast cancer.[5] This suggests that tumor spread may be influenced by the volume of circulating tumor cells that enter the blood stream via these tiny blood vessels.

HOW CANCER SPREADS

Before most cancers can spread, or metastasize, to distant organs, they have to invade tissues at the site of the tumor. In this section, we will look at the types of tissue the body is made up of, and see how cancer invades and then spreads from these tissues.

Types of Tissue

The human body consists of dozens of different types of tissue. *Epithelial cells* are among the most common. They cover all the free surfaces of the body. This includes the skin; the lining of the oral cavity; the intestines; the airways; and the ducts that carry milk, bile, digestive juices, and other fluids throughout the body. Some epithelial cell surfaces are constantly moistened with mucus, such as those of the oral cavity and intestinal tract. These are mucosal epithelial cells. Carcinomas arise from epithelial cells.

Epithelial cells rest on a very thin *basement membrane*, which supports the continuous production of epithelial cells. Beneath the basement membrane is a layer of connective tissue. *Connective tissue* provides a microscopic latticework throughout the body to support nerves, blood vessels, fatty tissue, hair follicles, and other structures, just as the skeleton provides a framework of bones to connect the tendons and muscles. There are several types of connective tissue. They include the elastic fibers that give skin its spring; the material that binds together fat cells; the material in the ligaments and tendons; and the lining of muscles, the brain, and the nervous system. Sarcomas arise from connective tissue.

Endothelial cells line the blood vessels. The various organs contain specialized cells that produce hormones, digestive enzymes, and other products. Bone, cartilage, and muscle are made up of still other kinds of tissue.

How Cancer Cells Invade Surrounding Tissue

Most of the cancers covered in this book start in the epithelial cells. Cancers that arise from these cells are not considered invasive until they escape beyond the basement membrane and into the connective tissue. Once into the connective tissue, they have better access to blood vessels and to the lymphatic vessels. (Lymphatic vessels carry lymph, the clear fluid that bathes all the body's cells.) In order to enter a blood vessel, a tumor cell must also penetrate the wall of the blood vessel, which itself includes both a basement membrane and a layer of endothelial cells.

A tumor cell produces a multitude of chemicals that enable it to move from one part of the body to another. These tissue enzymes, called proteases, can disrupt the basement membranes of tissues. Like the enzymes in the digestive tract, these enzymes can digest or break down protein and carbohydrates into small pieces. (The meat tenderizer we buy to soften steaks is an enzyme that disrupts tissue.) Tumor cells must disrupt these barriers to get into and out of blood vessels, and to invade normal organs.

The production of each tissue-dissolving enzyme is under genetic control. Specific genes and chromosomes have been identified for many enzymes. For example, a gene called *ras* was identified for its ability to transform normal cells into malignant cells. This gene allows the transformed cells to produce a certain type of tissue-dissolving enzyme called type IV collagenase, which dissolves a connective tissue called type IV collagen. Many other enzymes have been identified, a different enzyme for each of the different types of connective tissue. The blood and most tissues can produce proteins that inhibit the function of these enzymes. Inhibitors are there to protect the membranes of the body from damage. When cancer develops, these inhibitors are overwhelmed by the large amount of tissue-dissolving enzymes.

The ability of cells to break down membrane barriers and move through other types of tissue is not completely foreign to normal cells. Some of these activities occur during the nine months of normal fetal development. A human embryo must attach to and invade the wall of the uterus, form a placenta, and develop a network of blood vessels. Most of the enzymes that facilitate these tasks are no longer produced in normal cells after birth. The DNA that controls their production is switched off or a suppressor gene is switched on. Some tumors reactivate these enzymes by flipping the switch. These cancer cells produce fetal proteins that can be identified and measured in the blood.

How Cancer Cells Metastasize

In order to form distant colonies, or metastases, cancer cells from the original tumor must enter the blood stream. To do that, they must pass through two basement membranes: the basement membrane of the organ where the cancer arose, and the basement membrane surrounding the blood vessel. Each membrane is woven from several different types of connective tissue, and the membranes are different throughout the body. Although the cancer arose from a single cell, not all of the cells in a tumor are able to spread. Probably about one cell out of every million can manufacture all the enzymes and other proteins necessary to support tumor growth, invasion, and spread.

In order to invade nearby capillaries, the tumor cells must be able to recognize them. To do this, tumor cells have receptors on their surface that recognize the tissues around a capillary. The receptor is a chain of atoms, resembling a tangled string, that fits precisely with a matching chemical in the environment or on the membrane of another cell. (In recent years, scientists have been able to identify many receptors atom by atom. Computer-generated models can now recreate the precise shape of many chemical receptors.)

Tumor cells can also break away from the primary tumor and be carried to nearby lymph nodes via the lymph vessels. Lymph filters out through the thin walls of capillaries, carrying nutrients and other substances to the cells. (The red blood cells remain within the capillaries.) Once outside the blood vessel, the lymph flows toward lymph nodes located in the armpits, the groin areas, and the neck. These lymph nodes can filter out bacteria and cancer cells. Lymph eventually reenters the blood stream via a large vein in the neck.

Physicians used to believe that cancer cells drifted passively from the tumor to the nearby lymph nodes, where they would be trapped for months. It was thought that large tumors shed enough tumor cells to overload the filter capacity of the lymph nodes, allowing the cells to pass into the blood stream. Scientists now realize that tumor spread is an active process.

When cancer cells lodge in a lymph node, the patient's prognosis becomes much worse. The lymph nodes are said to be "positive" for cancer cells. As a tumor grows, the lymph nodes in the region are more likely to become positive. I believe that the increasing shower of tumor cells overwhelms the defense mechanisms in the lymph nodes. Lymph nodes can also become positive in patients with small tumors that do not appear aggressive. When tumor cells grow and thrive within a node filled with "tumor-fighting" lymphocytes, one may conclude that these lymphocytes are ineffective. Thus, positive lymph nodes may also be an indication of a weak host defense system. (This problem was studied in NSABP trial B-04, discussed in Chapter 1.)

All the while, cancer cells are constantly entering the circulatory system. Once inside the blood stream, tumor cells begin to flow toward the heart. While in the circulatory system, clumps of tumor cells are exposed to its pounding turbulence, thrown against blood vessel walls, and broken apart. The blood clotting mechanism may recognize the cells as abnormal and begin surrounding the tumor cell with a clot. (Over a hundred years ago pathologists saw tumor cells within blood clots. This led many doctors to conclude that living tumor cells could not spread to distant organs via the blood stream.)

The cells enter the right chamber of the heart and are pumped out into the lungs. Larger clusters of cells may be trapped there and form lung metastases. But small clusters pass back to the left side of the heart refreshed by oxygen from the lungs. The powerful left ventricle of the heart then pumps the cells into the rest of the body. Cancer cells circulate until they lodge in a narrow capillary in the liver or other organ. Tumor cells adhere to these tissues and secrete tissue-dissolving enzymes that disrupt the basement membrane of the capillaries. (These enzymes may be different from those that disrupted the basement membrane and blood vessels walls where the tumor began.) The organs affected by tumor spread are partially determined by the type of tissue-dissolving enzymes the tumor cells are able to manufacture. For example, cancer cells that are able to dissolve the tissues in the lung are likely to spread to the lung.

After passing outside of the capillaries in a distant organ, the cells may then migrate through the cellular matrix, the glue that holds the normal cells together. This barrier requires another type of tissue-degrading enzyme. Adhesion molecules—like the treads on a tire—are also needed to move the cancer cells through the tissue. A new web of capillaries must grow into the colony of spreading cancer cells before the metastasis can become established. The developing tumor does this by secreting homones, such as tumor angiogenesis factor, that lead to capillary production. Tumor cells are also nurtured by growth hormones from nearby tumor cells.

For many years, doctors debated whether tumor cells from a distant metastasis could cause additional metastases. Isaiah Fidler of M. D. Anderson Hospital in Houston designed elegant experiments in which the circulatory systems of two animals were united. Using this technique, he proved that tumor cells from distant metastases could also enter the blood stream and spread to other distant sites. Thus, metastases can metastasize.

We've seen what factors influence a tumor's ability to spread: tumor size, lymph node status, tumor grade, hormone receptor status, chromosome number, S phase fraction, and so forth. There are tests that allow us to measure these indicators of tumor activity. But there are no clinically available tests that provide equivalent information about the patient's side of the battle, such as the strength of a patient's immune system—how well the patient can kill cancer cells. This has led some clinicians to assume that tumor factors are the more important, and that patients are all about the same in the strength of their immune resistance. But some patients with large tumors and grave pathological signs manage to do well, and others with small tumors with favorable signs die quickly of their disease. Some scientists believe that this may be due to the immune system. Patients who do well may have an immune system that can protect them from a large tumor challenge.

As I will explain in the next chapter, the immune system is very complex. One aspect of the system may fail, and allow a tumor to develop. But other aspects of the system may be able to prevent the spread of disease.

3.

The Defense Against Cancer

Far better it is to dare mighty things to win glorious triumphs, even though checkered by failure, than to take rank with those poor spirits who neither enjoy much nor suffer much, because they live in the gray twilight that knows not victory nor defeat.

                                        Theodore Roosevelt, 1899

Doctors have long known that cancer provokes a response from the human immune system. In Chapter 2, we saw how cancer behaves in the body. In this chapter, we will look at how the body reacts to cancer.

AN IMMUNE SYSTEM ON GUARD AGAINST CANCER?

Scientists have wondered why humans have different types of red blood cells and white blood cells. These differences interfere with such life-saving treatments as blood transfusion and organ transplantation. Red blood cell types prevent the transfusion of type A blood into a patient with type B. White blood cell types can cause the rejection of a transplanted organ. Why did nature erect this artificial barrier to life-saving treatment? The principle of evolution—survival of the fittest—offers no ready answer. Immune defenses against bacteria make sense, but organ transplantation is hardly a naturally occurring threat. How have our bodies developed defenses against such an unnatural event?

In the early years of organ transplantation, biologist Lewis

Thomas proposed a theory. He thought that organ rejection was related to the body's ability to recognize and reject one of its own cells. Thomas suggested that a normal cell might become abnormal, even malignant. Markers on the cell's surface might change as the cell changed internally. The patient's immune system might recognize this change and treat the cell as a foreign invader. The cancer cell could then be attacked or rejected by the immune system. Perhaps we are killing cancer cells in this way every day. Thus, we may all have immune systems that are constantly on guard against cancer. Thomas suggested that we may form cancer cells frequently and that our immune system is constantly destroying these cells. This is called the theory of immune surveillance.

This theory has never been verified or disproved. Tests are simply not available to do so. But some evidence supports the theory. Cancer is more likely to develop in patients with a depressed immune response. This includes patients with an inherited immune deficiency, those with AIDS, and recipients of transplanted organs (who must take drugs that suppress the immune response). This association between a depressed immune system and an increased risk of cancer supports the immune surveillance theory. Of more importance than whether this theory is eventually confirmed or rejected is the need for patients and doctors alike to realize how little is known about the interaction between cancer cells and the patient's immune system.

As recently as 1986, a prominent textbook of cancer surgery observed: "The consensus at present is that by the time patients have clinically detectable cancers, whatever *hypothetical immunologic battles* were fought have been lost."[1] [emphasis added] In other words, if the immune system is unable to prevent the cancer locally, then it is unable to control the spread of disease. I do not agree with this statement. Although the immune system may have lost the battle within the primary tumor itself, the battle within the blood stream is far from over. The immune system is far too complex to be overwhelmed by the development of a single tumor.

HOW THE BODY REACTS TO CANCER

Since the nineteenth century, physicians have been aware that the immune system responds to cancer. In 1888, William

Coley of Memorial Hospital in New York was horrified by the death of a nineteen-year-old woman from bone cancer. In an effort to improve the treatment of this disease, he began to review the records of all the patients who had been treated for bone cancer in that hospital. He went back fifteen years and found the record of a patient who had been treated for terminal bone cancer seven years earlier. The patient had developed severe infections while in the hospital, but ultimately walked out in good health. Coley searched the tenements of the city and found the patient, who was still free of cancer. He then developed a vaccine, from a culture of streptococcal bacteria in the hospital laboratory, that was intended to stimulate the immune system. He used the vaccine from the late 1890s to the 1930s. Memorial Hospital's famous pathologist James Ewing said that there was substantial evidence that many patients with bone tumors benefited from the vaccine. (It is interesting to note that the therapy was not accepted because its results were unpredictable. The patients usually had a high fever. As is the case with much of today's so-called "unconventional therapy," physicians were not comfortable with the treatment.)

Scientists have known for years that animals could be immunized against specific tumors. When cells from the same type of tumor were later injected into an immunized animal, the cells would be rejected, and a tumor would not form. The immune response was only effective against the same tumor used to immunize the animal. This is an important feature of the immune system; it is highly specific. For example, patients who have been immunized against three types of flu virus are still susceptible to infection by a fourth type of flu virus.

For many years, there has been clinical and laboratory evidence that the immune system attempts to kill cancer cells. However, our understanding of the significance of immune defense is elusive. The battles between tumor cells and immune cells have been studied one at a time, primarily in the test tube. It is understood that both the tumor and the patient contribute to the overall battle. But the outcome of their conflict within a living patient is not predictable, just as no one can predict the outcome of an athletic contest based upon the statistics of the individual players.

Distinguishing "Self" From "Non-self"

The tumor-patient conflict is complicated because cancer cells may appear to be normal from the viewpoint of the immune system. A cancer cell may have a genetic switch turned to the ON position, but that does not make it a "foreign" cell. Early in life, the immune system is coded to recognized all cells in the body as "self." Bacteria, viruses, and other invaders are easily recognized as foreign—the enemy. But most cancer cells arise out of normal cells and may have no distinguishing marks that identify them as malignant. Cancer cells are very similar to their noncancerous parental cells. A change in a few atoms on a DNA molecule or in the protein that it produces may easily go undetected by the immune system.

This is a remarkable characteristic of the immune system—its ability to distinguish a normal substance in the body, considered "self," from an abnormal substance, considered "non-self." But a cancer that cannot be recognized as foreign may pose a serious threat. This is the primary reason that cancer is so difficult to detect and to treat. In order for the immune system to function at all, it must be able to recognize the enemy.

What Are Antigens?

An *antigen* is any substance that is able to arouse an immune response within animals (including humans). Viruses, bacteria, and pollen are familiar examples of external antigens. There are also internal antigens; for example, the blood types A, B, O, and AB are determined by the antigens on our red blood cells. We have many other antigens located on all the tissues of our bodies. Their purpose is to allow the immune system to identify bodily tissues as "self."

Identifying Malignant Cells

Scientists have tried to identify new antigens on tumor cells that identify the cells as malignant. These are called *tumor-associated antigens*. Cancer cells may produce antigens that were present during fetal development, but are normally suppressed during adult life. Carcinoembryonic antigen (CEA), produced by cells from some cancers, is an example. Cancer cells may also produce larger amounts of antigens that are produced normally. Prostate-specific antigen (PSA) is an example. Tumor-associated antigens can also be produced by viruses, such as the human papillomavirus, which may play a role in cervical cancer, or cancer-causing chemicals, such as methyl cholanthrene, which has produced tumors in animals.

Responding to Tumor Formation

Cancer may have won the initial battle by forming a tumor, but the patient's immune system may be able to prevent the spread of disease. There is mounting evidence, especially in animal research, of intense struggles between cancer and the defense forces of the patient. These struggles take place within the primary tumor, the lymph nodes, and the blood stream, and at distant sites. As the tumor enlarges, more cancer cells enter the blood stream. Some patients can destroy these circulating cells and prevent the establishment of distant metastases. Others may become overwhelmed by the growing number of circulating tumor cells, thus allowing tumors to grow in one or more organs.

When a tumor first begins to grow, very few tumor cells are shed into the blood stream. There are thousands of white blood cells for every tumor cell. Cancer cells are unable to survive in such a hostile environment. Even patients with advanced cancer have hundreds of white cells in their blood for every cancer cell. However, some cancer cells are eventually able to escape the system of immune protection and establish a living colony of tumor cells in a distant organ. The development of a distant metastasis is an event, usually irreversible, that usually contributes to the death of the patient. Thus, it is not surprising that the immune system has special defenses to prevent tumor spread.

COMPONENTS OF THE IMMUNE SYSTEM

We have learned a great deal about the intricate workings of the immune system. Step by step, scientists have unraveled an extraordinarily complex system of self-protection. In some ways, though, we can't see the forest for the trees. Knowledge of our defense against cancer is much like our knowledge of cancer itself. Thousands of specific details have been uncovered, but the big picture is far from clear.

We do know that the body fights cancer with a variety of mechanical, biochemical, and immunological weapons. Body tissues act as protective barriers against the spread of tumor cells. Blood turbulence may dislodge tumor cells from the inside of a capillary wall as they try to invade the tissue of a distant organ. Blood turbulence also disrupts clumps of tumor cells as they move through the blood stream.

But the primary protection against the spread of cancer is the immune system. The immune system includes many specialized white blood cells and dozens of chemicals that act to regulate the immune response. Before we look at these immune system components, we should look at the basic immune response.

The Immune Response

Consider a bacterial infection. Many bacteria in a wound may cause an infection. Infection-fighting white blood cells may pour into the wound, forming pus. Bacteria may enter the blood stream, causing chills and fever. But few people develop abscesses or infections in distant parts of the body. Presumably, most of the circulating bacteria are killed by the patient's immune system.

Surgeons know the danger of operating on a patient with an infection anywhere. A surgical wound is very susceptible to infection, even from the few germs circulating from a mild infection. Germs from a mildly infected toe may end up infecting a surgical incision in the neck. Also, patients with heart valve disease are asked to take antibiotics before having dental work. Manipulation of the teeth can introduce bacteria into the blood stream, which can infect a damaged heart valve. In these examples, small numbers of bacteria circulate in the blood stream of a patient from a small local infection. The bacteria may cause infection at susceptible sites, but the immune system kills the rest of the bacteria before they cause infection elsewhere.

Circulating cancer cells within the blood stream may be destroyed in a similar way. For many years, pathologists have seen white blood cells called lymphocytes infiltrating into tumors. Scientists showed that lymphocytes taken from patients with cancer could kill their own tumor cells. Further studies proved that lymphocytes taken from healthy patients were also able to kill some tumor cells. This means that the immune system does kill cancer cells in the same way that it kills bacteria. To do so, it employs two main groups of weapons: a cellular arsenal and a chemical arsenal.

The Cellular Arsenal

There are normally 5,000 to 10,000 white blood cells in each cubic millimeter of blood. (For comparison, a cubic millimeter of blood also contains about 5 million red blood cells.) An elevated white blood cell count of more than 10,000 per cubic milliliter is often a sign of infection somewhere in the body.

Most of these cells fight infections caused by bacteria. In the healthy person, these cells make up about 60 percent of all the white blood cells in the body. Another 5 percent consists of miscellaneous cells that fight infection or are involved in allergic reactions.

Cells called *macrophages* make up another 5 percent. They can recognize many cancer cells as abnormal or foreign. They then ingest the cells and process the cancer cell antigens.

Macrophages can then pass the processed antigens to *lymphocytes*. Lymphocytes make up the remaining 30 percent of the body's white blood cells. Although much of the immune system's activity occurs within the blood stream, most of the lymphocytes are located outside of the blood stream, in lymph nodes, the spleen, and the intestines. (Macrophages are also located in the liver, spleen, and lungs.) The body produces about 1 billion lymphocytes every day.

There are four basic kinds of lymphocytes: B cells, killer T cells, T helper cells, and natural killer cells.

B Cells

One type of lymphocyte produces antibodies; it is called a B lymphocyte or *B cell*. *Antibodies* are proteins that can attach to and neutralize antigens. There are thousands of different B cells, and each is programmed to produce a specific type of antibody. There are more different types of antibody than there are other types of protein combined. It has been estimated that the immune system is able to recognize 100 million different antigens; each lymphocyte is able to recognize only one antigen. Antibodies are most effective against threats from outside of cells, such as bacteria, parasites, and toxins.

Killer T Cells

Processed antigen can also be passed to T lymphocytes or *T cells*. T cells do not produce antibodies. Some of them can attach to a living cell and kill it by releasing toxic chemicals. These cells are also called cytotoxic or *killer T cells*. The chemicals they produce, called *lymphokines*, may punch holes in the cell membrane of the target (in this case, cancer) cells. Lymphokines can also signal the target cell to begin a program of self-destruction, a form of cell death called apoptosis. This aspect of the immune response is called *cell-mediated immunity*. Just as antibodies are most effective against threats from outside of the cell, cell-mediated immunity is most effective against threats from within other cells, such as viruses and DNA abnormalities.

T Helper Cells

Other T cells guide the immune response toward either antibody production or toward cell-mediated immunity. These are called *T helper cells*. Called helper cells because they help both halves of the immune response, they work with both B cells and killer T cells by producing chemicals that favor one response or the other. There are two types of T helper cell, T helper 1 (T_H1) and T helper 2 (T_H2). They have been called the drill sergeants that call other lymphocytes into action. T_H1 produces chemicals that activate killer T cells to engage in cell-mediated immunity. T_H2 produces chemicals that activate B cells to produce antibodies.

Natural Killer Cells

Other white blood cells that have demonstrated an ability to kill cancer cells in both animals and humans are the *natural killer (NK) cells* (not to be confused with killer T cells). NK cells are large lymphocytes that circulate in the blood stream. They contain tiny droplets of toxic chemicals, which give them a granular appearance under the microscope. The cells do not require prior exposure to a specific kind of tumor cell to function.[2,3] Mice that have had their NK cells removed become vulnerable to the spread of tumor cells. If NK cells are returned to these mice, their ability to prevent tumor spread is restored. These findings support the importance of NK cells in preventing tumor spread.[4] There is evidence that they play a similar role in humans.[5]

Do patients with cancer still have a functioning immune system? Amy Fulton of the Michigan Cancer Foundation in Detroit compared blood from healthy donors to that from breast cancer patients. She found no difference between them in the ability of the NK cells to kill cancer cells.[6] A tumor can suppress NK activity within the tumor itself or within adjacent lymph nodes without affecting the activity of circulating NK cells.[7] Thus, early cancers do not appear to affect the activity of NK cells in the blood stream beyond the actual tumor.

Some researchers have reported that a patient's prognosis is directly related to the level of NK activity.[8,9] Several studies have shown that NK activity is depressed by the stress of surgery and even by the painkiller morphine. Recent studies also suggest that one oncogene (cancer-causing gene) may also suppress NK activity by causing the tumor cell to produce a protein that prevents the NK cells from working properly.[10] Animal studies have also shown that a decrease in NK activity leads to an increase in tumor spread.[11]

Giorgio Trinchieri of the Wistar Institute for Anatomy and Biology in Philadelphia extensively reviewed the human and animal data on NK cells. He concluded, "Growing evidence indicated that NK cells play a role in vivo [in living organisms] in the resistance to certain types of tumors and their metastatic dissemination [spread]."[12] In his review of NK cells, John Ortaldo of the National Cancer Institute concluded, "Evidence now implicates NK active cells as major effectors in the natural defense against cancer."[13] Indeed, all aspects of the immune system have been shown to play a role in preventing the spread of disease. It will require additional decades of research to unravel this complex defense mechanism.

The Chemical Arsenal

White blood cells are regulated by an arsenal of chemicals that can either stimulate or suppress specific parts of the immune system. These chemicals are called *cytokines*. They are now being used to treat patients with advanced cancer. When they are used in treatment, they are called biological response modifiers (BRMs), discussed in Chapter 5.

In general, these chemicals can stimulate lymphocytes to multiply thousands of times. A small cluster of white blood cells, immunized against a specific antigen, can become an effective army of killer cells. Cytokines also stimulate these cells to function more effectively and to produce additional proteins that further fuel the intensity of the immune response. The overall immune response includes both the cellular arsenal and the chemical arsenal, working together. It may be decades before this interaction is completely understood. Thus, it is not surprising that scientists and physicians have been unable so far to find tests that can accurately measure a patient's ability to fight cancer.

The chemical arsenal is stocked with four main types of substances:

- *Interferon*. These substances are produced by lymphocytes to protect other lymphocytes from additional viral infection. They also stimulate all the types of immune cells discussed previously. They act by slowing the growth of both normal and tumor cells.
- *Interleukin*. These substances are primarily produced by T cells and macrophages. Over fifteen have been identified; each one stimulates only those cells that have receptors for that specific interleukin. They regulate the growth and function of lymphocytes.
- *Colony-Stimulating Factors*. These substances stimulate the growth of white blood cells as they mature within the bone marrow. They govern the proportions of different white blood cells that are produced.
- *Tumor Necrosis Factor*. Coley's toxin may have stimulated the production of this chemical. Produced by both immunized T cells and NK cells, it produces an inflammatory response that kills susceptible tumor cells.

The Immune Response in Action: An Example from AIDS

The importance of the immune system, and of the interplay

between its cells and its chemicals, has already been demonstrated for AIDS patients.[14] The AIDS virus is able to stimulate antibody production and retard cell-mediated immunity. This happens in part because the production of an interleukin, IL-12, is reduced. IL-12 governs the relative strengths of cell-mediated and antibody immunity. However, the antibodies are not effective against AIDS, because the virus is safely living inside of the lymphocytes.

Long-term AIDS survivors are able to overcome this unfavorable shift in their immune response. For reasons that are not entirely clear, their cell-mediated immunity remains strong. Their T_H1 cells can still produce large amounts of IL-12, which stimulates their killer T cells. These cells in turn suppress the multiplication of AIDS-infected lymphocytes. The T_H1 cells also produce a form of interferon that suppresses the T_H2 cells which aid in antibody production.

As you can see, the immune system is extremely complex, but scientists are learning its inner workings. The wide variation in survival rates of different patients with AIDS seems to depend in large part on their immune response to the virus. Long-term survivors are able to reduce the spread of the virus to uninfected cells. While the virulence of the AIDS virus may affect a patient's prognosis, survival may also depend on the patient's immune response to the virus. I believe that this is also true for cancer.

GENETIC CONTROL OF THE IMMUNE SYSTEM

Most of us are familiar with red blood cell types: A, B, AB, and O. Many of us know our own blood type. But we also have white blood cell types, called major histocompatibility antigens. There are many white blood cell types, far too many to list here.

The Genes That Control White Blood Cell Type

Clearly, blood cell types are genetically controlled. Certain genes control red blood cell type. Another set of genes controls white blood cell type. This latter set of genes is called the *major histocompatibility complex* (MHC). (*Histo-* means tissue.) Its DNA controls the production of every white blood cell antigen.

These are complex chemicals located on the surface of the white blood cells themselves and on all the other tissues in the body. These chemicals have two fuctions: to identify the MHC type of the individual (human or animal), and to grip and present an antigen to a macrophage or T cell for evaluation and possible destruction.

There are two MHC types, coded by genes that are located at positions near each other on the same chromosome: MHC I and MHC II. MHC I molecules are located on all cells that have a nucleus. If a cell becomes infected with a virus, the cell will deliver a portion of the virus to its surface. Here, the MHC I antigen combines with the viral particle. This combination is recognized as abnormal by a killer T cell, which kills the virus-infected cell.

How MHC II Antigens Work

MHC II molecules are only located on the immune cells. These cells search for both foreign invaders and tumor cells. Like the data on an identification badge, MHC II antigens identify each cell. These complex proteins also serve as receptors for antigens on other cells. They can distinguish a normal liver cell (self) from an intruder (non-self), such as a cell from a transplanted organ or a cancer cell.

The MHC II antigen behaves like a password. A white blood cell, such as a T cell or NK cell, carries its MHC II antigen on its surface. It makes contact with a second cell, or target. The immune cell asks for a password by comparing its MHC II antigen to that of the second cell. If the antigen on the second cell (or target cell) is not the same, it has failed the password test. It may be attacked. Immune cells do not attack each other, because they all carry the correct MHC antigen II (the correct password). Antigens from abnormal cells trigger the immune cells to release toxins, which kill the abnormal cells. Thus, MHC I molecules patrol the cell's interior, while MHC II molecules patrol the exterior.

The MHC and Immune Response Strength

The genes that code for white blood cell antigens also determine how these cells respond to immune challenges. Many diseases are determined by the way a patient's body responds to chemical substances from both outside and inside the body. Allergies are the result the body's immune response to chemicals in the environment. Sometimes a patient's immune system mistakenly reacts against normal tissue in the body. In other words, the immune system fails to distinguish properly between self and non-self. Severe illnesses such as systemic lupus and even some forms of diabetes are caused by an abnormality in the immune system.

Research has shown that other aspects of the immune response are controlled by MHC II genes.[15] The MHC determines the intensity of a patient's response to a particular antigen. For example, most patients respond to a hepatitis B vaccination with a healthy antibody response. A minority of patients have a very weak response. Scientists have proven that weak responders have a certain MHC type.[16] Other aspects of the immune response, such as antigen processing, tumor necrosis factor production, and NK cell activity, are determined by a patient's MHC type.[17,18]

Some MHC II lymphocytes have a greater affinity for certain types of antigens and a lesser affinity for others. Scientists have discovered that women with certain MHC genes are more likely to develop cervical cancer if they are also exposed to the human papillomavirus (HPV). These women may have an ineffective immune response against the virus. This research angle is very new.

Very little has been learned about the genetic control of our bodies' defenses against circulating tumor cells. But it is likely that the immune systems of different individuals vary widely in their ability to recognize, attach to, and destroy circulating tumor cells. This important facet of host defense is under genetic control.

USING THE IMMUNE SYSTEM TO FIGHT CANCER

Much attention has been paid to the therapeutic potential of immune system stimulation. One of the best known techniques has been the stimulation of lymphocytes with immune-activating hormones. Lymphokine-activated killer cells and tumor-infiltrating lymphocytes have been used primarily in patients with advanced disease. (It is considered too experimental to use on patients with less advanced disease.) Lymphocytes are removed from a patient and placed in a solution that allows them to increase in number by cloning themselves. They are then mixed with a stimulating hormone called interleukin-2 (IL-2). These activated lymphocytes are given back to the patient. This experimental procedure requires hospitalization and results in a severe fever, since IL-2 is toxic. Doctors have seen tumors shrink in about 20 percent of patients. This therapy has been most effective for patients with malignant melanoma and renal cell carcinoma (a cancer of the kidneys).

WHAT WE STILL MUST LEARN

Most of our knowledge about the immune system has come from experiments using special tumor cells that are grown in laboratories. These "test tube" cells grow on year after year, and are known as cell lines. It is likely that they change as time goes on. This raises the question of how reliable is the research that is carried out using these cells.

There are also questions as to exactly what happens inside the human body. Why does the immune system fail to kill all cancer cells? How do tumor cells resist the attack of the immune system? Is the immune system simply overwhelmed by great masses of circulating tumor cells? Research continues in these areas.

Both the development of tumor cells and a patient's defense against tumor cells seem to be genetically controlled. This perception of tumor-patient interaction is a departure from previous ideas. Tumor spread used to be considered a random event. The immune response was considered to be ineffective against tumor spread. The genetic control of this process adds stability to these events. Tumor spread may eventually become predictable, based upon information about the genetic makeup of the tumor and the patient's defense system. The fate of circulating tumor cells may eventually be found to be the outcome of a great battle – a battle controlled by the genetic machinery within the tumor cell, on one side, and that within the cells of immune protection, on the other. Based upon the information presented thus far, I will now discuss the reasons why conservative surgery seems to be so successful.

4.

The Seed and the Soil

When a plant goes to seed, its seeds are carried in all directions, but they can only live and grow if they fall on congenial soil.

Stephen Paget, 1889

Over a hundred years ago, Stephen Paget of England was puzzled by the spread of breast cancer. He observed that breast cancer frequently spread to the liver, but it almost never spread to the spleen. He concluded that the liver provided congenial soil for breast cancer cells, while the spleen provided a hostile soil.[1] Paget's seed-and-soil analogy is popular even today, because the overall outcome of the interaction between tumor and patient remains a mystery.

In the hundred years since Paget proposed his seed-and-soil hypothesis, scientists have learned about the chemicals and genetic information in tumor cells and in various organs that influence tumor growth and spread. As we saw in Chapters 2 and 3, scientists have learned much about many of the individual steps in the process of tumor spread. The relative importance of each of these steps is less clear. The entire process is very complex, and no single test or series of tests can accurately predict if a tumor will spread in a particular patient.

Cancer behaves in a unpredictable manner. Some patients develop distant metastases from a small cancer, while others can survive a large tumor without developing distant disease. The haphazard travel of circulating tumor cells seems to contribute to the unpredictable behavior of cancer. Many cancer specialists believe that any tumor cell with the proper cellular machinery has the potential to spread at any time. Many also believe that random chance plays a role in tumor spread.

During the past ten to twenty years, new evidence has emerged that has changed our perception of tumor spread. We now realize that tumor cell circulation may begin when the tumor is tiny, the size of a mustard seed. The idea that tumor cells start circulating early from a developing malignancy may sound frightening to you. But, in fact, it may be good news. It suggests that the defense system of each patient can effectively kill many cancer cells early in the course of the disease, wherever the cells may go. In other words, most patients provide a very hostile soil to small numbers of circulating tumor cells.

I would like to extend Paget's analogy somewhat. He focused upon the different organs of the body. But individual humans may also differ in their ability to promote or prevent the spread of tumor cells. Patients who offer a hostile soil to circulating tumor cells are unlikely to develop distant metastases. Patients who offer a fertile soil are more likely to do so. The spread of cancer is unpredictable, but it may not be random.

WHY IS CONSERVATIVE SURGERY SO SUCCESSFUL?

In 1980, I suggested an answer to this question.[2] I made two assumptions. One, patients vary widely in their ability to prevent the spread of disease from circulating tumor cells.[3,4] In Paget's terms, some patients are like fertile topsoil and others are like dry desert. Two, patients have a relatively stable defense against circulating tumor cells throughout life. In other words, the patient's soil, his or her internal environment, changes little during life. A patient doesn't change from desert sand to fertile topsoil.

A patient with a growing breast cancer, for example, is exposed to an increasing shower of circulating tumor cells. The immune defenses in the breast may have lost the local battle, but the immune system at large is able to destroy tumor cells in the blood stream and within distant organs. If the breast cancer is removed, the number of tumor cells circulating in the blood should decline. At the time of surgery, distant metastases have either started to grow or they have been prevented. If a few tumor cells are left behind after a conservative operation, these cells may grow and form a recurrent tumor. Tumor cells may begin to circulate again. But a patient who has survived her original cancer without developing distant disease can be expected to survive a similar volume of cancer cells arising from a recurrent tumor in the breast. Her blood stream and distant organs can be compared to unfertile soil. Promptly treated local recurrence is not a risk to survival, because surviving patients have a level of immune protection that exceeds the tumor challenge. This hypothesis may seem simple. But, as I hope you see, it explains why patients who are treated with conservative surgery seem to do so well.

I have found only two other attempts to explain the often innocent, or nonthreatening, behavior of local recurrence following conservative surgery, both of them from a breast-cancer research project called the NSABP.[5,6] Both are too complicated to include here, but I do not believe that either adequately explains this momentous observation.[7]

THE NATURE OF LOCAL RECURRENCE

As discussed in Chapter 1, surgeons have feared local recurrence for most of this century. Local recurrence following radical surgery is a very grave sign, far different from local recurrence following a conservative operation. A surgeon who performed a radical mastectomy would wince at the appearance of tiny red blotches on the patient's chest, the telltale sign of local recurrence. The surgeon knew with near certainty that distant metastases would soon appear.

Following radical surgery, the patient and her doctor may see an orderly series of events: surgery, local recurrence, and then distant metastasis. The local recurrence may appear several months before the distant metastasis. Since the local recurrence appears to be the only cancer anywhere in the patient's body, it may appear to be the cause the distant metastasis. But this conclusion is usually incorrect. In fact, distant metastases often occur first, but they are too small to be detectable. It has been shown that cancer cells can spread from a distant metastasis to another part of body. It is also known that scar tissue and other injured areas may be "fertile soil" for these circulating cells. Local recurrence appears when tumor cells return via the blood stream to the vulnerable surgical area.[8] For example, following a radical mastectomy cancer cells may spread from a liver metastasis back to the skin on the chest. Thus, local recurrence following radical surgery is usually a sign that distant metastases have already formed.

The following example illustrates my point. Conservative surgery pioneer George Crile, Jr., treated a female patient for melanoma on her leg. Two years later she had a radical mastectomy for breast cancer. Soon after the operation, she developed a large recurrence of tumor at the site of the mastectomy. A biopsy revealed the recurrent tumor to be melanoma. Circulating melanoma cells from an undetected metastasis had invaded the injured area on the chest wall and started to grow.[9]

I hope it is clear that local recurrence after a cancer operation can come in two entirely different forms. Since a radical operation seldom leaves any cancer cells behind, local recurrence is a very grave sign, evidence that cancer has spread from a distant site back to the surgical scar. Following a conservative operation, local recurrence may simply be the regrowth of a few remaining cells. As described above, this type of local recurrence does not come from a metastasis elsewhere in the body, but regrows from tumor cells that remain after surgery. I believe that this type of local recurrence can be expected to behave in the same way that the primary tumor behaved. In this case, promptly treated local recurrence is not an added risk to survival.

Following a breast-sparing operation, for example, both types of recurrence may appear, and it is usually possible to distinguish between the two. One type of recurrence can occur following only breast-sparing surgery. Persistent or residual tumor cells may form a mass within the breast. The second type may occur following either breast-sparing surgery or radical surgery. This form of local recurrence usually involves the skin of the chest wall. Tumor nodules may form beneath the skin or threads of tumor cells may form red blotches within the small lymph vessels of the skin.[10] Since it is seeded by cancer cells from a distant site, this type of recurrence is often disseminated throughout the breast. Richard Margolese studied local recurrence in the NSABP lumpectomy trial, discussed in Chapter 1, and identified both of these forms of recurrence.[11] He suggested that the first type, the growth of remaining tumor cells, be called a *type I recurrence.* The second type, the one that is seeded from a distant site, he called a *type II recurrence.*

For many years, surgeons have studied breast cancer and other tumors by comparing patients who developed local recurrence with those who did not. In the NSABP lumpectomy trial, patients who developed local recurrence were 4.3 times as likely to develop distant metastases as those who did not. Initially, this figure sounds worrisome. You may be tempted to say, "I don't want to be in the group with local recurrence. I want to do everything possible to prevent that." But consider this. The patients with type II recurrence (those arising from distant disease) created a great imbalance in the NSABP numbers. Their inclusion in the local-recurrence group meant that this group's statistics were already weighted toward distant metastasis. Here again, local recurrence does not cause distant spread. It is merely an indication that the disease has already spread-a condition that cannot be altered by aggressive treatment.

THE RISK OF LARGE RECURRENCES

However, Paget's seed-and-soil analogy doesn't always work. Local recurrence after conservative surgery is not always an innocent, or nonthreatening, event. It can be a type II recurrence. Or, the recurrent tumor may grow so large that it does become an added risk to the patient. The size of a malignant tumor can make a big difference. Farmers cannot grow plants in infertile soil simply by planting more seeds. But a growing tumor can release so many tumor cells into the blood stream that distant metastases will almost certainly appear.

It is well known that the risk of a primary tumor depends on its size. The larger the tumor, the more likely it is to spread. Similarly, a recurrent tumor may also pose an added risk if it becomes too large. It may grow to exceed the immune defenses of the patient, especially if its size exceeds that of the original tumor. Among patients who develop recurrent disease, the most important prognostic factor may be the volume of the recurrence. Several clinical studies support this conclusion. [12-20]

THE TUMOR-PATIENT BATTLE

Tumor growth exposes patients to an increasing shower of

circulating tumor cells. As the number of tumor cells increases, the chance that the patient will develop distant metastases also increases. The millions of tumor cells circulating in the body are being attacked by millions of immune cells. As more and more tumor cells enter the blood stream, they may overwhelm the defending cells of the immune system. This description of tumor-patient interaction resembles a struggle or battle, not the pastoral farming scene described by Paget. This battle between the immune system and the tumor is invisible to both the patient and the doctor.

Many scientists now view AIDS from a similar perspective. They noticed that as an HIV infection progresses, the number of AIDS virus particles in the blood slowly increased and the number of T cells gradually decreased. For many years, it was thought that this was a slow and steady process. In 1995, scientists at two AIDS research centers reversed this perspective. They found that up to one billion new virus particles are produced every day, and that the body in turn produces about one billion T cells to replace those killed by the virus. A newspaper article described this conflict as a "raging battle" in which the body loses a little ground every day.[21] One researcher said that scientific technology was churning out so much data that "people don't have time to think."

I believe there are lessons here for cancer specialists. Circulating tumor cells are also involved in a raging battle with T cells and other facets of the immune system. And, like many AIDS researchers, cancer researchers are also churning out so much data that they may have a hard time seeing the bigger picture.

In this bigger picture, both sides of the tumor-patient battle must be considered. The strength of the tumor is measured by the indicators of metastatic potential discussed in Chapter 2. The resistance of the patient is measured by the aspects of immune responsiveness discussed in Chapter 3. I believe that this struggle is reproducible and dependable. The patient who survives a tumor of a given size can be expected to survive the reappearance of a similar volume of tumor. I have found no cancers for which this simple analogy does not apply.

Testing The Soil

I believe that cancer researchers should try to develop tests that can identify patients with a high level of immune protection. There are hundreds of patients alive today who have already survived a large cancer. I believe these survivors should have their immune systems thoroughly tested. High levels of NK activity, T cell activity, or other immune factors may correlate with prolonged survival. It may also be valuable to perform white blood cell typing on some cancer survivors. Patients with certain white blood cell types may be better able to destroy circulating or metastasizing tumor cells, as discussed in Chapter 3. It is well known that some diseases, such as juvenile diabetes and rheumatoid arthritis, are more common among patients with certain types of white blood cells. We may find that immune protection against metastasizing tumor cells is also genetically determined and associated with certain white blood cell types.

Doctors need a series of reliable tests to evaluate the immune system. Information about both the cancer (the seed) and the patient (the soil) should greatly increase our ability to predict tumor spread. Such tests could be used to influence a variety of decisions about cancer treatment, including the selection of patients for chemotherapy and lymph node removal. Since both surgery and chemotherapy can temporarily depress some immune functions, such tests may also help doctors plan the best order of treatment. For example, patients with a weak immune system may need to avoid preoperative chemotherapy, or they may need to defer radiation therapy until their immune system has recovered from surgery.

Distant Metastasis: The Pivotal Event

The patient and the cancer are involved in a struggle. The outcome of that struggle is literally a life-and-death matter. It is a struggle decided by a single event—the spread of disease to another organ in the body. If the tumor is removed before the disease has spread, the patient is cured. If the cancer is removed after it has already spread, the patient is unlikely to be cured. Thus, the pivotal event in a patient's struggle with cancer is the appearance of metastases in another organ of the body. Paget realized that the spread of tumor cells is governed by more than random chance.

At the time of initial treatment, cancer cells have either

become established at distant sites or they have been held in check. If tumor cells are successfully growing in a distant organ, local treatment will have little or no effect on their growth. No operation, no matter how radical, will cure a patient who already has cancer cells growing in another part of his or her body. Few surgeons today would recommend disfiguring surgery for a patient with known metastatic disease. Unfortunately, there are few reliable tests to detect if a tumor has spread. Blood tests are beginning to be helpful. Many X-rays, even CAT scans and MRIs, are unable to detect a tumor smaller than 1 cm in diameter.

At the time of initial treatment, the primary question is, "How much surgery and other treatment are necessary?" Some doctors believe that a solitary cell left behind after an operation could be the cell that causes a metastasis. One cell, any cell, could be responsible for tumor spread. These doctors are likely to favor aggressive treatment to eliminate every possible cell in the region of the tumor. Others think that, like the growth of seeds in soil, tumor spread occurs in a regulated manner.

I speculate that immune protection against tumor spread is a complex matter involving many aspects of the immune system working in concert. Genetic factors are important to many aspects of immune responsiveness. Eventually, we will learn how a patient's white blood cell type determines how his or her immune system responds to many types of challenges. We will be able to predict that response. The spread of disease will eventually be understood so thoroughly that the outcome of every patient will be predictable. By that time, one hopes, we will be able to cure the disease.

Although metastasis superficially appears chaotic and random, it may result from an orderly and predictable battle. Doctors who view tumor spread as a controlled process are more likely to recommend conservative treatment. They realize that the primary factors contributing to tumor spread are beyond the influence of the surgeon's knife. They realize that local recurrence is not always a failure or complication of surgery. Scientists are a long way from describing all the events involved in tumor growth and spread. But there is enough information to strongly suggest that many aspects are under tight genetic control.

This perception of tumor-patient interaction is clearly accurate for breast cancer and soft tissue sarcomas. Many authorities have acknowledged that local recurrence following conservative surgery is not a risk to survival for either of these malignancies. There is emerging evidence that this principle also applies to malignant melanoma. For other cancers covered in this book, there is less information regarding the behavior of local recurrence. Most of these malignancies are less common than breast cancer and have been treated primarily with radical surgery. But most of the available information conforms to the ideas presented here. Indeed, I have found no studies pertaining to any malignancy that are contrary to the ideas presented here.

I hope this chapter has given you renewed confidence in your ongoing struggle against cancer. I hope that your immune system is victorious over an unwelcome invader. Regrettably, it may be several years before your victory can be declared. Paget's analogy is helpful in another way. The farmer who sows his crop must patiently wait for the seeds to germinate. Likewise, the patient and the doctor must patiently wait. All the participants would like to intervene, to influence the outcome. But after the tumor has been removed, the primary tasks are regular follow-up and waiting.

Part Two

Treating Cancer

5.

Principles of Treatment

Part Two of this book concerns the treatment of ten specific types of cancer: malignant melanoma, soft tissue sarcoma, and cancer of the bladder, breast, cervix, penis, prostate, rectum, vagina, and vulva. This chapter discusses the types of cancer that affect these organs, how they are graded, their routes of spread, screening procedures for early detection, signs and symptoms, diagnosis, staging, treatment, analysis, and follow-up. Chapters 6 through 15 divide treatment into types of treatment and treatment according to stage. The organization of this chapter into these sections serves as a model for all the other chapters in this part, each of which deals with a specific organ or tumor. Chapters 6 through 15 also contain anatomy and physiology sections. These provide information on the specific part of the body under discussion. This chapter covers each of these areas in a general way, but most of the emphasis here concerns various types of treatment.

TYPES OF CANCER

Environmental and hereditary factors can lead to the development of cancer in almost any cell in the body. By custom, all cancers are named for the organs where they arise. A liver tumor that originally came from the breast is still called breast cancer. The original tumor in the breast is called the *primary tumor*.

Cancer can be divided into three large categories: carcinomas, sarcomas, and lymphomas and leukemia. Within each catagory, there are dozens of specific types of cancer.

Carcinomas

Carcinomas arise from cells that cover or line the various parts of the body: the skin, the lining of the intestines, and ducts within various glands. These cells are called *epithelial cells*. Carcinomas are the most common types of cancer. When these carcinomas involve glandular or fluid-producing tissues, they are called *adenocarcinomas* (*adeno* is Greek for gland).

Sarcomas

Sarcomas arise from bone, cartilage, connective tissue, muscles, tendons, nerves, fat, fibrous tissue, or blood vessels. These tissue are present in almost all organs of the body, so sarcomas can occur anywhere. They are much less common than carcinomas. Bone and cartilage are both hard. The other tissues are soft. Therefore, sarcomas that arise from the latter are called soft tissue sarcomas. Both sarcomas and carcinomas usually grow as hard tumor masses called solid tumors.

Lymphomas and Leukemia

These are tumors of the white blood cells. Lymphomas, such as Hodgkin's disease, occur in organs with many white blood cells, such as the lymph nodes and the spleen. Leukemia occurs when the abnormal white blood cells circulate within the blood stream. Great success has been achieved treating these cancers with chemotherapy.

TUMOR GRADE

Pathologists can get an idea about a cancer's rate of growth by looking at the tumor under the microscope. As discussed in Chapter 2, the presence of many dividing cells suggests that rapid growth is occurring. This information determines a cancer's grade. Each cancer has its own grading system. Most commonly, cancers are graded as low, moderate, or high, or graded by number, such as grades 1 through 3. The lower the grade, the better the prognosis. There are a variety of other tests available to evaluate the aggressiveness of tumors. Tumor grade is very important for some cancers, such as soft tissue sarcomas, and less important for others, such as malignant melanoma.

ROUTES OF SPREAD

The stage of the disease and the prognosis are often determined by a tumor's depth of invasion, that is, the number of layers of tissue the tumor has penetrated. Tumors also spread to lymph nodes. In some areas of the body, enlarged lymph nodes can be felt. These are called *positive* nodes. They may be the first evidence that the tumor has spread. Spread of cancer to nearby nodes reduces the chances for cure, although some patients with positive nodes can be cured. Enlarged lymph nodes are often surgically removed. If the lymph nodes do not feel enlarged, they may still contain microscopic cancer.

Nodes that cannot be felt but that may contain microscopic cancer are called *clinically negative* nodes. Some surgeons believe these nodes should be removed right away, and others believe that nodes should be closely observed and removed only if they become enlarged. This topic is discussed more fully in the following chapters whenever it arises.

Cancer cells can also spread via the blood stream to distant organs. This process is called *metastasis*. The spread of cancer to a distant organ is more serious than spread to the lymph nodes.

SCREENING

Screening means testing individuals who have no symptoms or signs of the disease under consideration. Patients who see their doctor with a lump in the breast or with difficulty urinating are likely to be tested, but this testing is not screening.

There are many tests designed to detect cancer at an early stage, such as cell samples, blood tests, imaging procedures, and genetic testing. *Cell sampling* techniques, such as the Pap smear for cervical cancer, are excellent screening tests. Modern *blood tests* are not specific. They may appear positive in healthy patients and often appear normal in patients with cancer. *Imaging procedures* include X-rays, scans, and other techniques that produce a picture or image of the cancer. In order for a cancer to be detected with a scan, it must be about 1 cm in size (3/8 of an inch). (X-rays and mammograms are considerably more sensitive.) *Genetic testing*, or testing for inherited susceptibility to cancer, is in its infancy. It is suitable for selected patients with a strong family history of cancer.

The benefit of screening is primarily measured by one standard: does screening prolong life? It does in some cases, such as the Pap smear for cervical cancer or mammograms in women over fifty years of age. But there is much debate about the effectiveness of some screening procedures, such as testing for prostate-specific antigen to detect prostate cancer, discussed in Chapter 11, or mammograms for women under fifty, discussed in Chapter 7. There is no question that these tests and others can detect cancer at an early stage. However, it is not possible to determine whether or not screening is worthwhile for use on large populations by studying a few patients. Hundreds, perhaps thousands, of patients must be studied. Such tests are now underway for breast and prostate cancer.

In the meantime, doctors base their recommendations upon available, but inconclusive, information. It is likely that a few patients do have their lives prolonged by screening tests. But no one knows how small "a few" really is. Some patients may wish to undergo screening tests even if these tests are not recommended by an official organization.

SIGNS AND SYMPTOMS

A *sign* is an abnormality that a physician can discover; a *symptom* is any abnormality discovered by the patient. Early cancers usually have no symptoms because they often invade areas of the body with few nerve fibers. Even large tumors may be painless. Others symptoms vary according to the tumor. The cancer may have already spread by the time symptoms appear.

DIAGNOSIS

Almost all cancers are diagnosed by a pathologist examining a sample of tissue under a microscope. If a doctor feels a hard lump, he or she often suspects cancer, but only the pathologist can confirm the diagnosis. X-rays and other imaging studies are often more accurate than physical examination, but, again, only the pathologist can make a final diagnosis. Therefore, removal of a small amount of tissue—a *biopsy*—is necessary.

All of the tissue removed by the surgeon is examined by the pathologist. First, he or she looks at it with the unaided eye, measures the tumor with a ruler, and counts the lymph nodes. Then he or she examines the tissue under a microscope, including some of the edges of the tumor. If there are tumor cells in the margins, the pathologist concludes that the surgeon has cut through part of the tumor and may have left tumor cells inside the patient. The tumor margins are said to be *positive*. The pathologist may suggest that additional tissue be removed. Microscopic examination of the lymph nodes can determine whether tumor cells have spread to the nodes.

The pathologist must first stain the tissue in order to examine it under the microscope. For him or her to do so, the tissue must be firm enough to cut into very thin slices, slices that are only about one cell layer thick. Usually this is done via a *permanent section*. The tissue is placed in heated paraffin. The paraffin hardens as it cools. The tissue-paraffin block is then sliced, placed on a glass slide, and stained. This entire process may take two or three days. The sample is kept on file.

Occasionally, a biopsy is performed immediately prior to surgery, although surgeons no longer believe that cancer must be operated on immediately after being diagnosed. For example, the patient may have a mass in the abdomen. General anesthesia is needed for both the biopsy and the surgery. In this case, the pathologist may perform a *frozen section*. The tissue is frozen, cut, stained, and examined, all within a few minutes. Frozen sections can be prepared quickly, but are not as accurate as permanent sections. Frozen sections are discarded afterwards.

STAGES OF DISEASE

As a cancer grows and spreads, it goes through several stages. Stage is based upon the size of the primary cancer, its depth of invasion into the organ, and its spread to lymph nodes or distant organs. (This should not be confused with a tumor's grade, which is determined by the rate of cell growth.) Most cancers are divided into four stages: I, II, III, and IV, or A, B, C, and D. Each organ of the body has its own staging system. Many of these staging systems were named for their founders; the use of numbers or letters was the decision of the doctor who devised that system. Since 1959, a committee, now called the American Joint Committee on Cancer, has also played a prominent role in standardizing the staging systems. Here is a general description of most systems:

- *Stage I or A.* The cancer is small (often 2 cm or less), confined to the organ, and has only begun to invade into the organ.
- *Stage II or B.* The cancer is larger, often more than 2 cm, or has invaded deeper into the organ. Some cancers advance to stage II when regional lymph nodes are involved.
- *Stage III or C.* The cancer has spread outside the confines of the organ into nearby tissue and to regional lymph nodes.
- *Stage IV or D.* In most staging systems, this designation is reserved for patients who have developed distant metastases.

In the 1950s, there were a lot of staging systems, sometimes two or more for a single cancer. In an effort to bring uniformity to this chaos, the International Union Against Cancer began to develop a staging system called the *TNM system* that is based upon three criteria: the size of the tumor, the involvement of regional lymph nodes, and the presence or absence of distant metastases. The TNM system is widely used for all solid tumors. Table 5.1 shows a simplified version of the TNM system as it applies to several tumors.

The TNM system has many subcategories not listed in the table. The four stages of disease are made up of many combinations of the TNM categories. (You will find examples of this in later chapters.) In its complete form, the TNM system is difficult to use, since the doctor who treats several types of cancer must memorize many long lists of definitions and numbers. Therefore, the TNM system is more widely used in research than it is in practice.

Staging can be either clinical or pathological. *Clinical staging* is based upon the observations that the doctor makes while examining the patient. *Pathological staging* is based upon information obtained by the pathologist after surgery. For example, the lymph nodes of a patient may feel normal to the examining surgeon. The pathologist may find a few tumor cells in the nodes after surgery. The patient is said to be clinically stage I, but pathologically stage II.

Table 5.1 Simplified TNM Staging System

Tumor Size [T]	Nodal Metastases [N]	Distant Metastases [M]
T_1—2 cm or less	N_0—No cancer in the lymph nodes	M_0—No distant metastases are present
T_2—5 cm or less	N_1—A few enlarged lymph nodes involved on one side of the body	M_1—Distant metastases are present
T_3—Over 5 cm	N_2—Several enlarged lymph nodes or nodes are enlarged on two sides of the body	

TREATMENT

The ideal goal of cancer treatment is the removal or eradication of every malignant cell. This includes the primary tumor itself; those microscopic cells that may have grown, unseen, into the surrounding, normal-appearing tissue; and cancer cells growing in lymph nodes and distant parts of the body. Unfortunately, at the time of initial treatment, no doctor can be certain that all the tumor cells have been eliminated, either locally or elsewhere. Also, most cancer treatments have potential side effects and complications. Therefore, the practical goal of treatment is to balance the benefits of treatment against its risks—the elimination of cancer cells against the harm that the treatment itself may do to the patient.

Cancer treatment can be divided into two broad categories, local and systemic. *Local treatment* only eradicates cancer cells in a specific area of the body. Local treatment, such as surgery and radiation therapy, can only affect the local disease. A radical operation or large dose of radiation to the primary tumor cannot injure or destroy cancer cells that have already spread to another organ.

Systemic treatment is intended to kill tumor cells throughout the body, in the tumor, in the area of surgery and in distant organs. Chemotherapy and biological therapy are examples. If you've treated a wound by applying an ointment and taking antibiotics, you've used both local and systemic treatment.

Surgery

Surgery is the oldest form of cancer treatment and, even today, remains the most effective. The vast majority of cancer cures are achieved with surgery, and surgery alone. If your primary care physician suspects that you may have cancer, he is likely to refer you to a surgeon. Cancers of the prostate, kidney, or bladder are treated by urologists; cancers of the cervix, vagina, or vulva are treated by gynecologists. Many other cancers are treated by general surgeons, such as soft tissue sarcomas, malignant melanoma, and cancers of the breast, colon, and rectum.

Biopsy

Since a pathologist can only diagnose cancer by examining cells under a microscope, a surgeon usually obtains a small portion of the tumor in a minor surgical procedure called a biopsy. There are several types of biopsies.

The least traumatic form is the *skinny needle biopsy*. This is performed using a thin needle (smaller than the needle used for injections) that is passed through the tumor several times. Structures such as glands and ducts are not preserved, so the pathologist is only examining individual cells. When the diagnosis of cancer depends upon cellular patterns, not just the appearance of individual cells, the pathologist will ask for a larger biopsy specimen. The skinny needle technique is accurate over 90 percent of the time.

In a *needle biopsy*, a specially designed needle is used to remove a larger core of tissue. This maintains the tissue's organization and includes the various tissue layers. The pathologist can see the ways the cells are arranged as they attempt to form ducts, glands, or other structures. Cancer usually alters this pattern and the pathologist can more easily make an accurate diagnosis.

In an *incisional biopsy*, the surgeon cuts a wedge of tissue out of the tumor. This may be used to establish a diagnosis immediately before surgery, or if it is necessary to obtain a larger specimen for additional testing.

In an *excisional biopsy*, the surgeon completely removes the entire lesion. This technique is commonly used for skin and breast lesions, in which complete removal of the lesion is desirable, whatever its diagnosis.

You may wish to obtain the diagnosis first, and plan to have treatment later. Your surgical options depend upon the diagnosis. This gives you some time to consider your treatment. The complete tumor can be removed a few days after the biopsy. If you are having abdominal surgery, in which the functional or cosmetic consequences are less important, you may wish to have the biopsy and surgery in one operation.

Resection (Removal) for Cure

The surgeon's goal is to remove the entire tumor. A small tumor—2 cm or less—can often be removed with a margin or border of normal-appearing tissue. In general, to remove all, or nearly all, of the tumor cells, this margin should be 2 cm in width. The surgeon should be cutting through normal tissue at all times during the operation. Although this rule varies among the different types of cancer, removal of normal tissue beyond 2 cm does not usually improve results.

Surgeons have known that there is not always a clear dividing line between the tumor and surrounding normal tissue. Cancer cells may have spread in microscopic numbers into nearby tissue. Also, tumors are often surrounded by normal-appearing cells that are abnormal or premalignant under a microscope, cells that may become malignant if left alone. To successfully eradicate this surrounding tissue, surgeons have removed an extra margin of healthy-appearing tissue. Recently, this uncertain tissue has been treated with radiation therapy. The combination of limited surgery and radiation therapy has become popular for breast cancer, soft tissue sarcomas, and bladder cancer, among others.

For most cancers of intermediate size (2 to 4 cm), the surgeon can often perform a *wide excision*. A surgeon can perform this operation with a scalpel, but other techniques are also available:

- *Electrocautery*. This technique uses a handheld device resembling a ballpoint pen to direct an electric current at the tissue. An electric arc is often visible and the treatment often results in small areas of charring. Electrocautery can be used to cut tissues or to control bleeding (a purpose for which it is widely used).

- *Cryosurgery*. This technique uses a probe to freeze tissue.

Both cryosurgery and electrocautery may damage all or part of the tumor cells in a specimen, making it difficult or impossible for the pathologist to provide information about the margins around the tumor.

- *Laser surgery*. This technique uses a fine beam of high-intensity light to cut tissue. This light is of a precise wavelength that can be focused into a fine beam. It boils the water inside cells and causes them to explode. The laser beam cuts a very fine line of cells, equivalent to a scalpel cut.

Mohs micrographic surgery is a technique practiced by some dermatologists since the 1930s. The patient is given a local anesthetic and the lesion is removed. Additional fragments of tissue are then cut out and sent to the pathologist, who checks the margins for tumor cells. The dermatologist or surgeon continues to remove additional tissue until the margins are free of tumor cells. This technique has been used successfully to treat skin cancer, including malignant melanoma.

In *laparoscopic surgery,* tubes are placed into the abdomen and the abdominal cavity is distended with carbon dioxide. The surgeon manipulates tiny cutting tools through one tube; a tiny camera in another tube allows the surgical team to watch the operation on a television monitor. Laparoscopic surgery is being used for a wide variety of operations, including cancer surgery. It can also be used to remove lymph nodes. This is most commonly done in the pelvis for patients with cancer of the pelvic organs.

Staging Procedures

Sometimes tissue is removed just to see how far the tumor has spread. This is called a *staging procedure*. The removal of lymph nodes from the armpit in the treatment of breast cancer is an example. Scientific studies have proven that surgeons who feel no enlargement in these nodes can leave them alone, removing them later only if they become enlarged. But most surgeons remove them at the time of the original operation, because some patients who have tumor cells in their lymph nodes may benefit from chemotherapy. Thus, the nodes are removed to find out the stage of the disease, not to treat the patient.

Palliative Surgery

Palliative surgery is used to reduce or eliminate symptoms in a patient with widespread disease that cannot be cured. If cancer is pressing on the spinal cord, or obstructing the intestines, bile duct, or urinary tract, removal of the tumor can bring relief.

Debulking Surgery

Even large masses of tumor that cause no significant symptoms may be removed, at least in part.[1] Reducing the tumor mass through *debulking surgery* can lower a patient's burden of metabolic waste from dying tumor cells. Also, both radiation and chemotherapy rely upon good circulation of blood to the tumor to be effective. Radiation therapy requires oxygen in the tissues, and chemotherapy needs to be delivered via the blood stream. Most cells within a large tumor mass respond very poorly to both radiation therapy and chemotherapy because their circulation is so poor. A debulking procedure may improve the circulation to the remaining tumor and also improve its response to radiation and chemotherapy. It may also improve the well-being of the patient.

Second-look Surgery

It is difficult to diagnose the recurrence of tumors within the abdomen. Some tumors produce substances that can be measured in blood tests, such as prostate-specific antigen (PSA) in cases of prostate cancer. An increase in these substances suggests a regrowth of the tumor. If such an increase occurs, some doctors suggest a patient may benefit from a *second-look surgery*. As of now, there is little evidence that this approach saves many lives, but a second-look operation may occasionally allow the removal of a local recurrence before it spreads.

Removal of Metastases

The surgical *removal of metastases* is usually ineffective because new cancers appear soon after the first is excised. But some situations are amenable to such treatment. Patients with soft tissue sarcoma who have only a few lesions in the lung or liver may benefit from surgical removal of these lesions. To be effective, the primary tumor must be controlled, the surgeon must be able to remove all the metastases, and there must be no evidence of cancer anywhere else in the body.

Reconstructive Surgery

Reconstructive surgery includes such procedures as breast reconstruction after mastectomy. It was once thought that patients should wait several months before having reconstruction. The trend lately has been toward immediate reconstruction. For example, a patient can have a mastectomy and reconstruction performed as one continuous operation. Those who follow the recommendations of this book should reduce their need for reconstructive procedures.

Complications of Surgery

To learn how you can avoid surgical complications, talk to your surgeon. This will also give you a chance to ask any last-minute questions, and to make sure that you understand your preoperative instructions.

Most biopsies are performed under local anesthesia, in which a drug is injected to numb the treated area. For some operations, a spinal anesthetic is used, in which a drug is injected into the fluid surrounding the spinal cord. Major operations require general anesthesia, in which the patient is put to sleep. The most common side effect is an adverse reaction to the anesthetic. You can ask your anesthesiologist how the drugs will be administered and what effects you should expect.

The most common complication after local surgery is bleeding. Although advances in surgical techniques have considerably lessened the need for transfusions, you still may need blood during surgery. Some people have gotten hepatitis or AIDS from donated blood. The chances of this happening are very small, since donated blood is now tested for these diseases. It may be possible for you to bank your own blood before surgery.

After major surgery, pain can make it difficult for some people to take in a full breath. This can lead to small areas of partial collapse within the lungs. Treatment includes getting the patient to cough, walk, and breathe deeply. Patients can also develop blood clots in the legs if they lie in bed for long periods of time. A large clot can break loose and enter the heart, which can have serious consequences. Treatment consists of getting the patient to walk and move the legs.

The surgical wound can become infected. Most infections can be treated with antibiotics and are usually not serious, although some infections, such as intra-abdominal abcesses, can be life-threatening.

Radiation Therapy

Radiation was first used medically around the turn of the century by Marie and Pierre Curie, who were working in Paris. Unaware of the danger posed by X-rays, many practitioners (including Marie Curie) died of radiation exposure. By the 1920s, radiation could be produced artificially. Doctors did not have to depend upon natural sources of radiation. X-ray doses could be measured and controlled. Cobalt-60 was introduced in the 1950s and provided a source of high-energy radiation. Cobalt-60 units could treat cancer deep inside the body without burning the skin. In the 1960s, the linear accelerator offered radiation of even higher energy.

Radiation therapy can be used as primary therapy for some tumors such as lung cancer, Hodgkin's disease, or cancer of the voice box (larynx). Radiation also can be used to kill microscopic cancer that may remain following surgery. Some tumors are so large that they cannot be removed by surgery. Preoperative radiation may help shrink these tumors. Large tumors may grow very close to nerves, blood vessels, or other important structures. Postoperative radiation may allow the surgeon to preserve these vital structures.

What Is Radiation?

Visible light is a form of radiation. Radio waves and microwaves are invisible forms of radiation. But the radiation used to treat cancer is called *ionizing radiation*. It can disrupt the chemical makeup of atoms by knocking electrons out of place within atoms. This starts a series of reactions that disrupt chemical bonds in the DNA molecule, which leads to cell death. (See Chapter 2 for a discussion of how DNA is put together.) Rapidly dividing cells are the most affected because they are manufacturing DNA at a rapid rate. Tumor cells, white blood cells, the cells lining the intestinal tract, and those lining the mouth are all rapidly dividing cells, and are thus all affected by radiation.

Radiation beams vary widely in the energy they produce, from about 100 kilo-electron volts (KeV) to 25 million electron volts (MeV). The higher the energy, the greater is the depth of penetration. Low-energy beams deliver their highest dose at the skin. Beams with 25 MeV achieve their highest dose at a depth of about 2 inches.

Radiation is measured by the amount of energy absorbed by a tissue. The present unit of radiation is the gray (Gy). It replaces the rad; 100 rads equals 1 gray. A chest X-ray exposes the chest to about 1/20 of a centigray (cGy), which is a hundredth of a gray. A mammogram exposes the breast to less than 1/20 cGy. Therapeutic radiation doses are often about 50 Gy. Harmful effects of radiation can be reduced by dividing the treatment over several days, a process called *fractionating*. Therapy is usually administered weekdays, five days per week.

Types of Radiation Therapy

Radiation therapy can be delivered in several different forms.

External-beam radiation is directed at specific areas of the body, and affects only those cells touched by the rays. All tissues touched by the beam are affected, normal and malignant alike. The radiation therapist tries to maximize the effect on the tumor and reduce the effects on normal tissue. This can be done by selecting the appropriate type of beam, adjusting its strength, aiming the beam at angles that avoid sensitive organs, and protecting normal areas with lead shields. Radiation causes no discomfort while it is being administered.

Interstitial radiation is also called *brachytherapy*, because radiation can be administered in a short (*brachy-*) period of time. Radioactive seeds, such as those containing iodine-125, can be placed in the tumor. They deliver their dose over a period of several weeks. Also, hollow needles can be placed through a tumor. Radioactive seeds are later placed in the tubes, where they remain for several days.

Intracavitary radiation is most often used in gynecology. While the patient is asleep in the operating room, hollow applicators can be placed in the uterus or vagina. Once their correct position has been verified, radioactive material is placed in the applicators and left for forty-eight to seventy-two hours. This mode of treatment provides a high dose of radiation directly into the nearby tumor, while the energy level rapidly declines a short distance from the tumor. This minimizes radiation injury to the surrounding normal tissue. When used in the intestinal tract, it is called *endocavitary radiation*.

Adjuvant radiation therapy is administered to a patient whose visible cancer has been completely removed. The term adjuvant means "in addition to" and refers to therapy that is administered in addition to surgery. When doctors use the term adjuvant therapy, they almost always mean that the patient has no evidence of cancer anywhere, but may be at a high risk for developing recurrent cancer. Adjuvant radiation is generally able to reduce local recurrence, but seldom prolongs survival.

Side Effects of Radiation

The most common side effect of radiation therapy is fatigue, which occurs in most patients who receive therapy to a large area of the body. It lasts only during the weeks of treatment and shortly thereafter. Many patients experience some reddening of the skin, which behaves very much like a sunburn. Hair loss in the area of treatment is common. Radiation to the head and neck area can damage the salivary or tear glands, resulting in a permanently dry mouth or dry eyes. Radiation to the upper abdomen may cause nausea and vomiting. Radiation to the lower abdomen may cause diarrhea and urinary frequency.

Early changes in the breast after radiation treatment include redness, fluid retention, and pigmentation.[2] Over the next three years the breast may develop fibrous tissue with areas of shrinkage. Radiation therapy causes scarring in most of the tissues hit by the radiation beam. Should a mastectomy be required later, radiation therapy increases the complication rate of surgery and hinders surgical reconstruction.

Each part of the body can only tolerate a fixed amount of radiation. Once a therapeutic dose has been given, radiation is difficult to use again. It is my opinion that adjuvant radiation is used more often than necessary. If there is only a 10 percent chance of local recurrence, and if the recurrence can be easily detected and removed with no risk to survival, it may be preferable to defer postoperative radiation.

The long-term risks of radiation therapy have not been completely determined. There is evidence that radiation therapy may lead to a very slight increased risk of developing leukemia or a second cancer many years later. This risk has been estimated at about 3 to 4 percent.[3]

Chemotherapy

The use of chemotherapy to treat cancer began in the late 1940s. Nitrogen mustard, originally a chemical weapon, was the first drug approved for this purpose. Since then, tens of thousands of drugs have been tested on animals, and about fifty different drugs have been approved for use against cancer in humans. Many more are being investigated. These drugs are usually administered by physicians called oncologists, medical oncologists, or chemotherapists. Most of their training and experience centers on the administration of chemotherapy and the treatment of its side effects.

Chemotherapy can cure some childhood leukemias, Hodgkin's and non-Hodgkin's lymphomas, testicular and ovarian cancer, and choriocarcinoma (a cancer that arises from an abnormal pregnancy). The most common cancers cannot be cured by chemotherapy. *Chemosensitivity testing* is an experimental technique which attempts to determine which drugs are most effective against each patient's own tumor.

Types of Chemotherapy

Chemotheraputic drugs can be divided into several different categories.

Alkaloids, such as vincristine and etoposide, interfere with the cell's ability to make the spindles that are necessary for cell division. (Chromosomes are separated by these protein spindles as the cells divide.) Vincristine can cause nerve damage.

Antibiotics, such as doxorubicin (Adriamycin) and bleomycin, damage DNA in a variety of ways or prevent DNA from making RNA, which in turn helps to make protein. Bleomycin may cause lung damage.

Alkylating agents, such as cyclophosphamide and cisplatin, attach chemical compounds to strands of DNA that either break the strands or interfere with their division.

Antimetabolites, such as methotrexate and 5-fluorouracil, resemble normal vitamins or other cellular substances. They interfere with a variety of chemical reactions, ultimately hindering DNA synthesis. Methotrexate has been used with *leucovorin*, a chemical that reverses the effect of the drug. Since normal cells are more effective in absorbing leucovorin, patients can be treated with very large doses of methotrexate and then "rescued" with leucovorin.

Paclitaxel (Taxol) is a drug that interferes with the microtubules, structures that facilitate cell division and the transportation of substances within cells.

Bone Marrow Transplantation

All of the cells in the blood are produced in the bone marrow, the hollow core inside the bones. This includes red blood cells, white blood cells, and clot-forming platelets. The white blood cells are among those cells that are most sensitive to the toxic effects of chemotherapy. The maximum dose of chemotherapy that can be given is often limited by the fall in a patient's white blood cell count.

Recently, it has become possible to remove bone marrow cells from a patient and then administer high doses of chemotherapy. The patient's own bone marrow cells are later given back to the patient. This therapy has not greatly changed the outlook for patients with advanced cancer.

Bone marrow transplantation is also used to treat patients with some forms of leukemia. In this case, the cancer itself is within the patient's own bone marrow. Therefore, a donor with normal bone marrow cells must be used. This type of bone marrow transplantation is more effective than that used for breast cancer and other solid tumors because leukemia is more likely to respond to chemotherapy.

Resistance to Chemotherapy

Some cancers resist the effects of some drugs or develop resistance during treatment. Scientists are beginning to understand some of the ways that cells develop resistance, and are trying to develop drugs that counteract this resistance.

Attempts have been made to learn which cancers will respond to which drugs, in much the same way that doctors can now test bacteria from a patient and decide exactly which drugs will kill the infection. *Multidrug therapy* is seldom necessary for most bacterial infections. Such tests are not available for chemotherapy. Because tumors can change their sensitivity to chemotherapy and because reliable sensitivity testing is not available, oncologists usually give many drugs at once.

Resistance to chemotherapy has been associated with a gene called the multiple drug resistance gene (MDR-1). In addition to this gene, chemotherapy faces other barriers. The blood supply in a tumor is not uniform, since the growth of blood vessels within a tumor is no more organized than the growth of the tumor itself. Furthermore, cancers are often very hard because they are under great pressure. This also limits the flow of blood into a tumor and reduces the amount of chemotherapy that effectively reaches the tumor.

What Is "Disease-Free Survival"?

After surgery, small numbers of cancer cells in distant parts of the body may attempt to form metastases. *Adjuvant chemotherapy* is given to patients whose tumors have been completely removed, but who are at a high risk for developing recurrence. Chemotherapy is most effective on small clusters of tumor cells.

When doctors report the success of adjuvant chemotherapy, they often measure what is called *disease-free survival*. This refers to the amount of time that the patient lives without any evidence of cancer. Adjuvant chemotherapy has been very effective in prolonging patients' disease-free survival. Unfortunately, it has not been as effective in prolonging overall survival—real prolonged life. Chemotherapy suppresses the growth of microscopic cancer cells, so that the doctor and patient continue to consider the patient to be free of all cancer. After the chemotherapy is completed, the cancer cells can start growing again. If the cancer does recur, patients seldom live much longer than patients who received no chemotherapy. Patients receiving adjuvant chemotherapy should ask their doctors about its ability to improve real overall survival. Patients should understand how much of their added survival time may be spent enduring the side effects of the drugs.

Adjuvant chemotherapy for breast cancer is an example. Patients with cancer in their lymph nodes (stage II) may benefit from adjuvant chemotherapy. Some doctors think that treated women may have as much as a 7 percent better chance of surviving five years than untreated women. However, others doubt that the survival benefit is that great. One researcher says that about 6 percent of women have their lives prolonged by about fourteen to eighteen months,[4] while about 94 percent of treated patients receive no benefit.

In 1981, Gianni Bonadonna and colleagues at the National Tumor Institute in Milan, Italy, said that adjuvant chemotherapy had to be administered in full doses in order to be effective.[5] They came to this conclusion after some patients at their institute had received smaller doses of chemotherapy because they were experiencing side effects. These patients did not live as long as those treated with a full dose of chemotherapy. I do not believe that this study demonstrates the benefit of full-dose chemotherapy. It is likely that full-dose chemotherapy simply defined two groups of patients: a healthier group with reserved strength in their bone marrow and elsewhere, and a weaker group without these immunological reserves. Patients in the first group did better because their own immune defenses were also more effective in retarding the growth of the tumor.

What Are "Response Rates"?

Medical oncologists measure success in terms of *response rates*. This differs from disease-free survival in that response rate applies to a patient with a visible tumor, while disease-free survival applies to a patient whose visible tumor has been removed and there is no evidence of cancer anywhere in the body. A complete response or remission refers to a cancer that has completely disappeared. But imaging studies can fail to see some cancers 1 cm (3/8 of an inch) or less in diameter. The length of remission is unpredictable. A partial response refers to a tumor that shrinks to less than half of its original size. Another form of response is the relief of pain. If the physician observes any benefit from treatment, he may conclude that the tumor has responded to treatment.

The Effect of Chemotherapy on Cancer Treatment

The fact that a tumor responds to chemotherapy does not always mean that the patient's life is prolonged. Chemotherapy can temporarily slow a tumor's growth. Many patients who respond to chemotherapy do not gain any additional survival benefit. Patients should understand that chemotherapy is of little benefit for most patients with solid tumors. Every year, thousands of people endure the toxic side effects of therapy and receive little, if any, benefit. It is possible to get an overview of the effects of chemotherapy by looking at death rates in the United States for the most common cancers. See Figures 5.1 and 5.2.

During the past twenty years, dozens of new chemotherapeutic drugs have been used to treat patients with cancer. The number of specialists who administer these drugs has also greatly increased. Unfortunately, death rates from cancer have declined little in the past twenty years. Those changes in death rates that have occurred are not related to treatment. The declining death rate from uterine (cervical) cancer is due to the Pap smear. The declining death rate from stomach cancer may be related to changes in food preservation due to refrigeration. Dietary changes are probably responsible for fewer deaths from cancer of the stomach, liver, colon, and rectum. Lung cancer deaths have increased greatly due to smoking. (The information shown in Figures 5.1 and 5.2 explain why doctors continue to deplore smoking.)

Surgery is still responsible for most cancer cures now, just as it always has been. These stable death rates provide evidence that little therapeutic progress has been made toward curing or significantly prolonging the survival of most patients with solid tumors.

Side Effects of Chemotherapy

Because chemotherapeutic drugs are absorbed by normal cells, the difference between the treatment dose and the toxic dose is very narrow. Chemotherapy interferes with chemical processes within the cell. Since cancer cells use chemical reactions that are identical to those of normal cells, the drugs are also harmful to normal cells. Chemotherapy is effective against

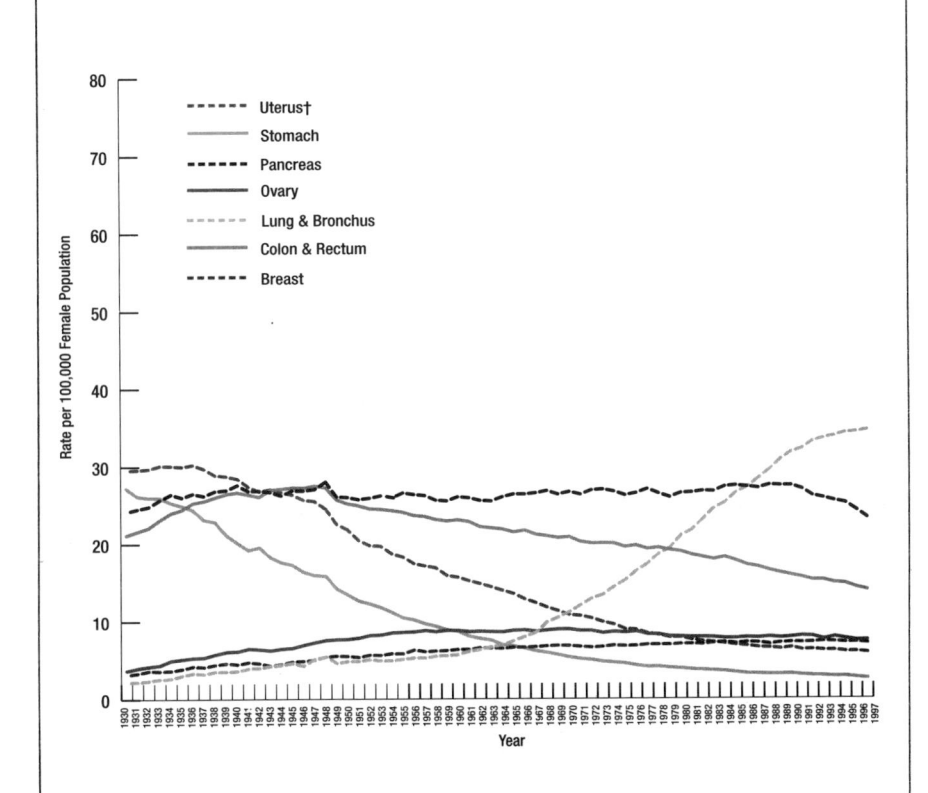

Figure 5.1 Age-Adjusted Cancer Death Rates for Selected Female Patients, United States.

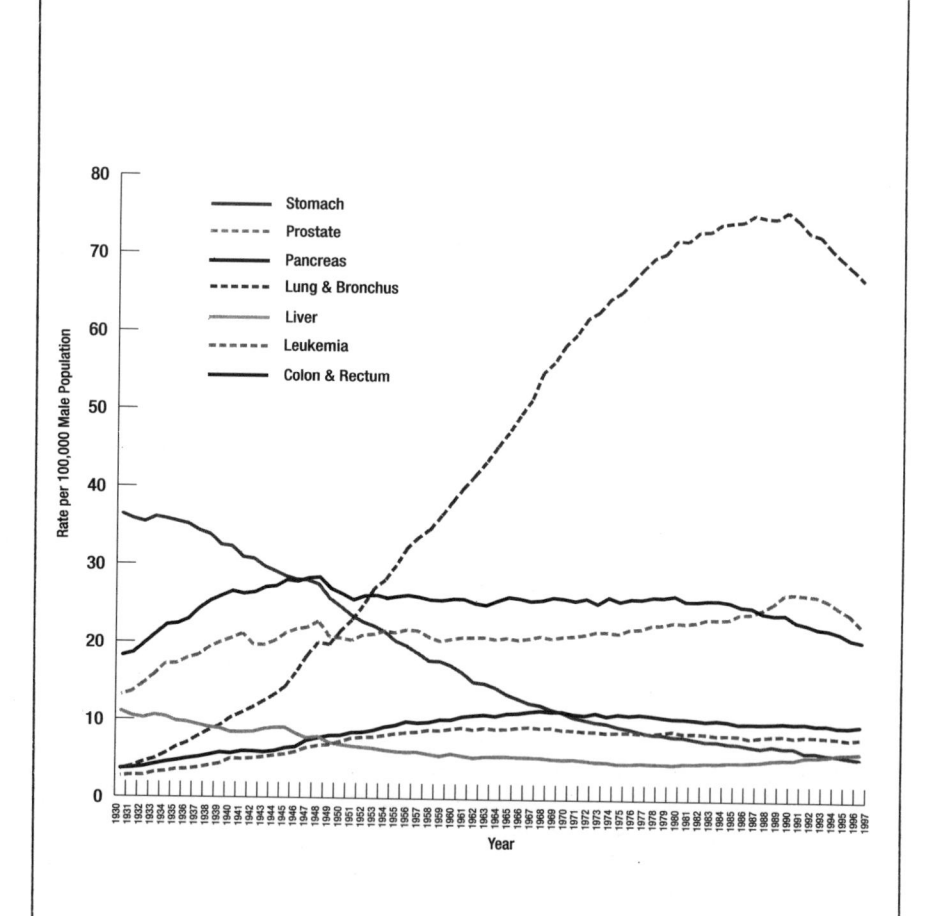

Figure 5.2 Age-Adjusted Cancer Death Rates for Selected Male Patients, United States.

those reactions associated with cell division, and therefore is most effective against rapidly dividing cells. The blood cells, both white and red, are among the most rapidly dividing. Damage to these cells leads to infections and anemia. Hair follicles and the cells lining the intestinal tract, from the moist mucosal lining of the mouth to the rectum, are also dividing rapidly. Hair loss, sores in the mouth, nausea and vomiting, and diarrhea are related to the injury of those normal cells. The most immediate side effects are nausea and vomiting during treatment, probably related to the action of the drugs on the stomach itself.

Hormonal Therapy

Some cancers are stimulated to grow by hormones—some breast cancers by the female sex hormones estrogen and progesterone, some prostate cancers by the male sex hormones testosterone and the other androgens. By altering these hormones, it is possible to alter the growth of cancer cells. Hormonal therapy is often more effective in treating solid tumors than chemotherapy, and usually has fewer toxic side effects. It can decrease the rate of tumor growth, reduce pain, and increase the quality of life. These effects may persist for several months or a few years. But hormonal therapy is generally not able to significantly prolong life, and is almost never curative. If one form of hormonal treatment stops working, another may be tried. But each new hormone treatment becomes less effective. Like chemotherapy, response rates for hormonal therapy do not translate into survival rates.

Hormone Production

Production of hormones is a multistage process that begins with two organs in the brain. The *hypothalamus* is a small, specialized area on the underside of the brain. It produces hormones that signal the nearby *pituitary gland*. The pituitary gland then produces secondary hormones that also act as a signals. These secondary hormones circulate throughout the body, acting directly on specific glands, such as the thyroid gland, the ovaries, and the testicles, stimulating these glands to produce hormones. These hormones then stimulate other target organs. Some hormones, such as cortisone and thyroid hormone, regulate metabolism—the way the body grows, repairs itself, and utilizes energy and nutrients. Steroid hormones include the sex hormones as well as cortisone. They regulate metabolism and sexual behavior, including the menstrual cycle and pregnancy.

Consider the production of testosterone in this multistaged process. The hypothalamus produces *luteinizing hormone-releasing hormone* (LHRH), the signal. LHRH is carried through a tiny system of blood vessels to the pituitary gland. The pituitary then sends another hormonal signal, *luteinizing hormone*, to the testicle. The testicle then produces the hormone, testosterone, that circulates in the blood and stimulates the target organ—the prostate gland. Testosterone also circulates back to the hypothalamus, and signals the hypothalamus to switch off, to stop making LHRH. Thus, the cycle is turned off. This is similar to how your home heating system works—you set the thermostat and the system produces heat until the thermostat senses that enough heat has been produced, and shuts the system off. The hypothalamus and the pituitary gland produce a separate set of signaling hormones for each gland in the body.

This complex process can be altered at any step along the way. The quantity of a particular hormone can be altered at different steps.

Types of Hormonal Therapy

Hormonal therapies can be divided into several different categories.

Diethylstilbestrol (DES) is a synthetic *estrogen* used to treat metastatic prostate cancer, instead of castration. DES is chemically similar to testosterone. The hypothalamus interprets the high level of DES as a high level of testosterone, and stops sending LHRH to the pituitary. Thus, the pituitary stops sending luteinizing hormone to the testicle, and testosterone production drops dramatically. The response rate depends upon the dose, but about 60 percent of patients will experience relief of pain from bone metastases. Patients may become impotent, and develop atrophy of the testicles and enlargement of the breasts. Blood clots, fluid retention, and other cardiovascular complications also limit its use.

Progestins, such as megestrol, have been used to treat breast cancer and prostate cancer. Their response rate is about 50 percent, and their mechanism of action is unknown. A common side effect of progestins is weight gain (40 percent). Fifteen percent of men develop impotence and 10 percent of women develop hot flashes.

Aminoglutethimide, an *inhibitor of steroid hormone production*, is used in the treatment of breast and prostate cancer. It blocks the production of a variety of steroid-type hormones, such as estrogens and androgens. The body functions as if the adrenal glands had been removed. About half the patients will experience some side effects, most commonly fatigue and skin rash. Ketoconazole is an antifungal agent that also inhibits the production of steroid hormones.

Leuprolide (Lupron) and goserelin acetate (Zoladex) are *releasing factor agonists*, very similar to LHRH, the hormonal signal from the hypothalamus to the pituitary gland. But these drugs are false signals and do not stimulate the pituitary. Thus, the pituitary gland does not send its hormonal signal to the testicles. The production of sex hormones is greatly reduced.

Tamoxifen is the most widely used *antiestrogen*, and is the world's best-selling cancer medication. This drug binds to hormone receptors within breast tumor cells. It is most effective on estrogen-receptor positive tumors, or tumors that contain estrogen receptors on the surfaces of their cells (see Chapter 2 for a fuller explanation of this concept). There is also evidence that tamoxifen directly interferes with the tumor's blood supply. In the case of estrogen-receptor positive tumors, there is a 50 to 60 percent response rate. Hot flashes, nausea, and vomiting are the most common side effects.

Flutamide (Eulexin) and bicalutamide (Casodex) are *antiandrogens*. They block the binding of androgen to hormone receptors with prostate cancer cells. They have a response rate of about 80 percent. The side effects include gynecomastia and hot flashes. Impotence is uncommon.

Estramustine is a drug that combines estrogen with a type of chemotherapy drug known as an alkylating agent. Its use is limited primarily to patients who fail to respond to other hormonal therapy.

Biological Therapy

The newest forms of anticancer therapy are the *biological response modifiers* (BRMs), which can alter the body's immune response to cancer. These agents have been used primarily in patients with far advanced disease. Therefore, they have been only slightly effective in some patients with solid tumors. They have been very effective in some forms of leukemia.

The results of biological therapy have been very disappointing. This disappointment has been enhanced by the great publicity given to these agents. Many of the therapies listed below may be familiar to you from the news media. But it is important to realize that this research has uncovered much about the biology of cancer and our defenses against it. Despite the disappointments, research into biological therapy does continue.

Types of Biological Therapy

There are several types of BRMs.

The *interferons* are a group of proteins that were discovered in the 1950s. Viral infections cause white blood cells called lymphocytes to produce interferon, which protects other lymphocytes from additional viral infection. Interferons have been very effective against some leukemias, and have been of limited benefit against cancer of the kidney. They act by slowing the growth of both normal and tumor cells, and by stimulating various white blood cells. Hailed as a breakthrough in the late 1980s, the interferons have not significantly altered the prognosis of patients with solid tumors.

The *interleukins* are a group of proteins produced primarily by lymphocytes and other white blood cells called macrophages. They regulate the growth and function of lymphocytes. Over fifteen interleukins have been identified, but IL-2 has been the most thoroughly studied. Lymphocytes stimulated by IL-2 are called lymphokine-activated killer (LAK) cells. They have demonstrated some activity against melanoma and cancer of the kidney. Doctors have also removed lymphocytes from a patient's own tumor, mixed them with IL-2, and reinfused the cells into the patient. These tumor-infiltrating lymphocytes have been effective against a few other types of cancer and are more active than LAK cells. All interleukin-based treatments are usually done in a hospital intensive care unit, as they result in severe fever and chills, and a drop in blood pressure that may lead to shock.

Naturally occurring substances known as *colony-stimulating factors* (CSF) have no direct effect against cancer. They stimulate the growth of white blood cells. Human granulocyte CSF and human granulocyte-macrophage CSF are in clinical use. The human gene that contains the code for CSF is inserted or combined into bacteria. The bacteria produce the CSF in large quantities. When patients suffer from low white blood cell counts following chemotherapy, CSF can help return these levels to normal.

Coley's toxin may have stimulated the production of *tumor necrosis factor*, a protein that produces an inflammatory response. Treated patients develop chills and fever. Early results have been disappointing.

Bacillus Calmette-Guerin is related to the bacterium that causes tuberculosis. It was once used to vaccinate children against TB, and it also causes a stimulation of the immune response that is not specific to any one disease. It was tested against melanoma, breast cancer, and other cancers without success. Now its only clinical use is to treat superficial bladder cancer.

Monoclonal antibodies attach to specific tumor antigens, which are tumor produced substances that stimulate an immune response. The antibodies can then be linked to drugs that can then be delivered directly to the tumor by the antibody. Monoclonal antibodies could also be linked to isotopes that could identify a tumor on a scan. There are many tumor antigens, and most of them are not specific to a particular tumor. This technology is still experimental.

Hyperthermia

This is another fairly new form of treatment. Cancer cells are more sensitive than normal cells to the killing effects of heat. Temperatures of 105 to 113 degrees have been used in experimental treatments. A tumor can be heated locally with microwaves. Whole body heating has also been performed using water blankets and other devices. Complications are limited primarily to the effects of the heat itself, such as blisters and burns. These can be reduced with careful monitoring.

Malignant melanoma is sometimes treated with *isolated regional perfusion*. The extremity to be treated is placed on a heart-lung by-pass machine, so that its circulation is cut off from that of the rest of the body. Then heated blood that contains a high concentration of a chemotherapy drug is introduced into the extremity. The heat enhances the effectiveness of the treatment. Possible side effects include a temporary sunburn-like effect and swelling, usually temporary. Bleeding and vein inflammation, which can lead to blood clots, can also result. In rare cases, these complications can lead to loss of the limb.

A form of hyperthermia used in the treatment of prostate cancer is *microwave thermal therapy*. A microwave heat applicator, inserted into the rectum, heats the prostate to between 109 and 111 degrees. The treatment is given in ten hour-long sessions. It can help patients with advanced cancer by lessening pain and relieving urinary blockage.

ANALYSIS

In the analysis section of each of the following chapters, I will try to explain when I think that conservative techniques should be used for the cancer under discussion. My analysis is backed up by the information presented in Appendix I. In the Appendix, I try to present the studies that provide information on local recurrence. I have not selected only those studies which agree with this hypothesis, but have tried to present all those studies that provide relevant information. I looked for studies that included the following information: the patient's stage of disease when first treated, the type of treatment, the schedule of follow-up visits, the size of the recurrent disease, and the overall survival rate. Often, the numbers of patients treated in each study are too small to reach firm conclusions. However, their harmony with the unified theory offered here gives them some additional significance. You can decide whether current clinical experience is sufficient to support conservative surgery for your illness.

Whenever I have recommended conservative treatment to patients, I have always recommended that they obtain a second opinion—a real second opinion. I don't send patients to doctors who will agree with me. I send them to doctors I know will not agree with me. Other doctors should do the same thing. Whatever your doctor's opinion, ask him to refer you to someone with different views. You can also obtain a referral by contacting a physician referral service at a local hospital, preferably a large teaching hospital in order to have access to the greatest number of doctors. Also think about joining one of the support groups listed in Appendix II. It is possible that you may not only find emotional support in such a group, but it may also be a good place to find people who can help you in your search for a doctor.

This search can be a difficult and frustrating process. But in such a vital matter as this, I would strongly urge you to keep trying until you find a doctor you are comfortable with and who will give you a true second opinion. See Chapter 17 for a list of questions you can ask on your visit.

FOLLOW-UP

Each chapter concludes with a suggested schedule for follow-up visits to your doctor and laboratory tests. These guidelines are very general. You and your doctor will want to prepare a follow-up schedule that is appropriate for you. A patient with a small, low-grade tumor that was removed with a wide margin may be followed less frequently than suggested. More vigilant surveillance may be needed in patients with very narrow margins of excision, regional lymph nodes that may contain cancer, or other risk factors that increase their risks of recurrence.

There has been a trend toward less diagnostic testing in the follow-up period. In 1980, I helped advance that attitude for malignant melanoma.[6] I also support it for other malignancies. The visit frequencies suggested here are widely used, but laboratory testing will probably become less vigilant. This is especially for cancers that respond poorly to treatment. David Schapira and Nicole Urban from the H. Lee Moffitt Cancer Center in Tampa, Florida, have argued that patients with breast cancer should be followed with physical examinations alone.[7]

I have tried to give you an overview of the evaluation and treatment of various types of cancer. This information will, I hope, give you a better idea about the characteristics of the cancer you may be dealing with and the types of treatment that are available.

6.

Bladder Cancer

Bladder cancer represents about 4 percent of all cancer cases in the United States. It is estimated that about 51,000 new cases appear each year and that about 11,000 patients die of this disease. Men have been almost three times as likely to get bladder cancer because of their exposure to carcinogens at work. Over 70 percent of patients with bladder cancer now live five years or longer due to the early detection of this disease.

About 30 percent of all bladder cancers are caused by exposure to industrial chemicals, such as aniline dyes. Cigarette smoking, the consumption of caffeine and of the painkiller phenacetin, and chronic bladder infections have also been related to bladder cancer. These environmental factors act on the cells lining the inside of the bladder. Usually, there is a twenty- to forty-year lag from the time of exposure to the development of the cancer. After a cancer is treated, the remaining cells are still damaged and often form another cancer. Thus, the rate of bladder cancer recurrence is much higher than that of other cancers.

Women who have had radiation therapy for cervical cancer have a twofold to fourfold increase in the risk for bladder cancer. In many cases, these women develop aggressive tumors.

This chapter will cover the following topics: the anatomy of the bladder, the types of cancer that affect the bladder, how this cancer is graded, how this cancer spreads, what screening procedures are available, what the signs and symptoms are, how this cancer is diagnosed, how this cancer is staged, what treatments are available, my analysis of how conservative surgery can be used to treat this cancer, my recommendations for the appropriate treatment at each stage, and what sort of follow-up is needed after treatment.

ANATOMY AND PHYSIOLOGY

Urine is carried from the two kidneys to the bladder via the ureters. It leaves the bladder through the urethra. These three tubes pass through an area in the floor of the bladder called the *trigone*. Urination is controlled by a complex system of voluntary (under willful control) and involuntary nerve reflexes.

The bladder is lined with *transitional epithelial cells*. These cells become large and umbrella shaped as they move toward the inside surface of the bladder. They line the entire urinary tract from the kidney to the bladder. These cells are designed to conform to the distension and contraction of the bladder, and to withstand their nearly constant contact with water. Beneath the layers of transitional cells is the lamina propria, a layer of fibrous tissue. It separates the transitional epithelial cells lining the bladder from the muscle layer, which is responsible for bladder contraction.

TYPES OF CANCER

Over 90 percent of bladder cancers involve the transitional cell layer. The cancers may begin as a flat lesion that only involves the topmost cell layer, known as *in situ* cancer. It may also begin as a mass that grows into the bladder cavity. Such an outgrowth of tissue is called a *papilloma*. Some patients have benign papillomas, and less than 10 percent of these patients ever develop malignant tumors.

Cancers of the squamous cells, another type of lining cell, represent about 5 percent of bladder cancers. They arise from the urethra. Other varieties of cancer account for less than 2 percent of all bladder cancers. They arise from glandular tissue or parts of the urinary tract that usually disappear after fetal development.

TUMOR GRADE

Tumors are graded according to how abnormal they appear under a microscope. A tumor with many dividing cells is abnormal and is presumed to be growing fast. In general, fast-growing cancers spread sooner. Pathologists may grade bladder cancers from grade 1, good prognosis, to grade 3, poor prognosis. The pathologist can also report if tumor cells are present in the blood or lymphatic vessels near the tumor. This may indicate that the cancer has spread.

ROUTES OF SPREAD

Bladder cancer first penetrates through the lamina propria and into the bladder muscle, at which point it is considered invasive. Within the muscles of the bladder are the lymphatic vessels, which carry lymph in the same way as blood vessels carry blood. The tumor cells can enter these vessels and spread to lymph nodes in the pelvis and higher in the abdomen, up the aorta, which is the main blood vessel from the heart to the intestines and legs. Tumor cells can also enter the blood vessels and spread to distant organs, such as the bone, liver, and lungs. Bladder cancer can also penetrate through the wall of the bladder into the surrounding fat or adjacent organs, such as the rectum, the vagina or uterus in women, or the prostate in men.

SCREENING

A routine urinalysis can detect blood in the urine. Bladder cancer is so rare that regular urine cytology, or examination of cells in the urine under a microscope, is not cost effective. Blood tests and additional urine tests are being developed.

SIGNS AND SYMPTOMS

Eighty percent of patients have no symptoms except blood in the urine. Blood gives urine a red or rusty appearance. Pain on urination, frequency, and urgency are usually associated with a number of small cancers throughout the bladder or with invasive cancer.

DIAGNOSIS

Bladder cancer can be diagnosed by examining the cells in the urine. Better specimens may be obtained by washing the bladder with saline solution. All patients who may have cancer of the bladder should undergo *cystoscopy*, in which a scope is placed up the urethra into the bladder. The bladder can then be examined. Malignant tissue can be removed and sent for pathological evaluation.

STAGES OF DISEASE

Today, there are two staging systems used for bladder cancer: the TNM system and the Jewett-Strong-Marshall system.

The TNM Staging System

The International Union Against Cancer and the American Joint Committee on Cancer Staging have developed a system based upon the TNM method, which is explained in Chapter 5. It is shown in Table 6.1.

The Jewett-Strong-Marshall Staging System

Shortly after World War II, urologists accepted the Jewett-Strong-Marshall system, which stages bladder cancer from stages A to D. Stage 0 was added later to account for very early disease. Table 6.2 shows the Jewitt-Strong-Marshall system. TNM abbreviations are included for comparison.

TYPES OF TREATMENT

Treatment options include surgery, radiation therapy, chemotherapy, and biological therapy. See Chapter 5 for more information about these treatments, including general information on the side effects associated with each treatment.

Surgery

Surgical options include the following procedures.

Radical Cystectomy

Radical cystectomy has been used to treat invasive bladder cancer. It involves removal of the entire bladder, the surrounding tissue and fat, and the pelvic lymph nodes. Additional surgery depends upon the sex of the patient. In women, the uterus, fallopian tubes, ovaries, urethra, and front portion of the vagina are removed. In men, the prostate gland and seminal vesicles are removed.

Table 6.1. TNM Staging System for Bladder Cancer

Tumor Size [T]	Nodal Metastases [N]	Distant Metastases [M]
T_a—Benign papilloma	N0—No cancer in the lymph nodes	M0—No distant metastases are present
T_{is}—Cancer *in situ*	N1–3—Lymph nodes contain cancer	M1—Distant metastases are present
T1—Tumor does not penetrate the lamina propria		
T2—Tumor invades the superficial muscle		
$T3_a$—Tumor invades the deep muscle		
$T3_b$—Tumor invades the fat around the bladder		
T4—Tumor invades a nearby organ		

The urinary tract can be reconstructed by creating an *ileal conduit*. A segment of small intestine is removed from the intestinal tract. One end is sewn closed, and the ureters implanted into it. The other end opens to the outside of the body through the abdominal wall. The ureters carry urine from the kidneys to the intestinal segment, which serves as a bladder. Patients urinate into a plastic bag attached to their side. Sometimes a pouch can be constructed inside the patient from a segment of intestine. In men, this pouch may be sewn to the urethra, allowing nearly normal urination. In women, the urethra is usually removed with the bladder and the internal pouch must be catheterized about three times a day.

Men used to become impotent because the nerves to the penis were cut. But since the late 1980s, some urologists have been using a technique that spares these nerves, and preserves erectile function in most men. In cases where impotence occurs, it can be improved with penile implants.

Partial Cystectomy

In this operation, all layers of the involved portion of the

Table 6.2. Jewett-Strong-Marshall Staging System for Bladder Cancer

Stage	Description	Five-Year Survival Rate
0	A superficial cancer. This includes benign papillomas (T_a) and cancer *in situ* (T_{is}).	Over 90%
A	A cancer that invades into the submucosa, the layer beneath the transitional cells, but not through the lamina propria (T1, N0, M0).	Over 75%
B1	A cancer that penetrates through the lamina propria and begins to invade the bladder muscle (T2, N0, M0).	About 60%
B2	A cancer that invades deeply into the muscle ($T3_a$, N0, M0).	About 40%
C	A cancer that invades into the fat around the bladder ($T3_b$, N0, M0).	About 30%
D1	A cancer that involves adjacent organs (such as the upper urethra, the lining of the bladder or rectum, or pelvic bones) or pelvic lymph nodes (T4 or N1–3).	About 5%
D2	Distant metastases are present (M1).	About 5%

bladder are removed with a 2-cm margin. Tests should be done to determine that the remaining bladder wall is free of tumor. The recurrence rates following this procedure are very high—70 percent in some studies. Most of this recurrence is due to new cancers that arise from the lining of the bladder. Fewer recurrences are due to bladder cancer that was incompletely removed by the partial cystectomy. Some studies make no attempt to distinguish between these forms of local recurrence. This distinction is important in order to help surgeons determine the optimum margin of removal.

Chemotherapy is often included as part of this treatment. Some urologists recommend low-dose radiation (10 to 12 Gy) prior to surgery to reduce the possibility of tumor cells implanting themselves into the bladder wall during the surgery. The pelvic lymph nodes are often removed.

Most urologists have strict criteria for partial cystectomy. Patients should have a solitary tumor limited to the bladder that can be removed with an adequate margin. There should be no prior history of bladder cancer or other cancer present, either as tumors or as atypical cells. The tumor should not invade the trigone or, in men, the prostate gland. These strict criteria are now being relaxed.

Transurethral Resection (TUR) or Fulguration

TUR involves the cutting or fulguration (burning) of tumors through a scope. Tumors must be accessible to the scope. Most urologists would require the tumor to be smaller than 2 cm and low grade. This is often combined with other treatment, such as radiation or chemotherapy. If the tumor is large, the pelvic lymph nodes can be removed through a laparoscope, which is a tube inserted into the abdomen. If the removed nodes are positive for cancer, the remaining nodes can be removed through the laparoscope. Most surgeons, though, prefer doing open abdominal surgery because they believe that the nodes can be more cleanly removed that way.

Laser Therapy

The laser can be placed into the bladder through a cystoscope using local anesthesia. It can destroy most small bladder tumors, with a recurrence rate of about 10 percent.

Hematoporphyrin is a chemical that can make some cancer cells more sensitive to the laser light. It is injected intravenously into the patient and is absorbed by most of the cells in the body. The chemical is quickly washed out of normal cells. Light of a specific wavelength is then trained on the cancer cells. The hematoporphyrin within the cancer cells is chemically altered by the light and becomes toxic to them. This is called *photodynamic therapy* and is considered to be experimental treatment.

Radiation Therapy

External-beam radiation therapy has been used for advanced tumors or as adjuvant, or additional, therapy following partial cystectomy. Bladder cancer responds poorly to radiation therapy. Therefore, some institutions do not use it as adjuvant treatment. Pain on urination, urinary frequency, and diarrhea are complications of radiation. They almost always subside, although symptoms may persist if the cancer remains. Iridium-192 implants are occasionally used to reduced local recurrence after partial cystectomy.

Chemotherapy

Drugs placed directly into the bladder can cure or control some patients with tumors that repeatedly recur. Drugs such as thiotepa, Adriamycin, and Mitomycin-C can be placed directly into the bladder for one to two hours at a time. Treatment is typically performed weekly for six to eight weeks, followed by monthly treatments for one year. Temporary bladder irritation occurs in most patients. This therapy is effective for about 20 to 40 percent of patients. Each drug is effective against different cancers. If the first drug does not work, a second or third can be tried. Chemotherapy can also be used to prevent recurrences after surgery.

Systemic chemotherapy—that given by injection—has been used in experimental programs designed to preserve the bladder. Intravenous chemotherapy can also be used prior to surgery to shrink large tumors and kill small distant metastases that may have formed. Cisplatin, methotrexate, vinblastine, and Adriamycin are the most effective drugs.

Biological Therapy

Bacillus Calmette-Guerin (BCG) is a bacteria that stimulates the immune system. BCG therapy is an effective treatment for 50 to 90 percent of patients. Interferon is a protein produced by the body's white blood cells that also stimulates the immune response. As with chemotherapy, these agents are instilled into the bladder on a weekly basis for six weeks. Temporary irritation of the bladder occurs in most patients.

ANALYSIS

Today, the main choice in treatment is between bladder-sparing procedures, such as TUR or partial cystectomy, and radical cystectomy. During the past two decades, over one hundred urologists have reported their experiences with bladder-sparing surgery. (See Appendix I for a complete discussion of these studies.) Most urologists agree that patients who are properly selected and treated survive just as long following conservative surgery as they do following radical cystectomy. But bladder-sparing procedures are used on a minority of patients with bladder cancers that have invaded the muscle of the bladder.

Bladder cancer is unique because of its very high recurrence rate of 70 percent or higher. Many urologists administer chemotherapy after partial cystectomy or TUR to kill remaining tumor cells and reduce the chance for recurrence. Recurrence is more likely to arise from cells previously exposed to damaging chemicals, rather than from cancer cells left behind after surgery. If radical surgery is of great benefit anywhere in the body it should be in the bladder, where local recurrence is so high. Radical cystectomy can reduce local recurrence from 70 percent to about 10 percent. In spite of this great reduction in local recurrence, radical cystectomy has not displayed a clear survival advantage over bladder-sparing operations. This observation also supports the speculation that locally recurrent bladder cancer and locally recurrent breast cancer, the cancer that has been most extensively studied, behave in a similar manner. Promptly treated local recurrence after conservative surgery does not appear to adversely affect survival.

No scientific trials have been performed to accurately define the type of treatment that is most effective or the types of patients who are best suited for bladder-sparing treatment. Several questions remain unanswered: How wide a margin of normal tissue should be removed in a TUR or partial cystectomy? How many failures should be allowed before the patient is treated with cystectomy? Should a third or fourth recurrence be treated with additional surgery or different therapy altogether? Without the benefit of randomized trials, there is only speculation.

However, I believe that partial cystectomy may be performed for stage B cancer with a margin of less than 2 cm, if necessary to save the bladder. Consider the added risk of local recurrence. If the risk from 70 percent to 80 percent, how much of a problem is that added 10 percent risk? I don't think it represents a great risk, especially since a recurrent tumor can be removed without jeopardizing patient survival.

This assumes, of course, that a recurrent tumor is found early as the result of good follow-up.

I would recommend conservative surgery if you are willing the accept the risk of recurrence and additional treatment. I agree with the following statement from J. Thrasher and E. D. Crawford of Duke University: "It is probably best to recommend transurethral resection therapy alone to patients in whom more radical therapy is precluded due to medical condition or *individual request*." [emphasis added][1]

TREATMENT ACCORDING TO STAGE

The following treatment options are recommended. Keep in mind that conservative surgery is best suited to the treatment of early cancer. Even so, I would still encourage you to ask your doctor about the most conservative options available to you in your specific case. Sometimes, radiation or chemotherapy is used before surgery to help shrink a large tumor. I think this is a good use for these therapies. However, radiation therapy or chemotherapy is sometimes used after surgery to help reduce local recurrence. They are mentioned here because they are options that you may be presented with. The way that chemotherapy is generally used in bladder cancer—as an agent placed inside the bladder, instead of as system-wide pill or injection form—results in minimal side effects. However, if radiation therapy or system-wide chemotherapy is prescribed, I would again encourage you to talk to your doctor to find out how much these therapies can actually help to prolong your life. "Standard treatment" refers to the treatment recommended as accepted medical practice.

Stage 0

At this stage, the tumor is very superficial, involving only the mucus membrane. The primary therapy is TUR or fulguration. Chemotherapy drugs or biological therapy agents can be placed inside the bladder to prevent recurrences. Radiation therapy is not effective. Photodynamic therapy is used experimentally for this stage of disease. Another treatment can be attempted if the cancer recurs. The same agents used to prevent recurrences are also used to treat recurrent lesions.

Stage A

At stage A, the tumor has penetrated into the tissue below the mucous membrane. The treatment is the same as for stage 0.

Stage B

At this stage, the tumor has invaded the muscle. It should be completely excised with a TUR or partial cystectomy. Radiation therapy or drugs placed inside the bladder may reduce local recurrence. Patients should have a pelvic lymph node removal. This can be performed through a laparoscope or as an abdominal operation, depending upon the treatment of the bladder and the status of the pelvic nodes. Positive nodes should be removed in an abdominal operation. If the tumor recurs, patients may wish to consider repeat local surgery or the use of different chemotherapeutic drugs inside the bladder.

Stage C

At this stage, the tumor has invaded into the fat around the bladder. Standard treatment is preoperative chemotherapy or radiation therapy followed by radical cystectomy.

Stage D

At stage D, the tumor involves adjacent organs or lymph nodes, or distant metastases are present. Standard treatment is the same as for stage C.

FOLLOW-UP

Regular and meticulous follow-up is the most important part of conservative treatment for bladder cancer. The patient should have a cystoscopy every three months for the first two years, then every six months for two more years, and annually thereafter. Cystoscopy can be performed as an office procedure. Some urologists rely more upon regular examination of the urine for abnormal cells. The amount of follow-up required varies with the situation. There can be a longer interval between visits if a wide surgical margin was used, and a shorter interval if a narrow margin was used.

7.

Breast Cancer

Breast cancer is the most common cancer among women, affecting about one woman out of every nine. In the United States, about 182,000 women each year are diagnosed with breast cancer; about 46,000 of them die of this disease. The diagnosis of breast cancer has been increasing during the past several years, primarily due to earlier detection with the increasing use of mammography.

No cancer has been more thoroughly studied than breast cancer. I believe that some of the biological lessons learned from this disease can be applied to other solid tumors.

This chapter will cover the following topics: the anatomy of the breast, the types of cancer that affect the breast, how this cancer is graded, how this cancer spreads, what screening procedures are available, what the signs and symptoms are, how this cancer is diagnosed, how this cancer is staged, what treatments are available, my analysis of how conservative surgery can be used to treat this cancer, my recommendations for the appropriate treatment at each stage, and what sort of follow-up is needed after treatment.

ANATOMY AND PHYSIOLOGY

The female breast is made up of lobules—small lobes—that produce milk. They are supported in a network of supporting tissue. Much of the mass of the breast is made up of fat. A network of ducts carries milk from the outlying lobules to the nipple. Visualize a cluster of grapes in which the grapes are lobules and the stem is the juncture of ducts at the nipple. The pigmented area surrounding the nipple is called the areola.

TYPES OF CANCER

The two primary types of cancer are *lobular carcinoma*, or cancer of the milk-producing lobules, and *intraductal carcinoma*, or cancer of the cells that line the ducts. About 85 percent of breast cancers are intraductal; about 10 percent are lobular. A patient may have both types of cancer at the same time.

Pathologists have identified dozens of other types of breast cancer that make up the other 5 percent. They develop from the surrounding support tissue of the breast. The treatment of these cancers is the same as that of intraductal and lobular cancers.

Several types of abnormal changes can occur in the cells that line the breast ducts. The buildup of extra cells is called *intraductal hyperplasia*. This is a callus-like formation. If these cells begin to look abnormal, they are called *atypical intraductal hyperplasia*. Patients with this condition have a fourfold increased risk of developing breast cancer. Doctors now believe that in some patients, these abnormal cells may eventually evolve into cancer. All parts of the breast may contain premalignant tissue, or tissue that is in the process of becoming malignant. This phenomenon is called "multicentricity," and is occasionally used to support the need for radical surgery or radiation therapy.

Cancers begin by growing into the space that would contain milk if the breast was lactating. The earliest cancer is limited to the most superficial cells and is called *in situ* cancer. This cancer involves only the duct lining cells. It has not penetrated any deeper and has not spread.

TUMOR GRADE

Tumors are graded according to how normal or abnormal they appear under a microscope. A tumor with many dividing cells is abnormal and is presumed to be growing fast. Fast-growing cancers tend to spread and have a more serious prognosis. Pathologists usually separate breast cancer into three grades, from grade 1, good prognosis, to grade 3, poor prognosis. The pathologist also can report if tumor cells are present in the blood vessels or lymphatic vessels near the tumor. These cancers are more likely to spread.

It is also possible to learn if a breast cancer is sensitive to the female sex hormone estrogen, using a test to measure estrogen receptors. Breast cancer cells that have estrogen receptors are called estrogen-receptor positive. They are slower growing and less likely to spread than are those which do not have estrogen receptors (estrogen-receptor negative). Estrogen-receptor positive tumors are more likely to respond to hormone-related therapy, such as tamoxifen. Tests may also be used to determine the cancer's sensitivity to another hormone called progesterone.

Pathologists also measure *DNA ploidy* to help determine how aggressively a breast cancer will behave. DNA ploidy refers to the number of chromosomes within cancer cells. Those with a normal number (twenty-three pairs) are less aggressive than are those with an abnormal number. This does not have an absolute influence on treatment decisions, but many doctors consider it when deciding how aggressively to treat their patients. For example, patients with threatening tumors are more likely to be treated with chemotherapy.

ROUTES OF SPREAD

Breast cancer becomes invasive when it penetrates the basement membrane that supports the cells which line the ducts. It takes about eight years for a single breast cancer cell to grow to 1 cm in diameter, a size that can be felt. Before this point, the cancer is unlikely to spread. When breast cancer spreads, it is often found first in the lymph nodes of the armpit, and then in other organs, such as the lungs, liver, brain, or bones.

Two factors are the most important in determining the prognosis of a patient with breast cancer: the size of the tumor, and the presence or absence of cancer in the lymph nodes. All of the other prognostic information taken together can alter a patient's survival by only 5 to 15 percent.

SCREENING

A monthly self breast examination is one of the best screening methods. Patients should examine themselves while lying in bed and while standing. Techniques are taught in many clinics. (Call your doctor or the American Cancer Society for information.) Almost 90 percent of all cancers are discovered by patients. Fortunately, 90 percent of all breast lumps are benign.

Risk Factors for Breast Cancer

While all women should perform monthly self exams, it is still not clear at what point any individual woman should begin having regular mammograms. Your decisions about mammograms may depend somewhat on your risk factors for developing breast cancer. If your mother or sister had breast cancer, your risk more than doubles. If two close relatives had breast cancer, your risk is ten times greater. Genetic testing may soon give you a better idea of your own risk.

Hormonal factors also play a role. Patients who have an early onset of menstruation or a late menopause have an increased risk of breast cancer. But an early pregnancy reduces the risk. Women who have a child before age twenty reduce their risk by 20 percent. Those who have a first child after age thirty increase their risk by 40 percent. Women who have never been pregnant increase their breast cancer risk by 60 percent. The reasons for these differences are not clear. It appears that a long period of estrogen-stimulated menstrual cycles increases the risk, but that pregnancy reduces it by interrupting these cycles. Surprisingly, birth control pills and estrogen replacement therapy for menopause do not affect the risk of breast cancer. The reason for this is unknown.

Mammograms and the Younger Woman

Low-dose mammograms are roughly 90 percent accurate and can detect cancers about one year before they can be felt. The National Cancer Institute recommends a mammogram every year in women over fifty years of age. The American Cancer Society and the American College of Radiology also recommend mammograms every two years in women between the ages of forty and fifty. At this age, the breast tissue is dense and a cancer is more difficult to see. Very rarely, a woman in this age group may benefit from a program of regular mammograms. But this benefit is so rare that no study so far has been able to dectect it. Routine mammograms in women under fifty years of age result in unneeded biopsies and unnecessary anxiety. Patients under fifty should consult their physicians about this subject. Women with one or more risk factors may want mammograms more often.

The X-ray dose for mammograms is much less than twenty years ago. One mammogram has about the health hazard of smoking a single cigarette.

SIGNS AND SYMPTOMS

On examination, breast cancer is usually a hard, painless, nontender round mass. The mass often stands out from surrounding breast tissue with a border that can be felt on all sides. In later stages, cancer may cause redness, dimpling, or even ulceration of the skin. On rare occasions, breast cancer first appears in an axillary lymph node or distant site.

It may be difficult to distinguish breast cancer from *fibrocystic changes*. Fibrocystic changes are exaggerated responses of breast tissue to female hormones. So many women develop tender breast lumps that the condition is hardly a disease. Lumps are less likely to be malignant if they are tender, blend into the surrounding breast tissue, or have irregular shapes.

These descriptions are general, however, and any new lump should be reported to your doctor.

DIAGNOSIS

After a physical examination or a review of the mammogram, the diagnosis may still be in doubt. Diagnosis is possible only with a biopsy. A small sample of the lesion can be obtained with a *needle biopsy*, an office procedure. Small lesions, whether found by self-examination or mammography, are often difficult to hit precisely with a needle. If they are suspicious, it may be worthwhile to use a technique called *needle localization*. The radiologist examines the breast while under X-ray view, and places needles in the lesion. The surgeon uses the needles to guide him to the suspicious area. Alternatively, the surgeon may take multiple needle biopsies using a very thin needle. This is called *skinny needle biopsy*, and is more fully explained in Chapter 5. Remember, a biopsy is only diagnostic when it is positive. A needle biopsy may miss the lesion or retrieve only cells that are benign. The presence of malignant cells assures the pathologist that cancer is present, but the absence of malignant cells in the biopsy does not guarantee that there is no cancer.

A newer technique is called *stereotaxic breast biopsy*. It may be more accurate than a skinny needle biopsy because a core of tissue is removed. Such a core preserves the structural integrity of the tissue and gives the pathologist more information. The abnormality on the mammogram can be precisely located and biopsied using sophisticated stereotaxic equipment.

A biopsy may not be necessary. This is especially true if the patient has few risk factors for breast cancer and the lesion itself is small with no signs that suggest a malignancy. Often the best solution is to repeat the mammogram in about three to six months. The decision to do a biopsy or to wait is often difficult for both the doctor and the patient. The decision should be clearly understood by the patient. A biopsy carries a small risk of complications, and a risk of missing a small tumor. Waiting carries a small risk that the cancer will grow and even spread. Fortunately, cancers that cannot be felt seldom spread. The patient and doctor should decide together whether to perform a biopsy or wait. If a cancer is found after a period of waiting, the decision to have waited was not in error.

STAGES OF DISEASE

Today, there are two principal staging systems used for breast cancer: the TNM system and the traditional system.

The TNM Staging System

The TNM staging system has been developed over the past forty years. (It is explained in Chapter 5.) Table 7.1 presents a simplified summary of this often complicated system.

The Traditional Staging System

This system has been developed over the past sixty years, and is popular among most practicing physicians in the United States. Table 7.2, which summarizes this system, also includes TNM abbreviations so that the two systems can be compared.

Table 7.1. TNM Staging System for Breast Cancer

Tumor Size [T]	Nodal Metastases [N]	Distant Metastases [M]
T_1—2 cm or less	N_0—No cancer in the lymph nodes	M_0—No distant metastases are present
T_2—5 cm or less	N_1—Lymph nodes contain cancer	M_1—Distant metastases are present
T_3—Over 5 cm	N_2—Lymph nodes are large and fixed together or to nearby tissue	
T_4—Tumor directly extends to the chest wall or skin	N_3—Lymph nodes near the collarbone contain cancer	

TYPES OF TREATMENT

Surgery and radiation therapy are the primary forms of treatment for breast cancer, as they have been for most of this century. Chemotherapy and biological therapy are promising additions to the arsenal, but their effects thus far have been limited. See Chapter 5 for more information about these treatments, including general information on the side effects associated with each treatment.

Surgery

Surgery can be divided into two basic groups: breast-removing surgery and breast-sparing surgery.

Breast-Removing Surgery

The most extensive surgery for breast cancer is the *radical mastectomy*. Breast cancer has traditionally been treated with removal of the entire breast, the lymph nodes in the armpit, and the pectoral muscles beneath the breast. This combination of procedures is called the radical mastectomy or the Halsted radical mastectomy, named after William Halsted who developed and popularized the operation. After a radical mastectomy, the skin lies directly on top of the ribs, giving a "washboard" appearance to the chest.

Slightly less extensive is the *modified radical mastectomy*. This

Table 7.2. Traditional Staging System for Breast Cancer

Stage	Description	Five-Year Survival Rate
0	A cancer that is limited to the topmost cell layer.	Over 90%
I	A cancer that is 2 cm or less in diameter with no evidence of spread to the lymph nodes or distant organs (T_1, N_0, M_0).	About 85%
II	A cancer that is 5 cm or less in diameter, or the patient has positive lymph nodes in the armpit (T_2, N_0, M_0; T_{0-2}, N_1, M_0).	About 60%
III	A cancer that is larger than 5 cm in diameter, or there are positive lymph nodes that are fixed to other tissue. The lymph nodes may adhere to one another or to the underlying muscle or overlying skin (T_{0-4}, N_{0-3}, M_0, excluding those combinations listed above).	About 40%
IV	A cancer that is fixed to the skin or chest wall, or there is lymph node spread above the collarbone, or there are distant metastases already present (T_{0-4}, N_{0-3}, M_1).	Less than 10%

operation is like the radical mastectomy except that the pectoral muscles are not removed. This gives the patient a smooth chest.

Breast-Sparing Surgery

All surgeons agree that patients with stage I and II breast cancer should have their entire tumor completely removed. This is called tumor excision, a general term that does not specify the amount of tissue that is removed. Breast-sparing procedures have more precise definitions, and are described below.

Lumpectomy is removal of the cancer without a wide margin of normal tissue. Some edges of the tumor are usually checked by a pathologist to be sure there are no tumor cells present. In the NSABP lumpectomy study discussed in Chapter 1, over 40 percent of patients treated with lumpectomy without radiation therapy developed local recurrence. This is the least aggressive type of tumor excision.

Wide excision is a general term for the removal of the tumor together with an undefined "wide" margin, usually at least 1 cm, of normal tissue. A wide excision removes more tissue than a lumpectomy, but less tissue than a partial mastectomy.

Partial mastectomy includes removal of the entire tumor with a wider margin of breast tissue. The goal is usually a 2-cm margin. The removal of the tumor and a surrounding margin of tissue creates a defect or hole in the breast. Surgeons have traditionally closed this hole by sewing the remaining breast tissue to itself. The NSABP trial determined that surgeons could sew together only the skin of the breast. This allows the cavity in the breast to fill with lymph fluid, which eventually becomes soft scar tissue. This technique create a more normal-appearing breast.

Quadrantectomy includes excision of an entire quarter of the breast surrounding the tumor. Margins of 2 to 3 cm are common. This procedure removes more tissue than a partial mastectomy.

An *axillary dissection* removes the lymph nodes in the axilla (armpit). This procedure determines the extent of tumor spread – the stage of the disease. This may influence the use of additional (adjuvant) treatment, such a chemotherapy or hormonal therapy. A *sentinel node* biopsy removes only those few lymph nodes most likely to contain tumor cells.

Radiation Therapy

Radiation therapy is used to eradicate microscopic cells that might remain after surgery. It is no longer used following modified radical mastectomy, even for patients with stage II disease. Radiation can reduce local recurrence with some patients, but it does not increase survival. Following breast-conserving surgery, radiation is usually administered to the remaining breast tissue, sometimes with a second dose of radiation concentrated on the tumor site. It is given five days per week for five to six weeks for a total dose of about 50 Gy.

Chemotherapy

The use of adjuvant chemotherapy—chemotherapy following surgery—is very controversial. In 1992, the British medical journal *Lancet* published a summary of 133 trials involving over 75,000 women who had been treated with adjuvant chemotherapy before 1985.[1] The summary was complicated by the many differences among the studies: the number of drugs used (including the hormonal therapy tamoxifen), the drug combinations used, and the duration of treatment. Most of the women had cancer in their lymph nodes (stage II). These patients are the ones most likely to benefit from adjuvant chemotherapy. *Lancet* concluded, "The effect of treatment on the average duration of survival will not be known for decades, and even estimates of median survival may be unreliable."

The following is my brief summary of the available information. Premenopausal and postmenopausal women must be considered separately, because their responses to treatment are very different.

Stage I Breast Cancer

Some doctors suggest adjuvant chemotherapy for selected premenopausal patients with negative lymph nodes (stage I). Patients with stage I disease receive less benefit from adjuvant therapy than patients with stage II disease because fewer patients at stage I are likely to die of breast cancer. Patients with a poor prognosis may benefit from treatment. Patients with a good prognosis are usually not treated. Because tamoxifen has fewer side effects than standard chemotherapy, postmenopausal women with stage I disease may benefit from this treatment.

Stage II Breast Cancer

Premenopausal women are sometimes treated with a combination of three to five drugs. Treated women may have as much as a 7 percent better chance of surviving ten years than untreated women. However, some specialists believe that the survival benefit is not that great. Barber Mueller of McMaster University in Hamilton, Ontario, argues that about 6 percent of premenopausal women have their lives prolonged by about fourteen to eighteen months.[2] Conversely, he says, about 94 percent of treated patients receive no benefit. The treatment does cause side effects, such as hair loss, nausea, and vomiting. (The number of months spent enduring the side effects is probably as important a consideration as the number of months of added survival.) Some oncologists base their decision to use chemotherapy upon the presence or absence of such risk factors as tumor size and estrogen-receptor status.

The studies published in *Lancet* showed that postmenopausal women benefit even less from multidrug adjuvant chemotherapy. Nevertheless, those with estrogen-receptor positive tumors usually benefit from a two- to five-year course of tamoxifen. Women with stage II cancer improve their chances of surviving five years by about 6 percent. The side effects of tamoxifen are much less than those of conventional chemotherapy, but can include hot flashes, nausea, and vomiting. Dosage adjustments can sometimes reduce these symptoms.

Advanced Breast Cancer

Multidrug chemotherapy is able to cure some patients with advanced, localized breast cancer.[3] Now as many as 50 percent of patients with stage III disease are living ten years or longer. The most aggressive form, known as inflammatory breast cancer, was once fatal in 95 percent of patients within one year. Survival rates among these patients have also improved.

ANALYSIS

Breast-sparing surgery is becoming the standard treatment for most patients with early breast cancer. Unfortunately, many patients still elect to have a mastectomy simply because they are not able to undergo several weeks of radiation treatment. Others choose mastectomy because they fear local recurrence. Today, fewer than half of patients with early breast cancer are being treated with breast-sparing techniques. Several studies have shown that a patient's decision to have a mastectomy is influenced by the surgeon's preference for more radical treatment.

Breast-Sparing Surgery:
Is Radiation Therapy Always Necessary?

Let us now examine the routine use of radiation therapy following breast-sparing surgery. In June 1990, a group of medical specialists, researchers, a nurse, and a laywoman met at the National Institutes of Health.[4] This Consensus Development Conference on the Treatment of Early-Stage Breast Cancer concluded, "Although local control can be obtained in some patients with local excision alone, no subgroups have been identified in which radiation therapy can be avoided." This recommendation says that all patients who have breast-sparing treatment should receive postoperative radiation therapy.

I do not agree with this recommendation. It reflects a disadvantage of consensus conferences—their goal of a single therapy on which most or all of the participants agree. I believe that this conference should have offered a range of alternatives—called practice parameters—that consider the wishes of the patient and the opinion of her doctor.

In England, over one third of the surgeons treat their patients with wide tumor excision without postoperative radiation therapy.[5] I believe that many patients with stage I cancer can be spared postoperative radiation therapy. Radiation does reduce local recurrence following narrow excision, but there is no data suggesting that it adds a single day to the survival of the average patient with breast cancer.

Surgery and Local Recurrence

Local recurrence can be minimized by surgery alone. Recent experience shows that surgeons who perform a careful partial mastectomy can achieve results equal to those achieved by lumpectomy and radiation therapy. Surgeons in England, Sweden, and Canada have achieved local recurrence rates of 10 to 11 percent with surgery alone.[6-8] In this country, surgeons at the Cleveland Clinic, the Roswell Park Cancer Institute, and the University of Miami have achieved similar results by removing the tumor with a wide margin (1 to 2 cm).[9-11] As discussed in Chapters 1 and 4, local recurrence following conservative surgery is not a grave event. Reexcision does not impair survival.

There are several factors that influence recurrence rates after surgery. They are the size of the primary tumor, the margins of excision (both their width and whether or not they contain cancer cells), the lymph node status, and patient age, as well as factors relating to the tumor itself, such as its grade. As the number of adverse factors increases, the chances for local recurrence and/or distant spread also increase. If patients are carefully selected based upon these factors, satisfactory local control can be achieved in many patients with surgery alone.

TREATMENT ACCORDING TO STAGE

The treatment of breast cancer has been changing significantly in the United States. Breast-sparing surgery is widely practiced, although not widely enough. Reconstructive procedures have improved markedly. Radiation therapy techniques have changed to increase the local effectiveness and reduce complications, although radiation therapy is still used more than necessary.

Keep in mind that conservative surgery is best suited to the treatment of early cancer. Even so, I would still encourage you to ask your doctor about the most conservative options available to you in your specific case. Sometimes, radiation or chemotherapy is used before surgery to help shrink a large tumor. I think this is a good use for these therapies. However, radiation therapy or chemotherapy is sometimes used after surgery to help reduce local recurrence. They are mentioned here because they are options that you may be presented with. However, I would again encourage you to talk to your doctor to find out how much these therapies can actually help to prolong your life. "Standard treatment" refers to the treatment recommended as accepted medical practice.

Stage I

At this stage, there is a tumor of 2 cm or less without spread to the lymph nodes in the armpit. Wide excision and lymph node removal with radiation therapy is becoming standard treatment for most stage I patients. I believe that many patients at this stage can prudently decline postoperative radiation therapy, if the tumor can be excised with a 1- to 2-cm margin of normal tissue, while preserving a cosmetically acceptable breast. The margin is influenced by the tumor size compared with the breast size. The surgeon must balance the functional loss and cosmetic defect of the surgery against the risk of recurrent cancer. To underline an important point: if local recurrence were a great survival hazard, then the added security of radiation might be justified. But the NSABP lumpectomy trial proved that recurrent disease can be safely removed without compromising patient survival. Removal alone spares patients the five weeks of daily radiation therapy and its unpleasant side effects, as well as the possible long-term complications of radiation. Since each area of the body can tolerate only a limited quantity of radiation, it may be prudent to keep this therapy in reserve.

Removal of the lymph nodes under the arm may be performed if the results affect subsequent therapy. Most patients with a tumor 1 cm or smaller can prudently decline this procedure, since more than 95 percent of these patients have an excellent prognosis without adjuvant treatment.[12] A postmenopausal patient may elect to take tamoxifen, whatever the lymph node status. (This is another reason to avoid removing the lymph nodes.) A premenopausal patient with a 2-cm tumor may elect to receive adjuvant chemotherapy if the lymph nodes are positive. Therefore, the surgeon may remove the lymph nodes after the tumor has been thoroughly tested.

Stage II

At stage II, the tumor is 5 cm or less in size, or there is a spread to the axillary lymph nodes. Wide excision and lymph node removal with radiation therapy is becoming standard treatment in many stage II patients. If the surgeon is able to remove a wide margin of healthy tissue, I believe that radiation therapy may be omitted in selected patients. If the patient has a tumor that is large compared with the size of the breast, she may achieve better cosmetic results with mastectomy. Tamoxifen is given to some postmenopausal patients with estrogen-receptor positive tumors. Combination chemotherapy may be appropriate for premenopausal women.

Stage III

At stage III breast cancer, the tumor mass is larger than 5 cm, or the axillary lymph nodes are fixed to one another or to surrounding tissue. Preoperative chemotherapy followed by either partial mastectomy or modified radical mastectomy are recommended here. By reducing the size of the tumor, treatment probably reduces the volume of circulating tumor cells, allowing the patient's own immune system a chance to prevent the formation of distant metastases. Postoperative radiation therapy may reduce local recurrence. Postoperative chemotherapy may also be used. This treatment is enhancing the survival of those patients who have localized breast cancer.

Stage IV

At this stage, the tumor is fixed to the chest wall, or there are positive lymph nodes above the collarbone, or distant metastases are present. Treatment recommendations are the same as for stage III.

Special Considerations

Some doctors would prefer to use more aggressive treatment if any of the following conditions exist. However, I believe that more conservative treatment may be possible even under these conditions.

Tumor Size

If the surgeon can remove a large tumor—greater than 5 cm—and leave a cosmetically acceptable breast, conservative surgery may be possible. Investigators at M. D. Anderson Hospital in Houston have treated patients with tumors over 5 cm in diameter using preoperative chemotherapy and breast-conserving surgery.[13] If breast preservation is reasonable for some patients with 5-cm tumors or stage III disease, it should be prudent for many patients with less advanced disease.

Extensive Intraductal Component (EIC) Presence

Many studies have shown that patients with intraductal cancer throughout the breast, known as extensive intraductal component, are at a greater risk of developing local recurrence, especially if they are not treated with radiation therapy. Patients with this condition should usually receive radiation therapy following a partial mastectomy.

Tumor Location

It is more difficult to obtain a good cosmetic result if the tumor is beneath the nipple. If the tumor itself is directly against the nipple, the nipple itself may need to be excised. In special cases, you and your doctor might elect to save the nipple and rely on radiation therapy to kill a few remaining tumor cells.

Number of Tumors

Two or more tumors can be excised separately. Again, the important consideration is removal of all the cancerous tissue.

Superficial Tumors

Cancer of the topmost cell layer, called *in situ* cancer, is very early disease. It has not yet begun to invade surrounding tissues. But some investigators have found patients with this disease to have a higher incidence of multiple small cancers in the breast. In an NSABP trial, B. F. Fisher and colleagues concluded that radiation therapy reduced the rate of local recurrence following lumpectomy for patients with superficial cancer.[14] But it does not increase survival. *In situ* cancer does represent a small risk to your survival. You might survive your first early lesion, but then allow a recurrence to go untreated until it is larger and perhaps invasive. A recurrence that grows larger than the primary lesion could represent a risk. In terms of percentages, this risk is small, and you have to be the judge. Your treatment is a very personal matter. It must be tailored to your cancer and your concerns about your body image, as well as to the results of treatment.

FOLLOW-UP

Regular and meticulous follow-up is the most important part of conservative treatment for breast cancer. Patients should be examined every three months for the first two years, then every six months for three more years, and annually thereafter. Blood chemistries, mammograms, and chest X-rays should be performed annually. Scans and other X-rays should be performed if symptoms develop. The amount of follow-up required varies with the situation. There can be a longer interval between visits if a wide surgical margin was used, and a shorter interval if a narrower margin was used.

8.

Cancer of the Cervix

Cervical cancer is the seventh most common malignancy among women in the United States. About 16,000 women are diagnosed with cervical cancer and 5,000 die of this disease each year. Since 1940, cancer of the cervix has gone from being a common female malignancy to being among the least common. This success is largely due to the widespread use of the Papanicolaou (Pap) smear, which successfully detects abnormal cells before they become malignant. This disease affects primarily older women who are out of their childbearing years. Thus, there are few patients who are suitable candidates for conservative, fertility-sparing surgery. Nevertheless, younger women are increasingly affected. Most cases of cervical cancer are associated with the human papillomavirus (HPV). This virus causes both skin and genital warts; genital warts are sexually transmitted.

This chapter will cover the following topics: the anatomy of the cervix, the types of cancer that affect the cervix, how this cancer is graded, how this cancer spreads, what screening procedures are available, what the signs and symptoms are, how this cancer is diagnosed, how this cancer is staged, what treatments are available, my analysis of how conservative surgery can be used to treat this cancer, my recommendations for the appropriate treatment at each stage, and what sort of follow-up is needed after treatment.

ANATOMY AND PHYSIOLOGY

The cervix is a muscular organ that lies below the uterus. It keeps the developing fetus inside the uterus during pregnancy and dilates dramatically at the time of delivery. It is lined by cells that are similar to those of the skin and are called *squamous cells*. The opening into the uterus is called the *endocervical canal*. A portion of the endocervical canal is usually lined by glandular tissue.

TYPES OF CANCER

About 85 percent of all cervical cancers arise from the squamous cells lining the cervix and the lower portion of the endocervical canal. A less common cancer, which starts in the glandular tissue inside the canal, is called *adenocarcinoma* and represents about 15 percent of all cervical cancers. Some gynecologists believe that adenocarcinoma has a higher incidence of spread to the lymph nodes and a worse prognosis.

TUMOR GRADE

Cancer of the cervix often arises from cells infected with HPV. Initially, changes in these cells are premalignant and are called *cervical intraepithelial neoplasia* (CIN) grade 1. Over a period ranging from months to many years, a minority of patients with this condition can progress to *cervical intraepithelial neoplasia* grade 3 (CIN-3), the highest CIN grade. This is known as cancer *in situ*, or cancer limited to the topmost layer of cells. On the average, this entire process takes about ten years. Note that these grades represent the earliest changes in the malignant process.

ROUTES OF SPREAD

Cancer of the cervix becomes a real malignancy when it penetrates the basement membrane, which is the layer between the squamous cells and the underlying tissue. The deeper the cancer penetrates, the greater the chance for it to enter the lymphatic and blood vessels. Vessel invasion increases the potential spread of this cancer. Early invasion occurs when the tumor is about 1 mm thick. Metastases, or groups of cells from the original cancer, travel to lymph nodes and distant organs in about 5 percent of patients whose lesions have invaded between 3 mm and 5 mm of tissue.

Cervical cancer usually spreads first to the lymph nodes in the pelvis. In patients with advanced disease, it can spread down to the groin or up to the lymph nodes beside the aorta, the large blood vessel that carries blood from the heart to the intestines and the legs. Distant spread occurs primarily to the lungs, and rarely to the brain, liver, and bone.

As the tumor grows, it can spread locally onto the upper vagina, and into the *parametrium*, which is the tissue around the cervix. It can then spread into the pelvis, invading the bladder and rectum, obstructing the tubes that carry urine from the kidneys to the bladder (ureters), and onto the side walls of the pelvis.

SCREENING

Women should begin having Pap smears when they are eighteen years of age or become sexually active. Women who have multiple sex partners should have annual Pap smears. Women who are at low risk, such as those in monogamous relationships, may be examined less frequently after they have had three negative smears. Women should consult with their gynecologists for current recommendations.

SIGNS AND SYMPTOMS

For signs that a doctor can discover, see the following section on diagnosis. Symptoms noticable to the patient would not develop until the cancer was quite advanced.

DIAGNOSIS

Patients with abnormal Pap smears usually have a *colposcopic examination*. The gynecologist looks at the cervix using a scope that magnifies the appearance of the cervix about ten times. Any abnormalities on this visual inspection may lead the gynecologist to perform a *cone biopsy*. This is the removal of a cone-shaped core of cervical tissue. The biopsy is usually done in the office or other outpatient setting under local anesthesia.

STAGES OF DISEASE

If cervical cancer is allowed to grow untreated, it will progress through five clinical stages, stages 0 to IV. This staging system, one of several in use, has been approved by International Federation of Gynecology and Obstetrics (FIGO) and is summarized in Table 8.1.

Another system, that of the Society of Gynecologic Oncology, defines stage Ia more narrowly. In that system, any lesion with more than 3 mm of invasion or any lymph node involvement is classified stage Ib. This distinction is important because patients with stage Ia disease are more likely to be treated conservatively, and thus have their fertility preserved. Patients with stage Ib disease are likely to be treated with radical hysterectomy. Some gynecologists in Europe, where FIGO is used more often than in the United States, have argued that stage Ia should be expanded even farther. This means that even more patients would be eligible for conservative treatment.

TYPES OF TREATMENT

Almost all patients with early cervical cancer are treated by some form of surgery. Surgical therapy ranges from removal of a portion of the cervix, to removal of the uterus, to the removal of most pelvic structures. Few studies have attempted to compare the efficacy of hysterectomy versus conservative surgery, known as conization. Radiation therapy is generally used for more advanced disease, stages II to IV. Chemotherapy is of little help, although preoperative chemotherapy is being tried in several centers to shrink large tumors. Some tumors that respond to this treatment may then be surgically removed; others are irradiated. See Chapter 5 for more information about these treatments, including general information on the side effects associated with each treatment.

Surgery

The treatment of cervical cancer has remained stable in the United States. Radical hysterectomy has been the primary treatment for most of this century. The use of conservative surgery to treat patients with superficial cancer, that which has invaded less than 3 mm, is the primary advance. Most other experimental surgery is conducted in Europe.

Surgery can be divided into two basic types: that which does not spare fertility and that which does. A *staging procedure* can determine whether the cancer has spread to the lymph nodes or not.

Table 8.1. FIGO Staging System for Cervical Cancer

Stage	Description	Five-Year Survival Rate
0	A cancer that is limited to the topmost layer of cells.	Over 95%
I	A cancer that is limited to the cervix.	
Ia	A cancer that is diagnosed microscopically.	
Ia$_1$	A cancer that invades less than 1 mm below the surface.	Over 95%
Ia$_2$	A cancer that invades less than 5 mm over an area of less than 7 mm.	85%
Ib	A cancer that is greater than Ia$_2$, but is still confined to the cervix. It is generally obvious to the naked eye.	85%
II	A cancer that extends onto the upper two-thirds of the vagina or involves the parametrial tissue around the uterus.	
IIa	A cancer that does not involve the parametrial tissue.	85%
IIb	A cancer that involves the parametrial tissue.	70%
III	A cancer that is locally advanced.	
IIIa	A cancer that involves the lower third of the vagina.	45%
IIIb	A cancer that involves the pelvic side wall or obstructs the kidneys.	35%
IV	A cancer that is very advanced.	
IVa	A cancer that involves the inside lining of the bladder or rectum.	25%
IVb	Distant metastases are present or the disease extends beyond the pelvis.	15%

Surgery That Does Not Spare Fertility

The *radical hysterectomy* removes the entire uterus, including the cervix and the upper third of the vagina. It also removes all the supporting ligaments and the parametrial tissues all the way to the pelvic side wall, as well as the surrounding lymph nodes.

Radical hysterectomy has many complications. Bladder dysfunction is the most common; it persists in about 3 percent of patients. Injury to the vagina and urinary tract can lead to an abnormal channel called a *fistula* between the ureter or bladder and the vagina. Fistulas occur in about 2 percent of cases. The ureter can be accidentally tied with a suture or otherwise blocked. This must be corrected to avoid a backup of urine and injury to the kidney.

All of these complications can occur with any type of hysterectomy discussed here. The larger the operation, the greater the chance of complications.

The *modified radical hysterectomy* spares portions of the supporting ligaments, which also contain some of the nerves necessary for proper bladder function. Thus, there is less bladder dysfunction than with a radical hysterectomy. The lymph nodes may also be removed.

The *total hysterectomy* removes only the uterus and cervix, either through the abdomen or the vagina. There is less bladder dysfunction than with either the radical or the modified radical hysterectomy.

The most aggressive of all these operations is the *radical pelvic exenteration,* which removes most of the important structures in the pelvis, including the uterus, cervix, vagina, bladder, and rectum. This requires reconstruction of the vagina. Urine and intestinal contents may be permanently diverted through separate openings in the abdominal wall. This operation often results in complications. About 5 percent of patients do not survive the operation. It is performed on patients who develop recurrence after other forms of treatment.

Surgery That Spares Fertility

The *trachelectomy* removes most of the cervix. The uterus is sewn to the vagina. An episiotomy, or incision between the vagina and the anus, is sometimes required. Patients should be able to bear children after this procedure, although they should be carefully watched. Possible complications include bladder injury and the development of a fistula between the bladder and the vagina.

The *loop electrosurgical excision procedure* (LEEP) is like electrocautery, described in Chapter 5, but uses a wire loop instead of a metal tip to cut tissue with an electric current. It is often used to remove the *transition zone*—the area within the endocervical canal where the squamous cells of the cervix meet the glandular tissue that lines the inside of the uterus. The depth of incision is about 1 cm. This procedure destroys the cells at the margins of the excision. Therefore, the pathologist may be unable to determine if the margins are free of tumor cells. LEEP causes discomfort, but no serious complications. *Cryosurgery* is similar to LEEP, except that it uses a cold metal probe to freeze the tissue.

Conization is the excision of a cone-shaped area of tissue from the cervix, performed with either a scalpel or a laser. Like the LEEP, the laser destroys the cells at the margin, while the scalpel preserves them. It is used to both diagnose and to treat early cancer.

Staging Procedure

It is impossible to learn if lymph nodes are involved with cancer without removing them and examining them under a microscope. Thus, these nodes are sometimes removed to learn the extent of the disease. Patients with advanced disease may live longer if their lymph nodes are removed. Recently, the use of a laparoscope, a tube through which abdominal tissue is removed, has been used for sampling lymph nodes prior to radiation therapy. It is the least invasive method.[1] It is a new procedure, and its risks and efficacy have not been determined.

The risk of pelvic lymph node metastasis (spread) increases with the volume of the cancer:

- For a tumor volume less than 0.5 cc, the risk is 0 percent.
- For a tumor volume of 0.5 to 1.5 cc, the risk is 12 percent.
- For a tumor volume of 1.5 to 3.5 cc, the risk is 22 percent.
- For a tumor volume of 3.5 to 6.5 cc, the risk is 27 percent.
- For a tumor volume of 6.5 to 10 cc, the risk is 40 percent.

Conservative surgery of cervical cancer should include evaluation of the pelvic nodes.

In performing a hysterectomy, the pelvic lymph nodes are usually examined first. If the cancer has spread to these nodes, many gynecologists will terminate the operation without removing the uterus. They believe that radiation therapy can be delivered more effectively if the uterus is in place.

Radiation Therapy

Radiation therapy can be delivered with either an external beam, or with the insertion of radioactive material into the cervix, or both. It is used primarily to treat more advanced disease, stage Ib and higher, or in cases where surgical removal is difficult.

Therapists usually administer 40 to 50 Gy over a four- to five-week period using an *external beam*. Radiation can sterilize the ovaries, and cause atrophy and narrowing of the vagina. Most patients experience temporary diarrhea, which may become chronic in some patients. Abdominal pain is another chronic side effect of external-beam radiation. Drugs such as sucralfate and glutamine may protect the intestines from radiation injury.

Additional radiation can be administered with devices placed inside the patient in a process called *intracavitary radiation*. The patient is put under anesthesia. Then, specially-shaped containers called tandem and ovoids are usually placed in the upper vagina and inside the uterus, respectively. Later, a radioactive material, usually cesium, is placed into these devices after the patient has returned to her hospital room. The radioactive material remains in place for two to three days.

Radioactive needles maybe placed directly into the tumor itself. This is called *interstitial radiation*. Complications include inflammation of the bladder, intestines, and rectum.

When radiation is administered as the principal or only therapy, it can effect a cure in some patients with early disease. Radiation therapy given following surgery to kill microscopic disease in the lymph nodes can reduce local recurrence, but usually does not prolong overall survival.[2]

Chemotherapy

Chemotherapy is largely experimental. Mitomycin, bleomycin, 5-fluorouracil, and cisplatin can shrink tumors or relieve pain in some patients. These responses usually last for a few months. Rarely, a remission will last several years. Some studies have suggested that preoperative chemotherapy may shrink large tumors.

Hydroxyurea is a drug that is toxic to dividing cancer cells that are synthesizing DNA. These cells resist radiation therapy. Several studies that combined radiation therapy and hydroxyurea have achieved prolonged survival.

ANALYSIS

Many gynecologists are performing conization for stage Ia_1 disease. Experience with conization for more invasive stage Ia_2 cancer is limited. I have found no studies suggesting that conization adversely affects the survival of patients with stage Ia disease. See Appendix I for a more complete discussion.

I believe that some women of childbearing age may be safely treated with fertility-sparing procedures. The limits of this approach are determined by the extent of disease. The surgeon must be able to remove the tumor with a margin free of microscopic cancer several millimeters wide. However, patients with pathologically negative margins have been reported to have a 25 percent chance of having residual disease in the cervix.[3] This should be reduced if the surgeon performs a wider excision with a 1- to 2-cm margin. Since postoperative radiation therapy would sterilize many patients, this margin should be generous. On the other hand, too great an excision may lead to cervical failure during pregnancy. This, in turn, would make it difficult, if not impossible, to carry a pregnancy to term.

The patient who desires fertility-sparing surgery and the physician recommending it should understand the added risks of this treatment: the risk of local recurrence and the risk of a poor outcome that increases with the number of grave prognostic signs. The patient must understand that laparoscopic removal of lymph notes is a new procedure. She should understand that promptly treated local recurrence does not adversely affect the survival of patients with breast cancer, which is the cancer that has been the most thoroughly studied, but that this conclusion is not proven for cervical cancer. As with breast cancer and other solid tumors, there is currently no evidence that promptly treated recurrent disease following conservative surgery adversely affects survival. I am not proposing this treatment for widespread use, but it deserves to be tested in clinical trials. It should be offered to selected patients who have a strong desire to maintain their fertility. Problems with conservative treatment have been limited primarily to those patients whose recurrent disease was allowed to grow to a large size before being detected.

TREATMENT ACCORDING TO STAGE

Conservative surgery is best suited for patients with early cancer. Dr. Daniel Dargent in Lyon, France has been performing a type of "lumpectomy" for cervical cancer since 1989. Read about his pioneering work in Appendices I and II. Gynecologists in the U.S. are unlikely to support this conservative approach.

Stage 0

Cancer at this stage involves only the topmost layer of cells. It can be cured with a conization that has negative margins. Laser vaporization or excision is also successful for larger lesions. Other techniques include LEEP and cryosurgery. These procedures can be performed in a doctor's office. It is usually preferable to totally remove the lesion without destroying the cells at its margin in order to determine that all the disease has been removed and that no invasion has occurred. This is best done with a scalpel.

Stage Ia$_1$

At this stage, there is less than 1 mm of invasion. Standard treatment is conization or total hysterectomy. Conization should be the preferred procedure for women of childbearing age who wish to preserve their fertility.

Stage Ia$_2$

A stage Ia$_2$ tumor involves less than 5 mm of invasion, and less than 7 mm of the cervix is covered by the tumor. Abdominal hysterectomy is the standard treatment. Conization is used on patients with less than 3 mm of invasion. I believe that conization or trachelectomy for deeper lesions should be considered for women who wish to preserve their fertility.

Stage Ib

At this stage, the tumor is bigger than at Ia$_2$, but is still confined to the cervix. Standard treatment is radical hysterectomy or radiation therapy. For patients with tumors of a volume less than 15 cc, I believe that consideration may be given to trachelectomy and laparoscopic lymph node removal.

Stage IIa

A stage IIa tumor extends onto the upper two-thirds of the vagina without involving the surrounding tissue. Standard treatment includes radical hysterectomy or radiation therapy. The latter is usually the preferred treatment and includes both external-beam and intracavitary treatment. In France, D. Dargent has treated at least two patients with a trachelectomy. I know of no gynecologists in the United States who would consider conservative surgery for this stage.

Stage IIb

At stage IIb, the tumor involves the tissue surrounding the cervix. Standard treatment is radiation therapy.

Stages III and IV

At these stages, the tumor is either locally advanced or it has metastasized. Radiation therapy is the preferred therapy. Surgery is occasionally helpful to relieve symptoms. Chemotherapy is often added.

Cancer During Pregnancy

Cervical cancer is diagnosed in about 0.01 percent of pregnant patients. Some gynecologists used to believe that pregnancy makes the cancer worse, but reliable studies have challenged this belief. Gynecologists usually allow patients who are twenty-four weeks or more into gestation to wait until fetal viability, or the point at which the baby could live outside of the mother. But patients in the first and second trimester are usually encouraged to terminate their pregnancy and begin conventional therapy. Exceptions have been made for patients with stage Ia disease whose lesions have been completely removed.

I believe that termination of the pregnancy is not always necessary. Patients whose disease can be controlled can probably maintain their pregnancy. Some women may wish to accept some risk in order to bear children and should understand the risks involved. They should not be denied the option of fertility-sparing surgery. Patients must understand that conization during pregnancy has a 20 percent complication rate, including bleeding, abortion, and premature delivery. The studies that have been done in this area are discussed in Appendix I.

FOLLOW-UP

Regular and meticulous follow-up is the most important part of conservative treatment for cervical cancer. A Pap smear and physical examination of the pelvis, abdomen, and lymph nodes should be performed every three months for the first two years, then every six months for at least the next three years, and annually thereafter. The amount of follow-up required varies with the situation. You and your doctor will come up with a follow-up plan that is best for you.

9.

Malignant Melanoma

Each year in the United States, there are about 630,000 cases of skin cancer. Most of these are low-grade cancers that seldom threaten life. Malignant melanoma makes up about 30,000 of these new cases. This disease causes about 7,000 deaths annually. Unfortunately, the incidence of melanoma is increasing at about 4 percent each year. By the year 2000, an estimated one person out of every ninety will develop melanoma sometime during his or her lifetime.[1] The good news is that deaths from melanoma are increasing far more slowly than new cases. This is due to early detection by patients and doctors alike.

Melanoma is frequently seen in patients who have previously had a blistering sunburn. (Chronic exposure to sunlight does not seem to be a great risk.) The decrease in the ozone layer is probably contributing to the increase in melanoma, although some melanomas are hereditary. People with red or blond hair and fair complexions, and those with many moles, are at some increased risk. It is rarely found in African-Americans, but when present is usually on the palms or the soles of the feet.

Melanoma is the most common cancer among women who are from twenty-five to twenty-nine years of age. Most patients, though, are in the forty- to sixty-year age range.

Unlike most other skin cancers, which are easily cured by surgery or chemotherapy ointments, malignant melanoma is very dangerous. It is one of the most malignant of all cancers. While it is still quite small, melanoma can spread to other parts of the body, sometimes appearing in unusual sites such as the spinal cord or intestines. Even years after a melanoma has been removed and considered cured, it can recur locally or at a distant site.

This chapter will cover the following topics: the anatomy of the skin, the structures from which melanomas arise, how this cancer is graded, how this cancer spreads, what screening procedures are available, what the signs and symptoms are, how this cancer is diagnosed, how this cancer is staged, what treatments are available, my analysis of how conservative surgery can be used to treat this cancer, my recommendations for the appropriate treatment at each stage, and what sort of follow-up is needed after treatment.

ANATOMY AND PHYSIOLOGY

The skin contains two primary layers: the *epidermis* and the *dermis*. They are separated by the basement membrane. New epidermis cells grow at the basement membrane and slowly move to the surface. The cells that contain the skin's pigment are located on the basement membrane; skin color is determined by these cells. The epidermis has five sublayers, called strata. Each of these sublayers contains a few layers of cells each, so it is difficult to determine how many layers the skin actually contains.

Beneath the epidermis is the dermis, which is divided into two layers. The top layer, called the *papillary dermis*, contains papillae, or small, nipple-like formations of connective tissue or collagen. These push their way up against the basement membrane, giving it a wavy appearance. Beneath the papillary dermis is the bottom layer, called the *reticular dermis*, which contains hair follicles. Beneath that is the *subcutaneous tissue*, which is made up mostly of fat.

TYPES OF CANCER

Melanomas usually arise from *melanocytes*, the cells of the body that produce the pigment melanin. Although most occur on the skin, about 10 percent appear in the eye.

TUMOR GRADE

Tumor grade is not a major factor in melanoma. It is more precise to speak of tumor invasion. Growth patterns, either superficial spreading or nodular, are of greater importance, although these terms have been replaced by two precise systems of measurement, shown in Figure 9.1. Clark's levels measure the number of layers of the skin invaded by the malignant melanoma. But skin varies in thickness in different parts of the body. Compare, for instance, the skin on the eyelid to the skin of the back. Therefore, another system was developed by Alexander Breslow. It measures in millimeters the depth of penetration of the melanoma into the skin. Breslow's system gives a better indication of the patient's prognosis.

ROUTES OF SPREAD

Melanoma cells travel via both blood stream and the lymphatic system, the vessels that carry lymph in the same way that blood vessels carry blood. It can spread to the lymph nodes in the neck, armpits, and groin. While in the lymphatic system, melanoma cells can stop and develop metastases within the skin called *in-transit metastases*. These are very ominous, and usually suggest that the cancer has already spread elsewhere in the body. Melanoma usually spreads to the liver, lungs, or brain, but every organ in the body is a possible target.

SCREENING

The best screening is careful and deliberate inspection of the skin. The American Cancer Society recommends that individuals examine themselves every year using both full-length and handheld mirrors if by themselves, or to get someone else to check the skin on the back.

SIGNS AND SYMPTOMS

Any change in an existing mole or the appearance of a new one deserves attention. Changes such as darkening, increase in size, itching, scaling, or bleeding should be seen by a doctor. Moles can change in one small spot by losing pigment or developing a blue tint. Some melanomas produce no pigment. Doctors also look for elevations within a mole or an irregular margin. Fortunately, most moles that change are not melanomas.

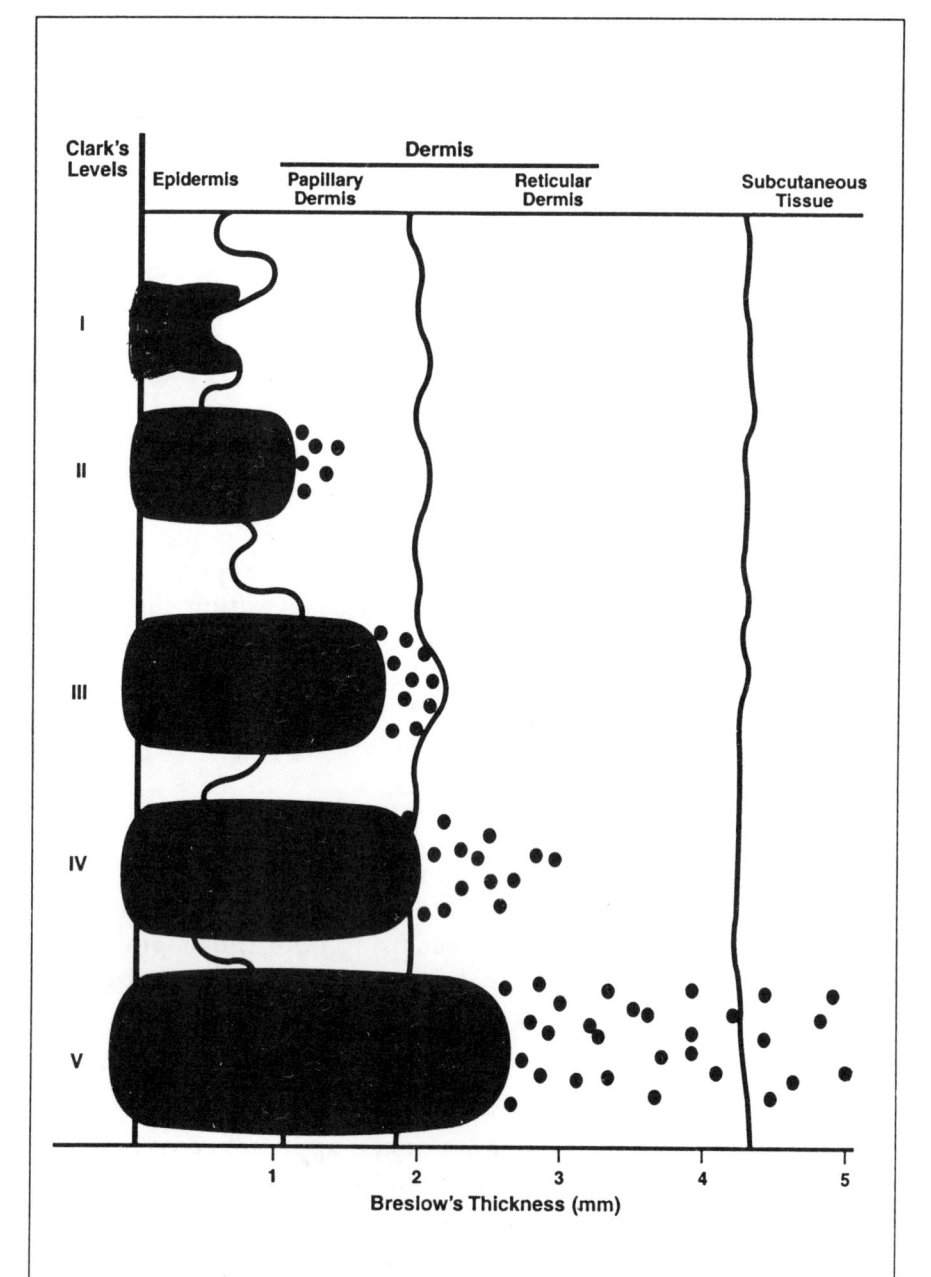

Figure 9.1 Measuring Melanomas, Clark's Levels and Breslow's Thickness

DIAGNOSIS

Melanomas can only be diagnosed with a *biopsy*. The lesions should be completely excised. Shave biopsies and cauterizations, or burning away of the lesion, should not be done. For patients who have no obvious evidence of tumor spread to regional lymph nodes or other organs, additional tests are not necessary. Liver scans, brain scans, CAT scans, and MRIs should not be routinely performed.

STAGES OF DISEASE

There have been several different staging systems for melanoma. The simplest includes only three stages: I, localized disease; II, positive regional lymph nodes; and III, distant metastases. Since most staging systems reserve stage IV for the presence of distant metastases, this system is seldom used. Recently, the American Joint Committee on Cancer (AJCC) recommended the staging system shown in Table 9.1.

TYPES OF TREATMENT

Treatment options include surgery, chemotherapy, biological therapy, and hyperthermia. Radiation therapy may help shrink large tumors and relieve pain in advanced cases, but it plays a very small role for most patients with this disease. See Chapter 5 for more information about these treatments, including general information on the side effects associated with each treatment.

Surgery

The treatment of a primary malignant melanoma has always been complete surgical removal. Skin grafts are seldom used. Removal of a wide margin of normal tissue around the tumor may leave a disfiguring scar. *Mohs micrographic surgery* removes just the cancer and a thin margin of normal tissue.

If the lymph nodes are enlarged with cancer cells, these nodes should be removed. If the nodes do not feel enlarged, a *sentinel node biopsy* can be performed to examine those nodes most likely to contain cancer. This determines the extent of tumor spread. For this reason surgeons believe that lymph nodes

Table 9.1. AJCC Staging System for Malignant Melanoma

Stage	Description	Five-Year Survival Rate
I	A cancer that is from 0 to 1.5 mm thick without spread to either the lymph nodes or to distant organs.	About 90%
II	A cancer that is thicker than 1.5 mm without spread to the lymph nodes or to distant organs.	About 70%
III	The lymph nodes contain cancer or there are in-transit metastases.	About 40%
IV	Distant metastases are present.	Less than 10%

nodes in the area of the melanoma should be removed even if they do not feel enlarged. Complications do occur frequently. They include breakdown of the wound, wound infection, death of the overlying skin, and swelling of the arm or leg. These complications are all worse when the groin lymph nodes are removed, because of the large area of the leg and the effects of gravity. Less extensive surgery can reduce complications.

Chemotherapy

Chemotherapy for melanoma is limited to those drugs used in hyperthermia treatment for stage III and to a single drug, DTIC, for stage IV. DTIC has a response rate of about 10 to 20 percent.

Biological Therapy

During the 1970s and 1980s, Bacillus Calmette-Guerin, which produces a general stimulation of the immune system, was scratched into the melanoma or surrounding skin. Results appeared promising at first, but ultimately there was no increase in survival.

Attempts have been made to treat patients with their own white blood cells. These cells have been concentrated from the patient's blood or removed from tumor specimens. The cells are cloned in a lab, stimulated to multiply many times, and infused back into the patient. Side effects include severe fever and chills, and a drop in blood pressure. The response rate for this treatment is about the same as for chemotherapy, which has not translated so far into increased survival rates for many patients. However, studies continue, and this might become a more effective form of treatment.

Hyperthermia

Isolated regional perfusion has prolonged life for some patients with advanced disease. Tubes are inserted into the artery and vein of the involved arm or leg. A tourniquet is applied and the extremity is placed on a heart-lung by-pass perfusion machine. This isolates the arm or leg from the rest of the body's circulation. The extremity is perfused with heated blood that contains a high concentration of a drug. Heat enhances the effectiveness of this treatment and helps to prolong survival. Possible side effects include a temporary burn, like a sunburn, and swelling, usually temporary, of the affected limb. There could also be bleeding and vein inflammation, which may lead to the development of blood clots. Complications severe enough to result in loss of the limb occur rarely.

ANALYSIS

In this section, I will discuss the primary lesion where the cancer first arose and then the lymph nodes. See Appendix I for further discussion on both of these topics.

The Primary Lesion

Most surgeons agree that lesions of less than 0.75 mm may be excised with a 1-cm margin, but use a wider margin (2 to 3 cm) for thicker lesions. Some studies have demonstrated that patients treated with a narrow margin of excision (less than 2 cm) have a 12 to 13 percent chance of developing local recurrence. This compares with a 3 percent chance of local recurrence following a 3-cm excision. Local recurrence may increase to 20 percent among patients with lesions 4 mm or thicker excised with margins of 1 cm or less.[2] Nevertheless, investigators from both Australia and the Netherlands found no increase in local recurrence following excisions of less than 1 cm.[3,4]

Fortunately, none of these studies suggests that an increase in local recurrence causes a decrease in survival. I have found no published paper which demonstrates that narrow margins of excision reduce survival. There has also never been a study demonstrating that wide margins improve survival. If aggressive surgery would impair bodily function or leave a disfiguring scar, you may want to consider having a narrow margin of excision. This margin should be checked by a pathologist to be sure that it is free of tumor cells.

The Regional Lymph Nodes

The purpose of elective lymph node dissection (ELND), or lymph node removal, is to remove the tumor cells before they spread to distant organs. Patients with lesions of less than 1 mm are not usually treated with ELND because the chances of tumor spread are low. Patients with lesions thicker than 4 mm are also not treated with ELND because the chances are great that the disease has already spread to distant organs. It is too late for this precautionary procedure to be of help.

Today, the uncertainty centers upon patients with lesions from 1 to 4 mm in thickness. Two scientifically controlled studies have failed to find a benefit for ELND in this group of patients, although the studies may have been too small to show a benefit that was slight.[5,6] A 1994 retrospective study from Duke University also failed to find a survival benefit for ELND.[7]

Many surgeons have reported that patients with this disease live longer if their lymph nodes are removed when the melanoma is removed. Their retrospective studies have exaggerated this benefit, though, because some patients treated with a delayed lymph node removal developed large recurrences in the nodes. They died because the volume of recurrent disease in the nodes was so large. Many of them could have been cured if they had returned to their doctors earlier, when their lymph nodes first began to enlarge. The problem was not failure to remove the lymph nodes at the first operation. The problem was failure to remove them before they enlarged to the point of pouring many melanoma cells into the blood stream. This was the cause of tumor spread.

Malignant melanoma is a highly aggressive malignancy that can spread from a small primary tumor or regional lymph node. I believe that wide excision alone should be limited to patients who can be seen by a doctor every two to three months, and who can perform regular, effective self-examinations. Doctors must be prepared to contact those patients who miss their follow-up visits. Doctors and patients alike must be willing to accept the potential threat to survival posed by disease in the lymph nodes. If this strict follow-up regimen cannot be followed, the patient should seriously consider having an ELND.

TREATMENT ACCORDING TO STAGE

The following treatment options are recommended. Keep in mind that conservative surgery is best suited to the treatment of early cancer. Even so, I would still encourage you to ask your doctor about the most conservative options available to you in your specific case.

Stage I

This stage involves a primary melanoma that is 0 to 1.5 mm thick, with regional lymph nodes that do not feel enlarged. Authorities agree that melanomas less than 0.75 mm thick can be safely removed with a 1-cm margin on each side of the melanoma. I believe that thicker lesions may also be prudently removed with a margin of 1 cm. Some areas of the body have cosmetic or functional significance, such as the face, fingers, toes, genitals, anus, and so forth. In these cases, a narrow excision with a margin free of microscopic cancer may be appropriate.

Routine ELNDs are not required because lymph node spread is very unusual. Patients who elect not to have an ELND must learn careful self-examination and be followed by their physicians every two to three months. They must understand that they may be living with a time bomb.

Stage II

At this stage, the melanoma is thicker than 1.5 mm, and the regional lymph nodes do not feel enlarged. Local recurrence rates are likely to increase among patients with thick tumors that are removed with narrow margins. The width of excision is usually a cosmetic decision, which you will have to balance against the recurrence risk. There is no reliable evidence that narrow margins of excision adversely affect survival. A 2-cm margin is becoming accepted practice. I believe that a narrower margin free of tumor cells may be appropriate in cosmetically or functionally sensitive areas.

The role of ELND is discussed in the Analysis section.

Stage III

At stage III, enlarged lymph nodes can be felt or in-transit metastases are present. The primary lesion should be excised as suggested for stages I and II. The regional lymph nodes should be removed. An isolated in-transit metastasis can be removed. Patients with multiple in-transit metastases or local recurrences should have chemotherapy given via regional perfusion.

Stage IV

At this stage, the disease has spread to distant organs. Only one drug, DTIC, has been approved for use in treating melanoma. Various forms of biological therapy are also available, but their use is largely experimental.

FOLLOW-UP

Regular and meticulous follow-up is the most important part of conservative treatment for malignant melanoma. This is especially true for those who have not had an ELND. Patients should be carefully instructed in self-examination, both in the area of the primary melanoma and of the regional lymph nodes. Patients should be followed every two to three months for the first two years, and then every four to six months for the next three years. Blood chemistries and a chest X-ray should be done annually. Scans should be done for patients who develop symptoms. Patients who do not return regularly should be advised to have an ELND. The amount of follow-up required varies with the situation. There can be a longer interval between visits if the risks of recurrence are low, and a shorter interval if the risks of recurrence are high.

10.

Cancer of the Penis

Cancer of the penis is very rare, occurring in only one or two men out of every 100,000 in the United States. It is found more frequently in less developed countries, where circumcision and good hygiene are less common. It occurs late in life, and almost exclusively in uncircumcised males.

This chapter will cover the following topics: the anatomy of the penis, the types of cancer that affect the penis, how this cancer is graded, how this cancer spreads, what screening procedures are available, what the signs and symptoms are, how this cancer is diagnosed, how this cancer is staged, what treatments are available, my analysis of how conservative surgery can be used to treat this cancer, my recommendations for the appropriate treatment at each stage, and what sort of follow-up is needed after treatment.

ANATOMY AND PHYSIOLOGY

The penis is made up of three columns of spongy tissue, two on each side and one below. During erection, this tissue fills with blood. The urethra passes through the bottom column, which expands toward the end of the penis to form the glans. The skin of the penis consists of *squamous cells*.

TYPES OF CANCER

Almost all cancers of the penis involve the skin itself and are therefore squamous cell cancers. The penis can also be the site of malignant melanoma (see Chapter 9) or, rarely, sarcomas of the underlying tissue (see Chapter 13).

TUMOR GRADE

Penile cancer can be low, intermediate, or high grade. Most penile cancers are of low grade. Prognosis does not correlate well with grade, as it does with other tumors. However, *DNA ploidy* may correlate with survival. DNA ploidy refers to the number of chromosomes within the cancer cells. Those with a normal number (twenty-three pairs) are less aggressive than those with an abnormal number.

ROUTES OF SPREAD

Penile cancer becomes invasive when it penetrates the basement membrane beneath the squamous cells on the surface. It spreads first to the groin lymph nodes. It can later spread to the lymph nodes inside the pelvis. About 20 percent of patients with lymph nodes that are not enlarged will have microscopic cancer in the nodes. This percentage increases as the tumor size increases. The groin nodes are enlarged in 25 to 50 percent of patients. This depends mainly on the size of the primary tumor. About half of these nodes contain cancer and about half are only inflamed. Distant sites of spread include the lungs, bones, brain, and other organs.

SCREENING

There are no blood tests or other screening procedures for cancer of the penis. Men should be able to retract the foreskin and should examine themselves monthly.

SIGNS AND SYMPTOMS

Penile cancer usually appears as a painless ulcer on the glans or foreskin. It may become infected.

DIAGNOSIS

Diagnosis is made by a *biopsy*.

STAGES OF DISEASE

In 1966, S. M. Jackson proposed a staging system that runs from stage A to stage D. Doctors are increasingly using Roman numerals to stage cancer, so both letters and Roman numerals are included in Table 10.1. It is the most commonly used system in the United States. There is also a system based on the TNM system, which is discussed in Chapter 5. This is used less often.

TYPES OF TREATMENT

Treatment options include surgery, radiation therapy, and chemotherapy. See Chapter 5 for more information about these treatments, including general information on the side effects associated with each treatment.

Surgery

Total or partial removal of the penis, or *penectomy*, is the standard surgical procedure for cancers of the penis that have gone beyond stage 0. Urologists who perform local excision usually recommend a 1.5- to 2-cm margin of normal tissue. Laser excision has also been used.[1]

Mohs micrographic surgery is a very limited excision of the tumor. The patient is given a local anesthetic and the visible tumor is removed. Additional small fragments are removed and sent to the pathologist for microscopic examination. This is continued until all fragments are free of cancer.

If the lymph nodes are enlarged and contain cancer, they are removed in an operation called a *therapeutic lymph node dissection*. If the lymph nodes are not enlarged, their removal is a precautionary operation. It is then called an *elective lymph node dissection* (ELND). Complications occur frequently. They include breakdown of the wound, wound infection, death of the overlying skin, and swelling of the leg. These complications can be reduced with less extensive surgery.[2]

Radiation Therapy

Squamous cell cancer responds poorly to radiation therapy. Therefore, high doses (such as 60 Gy) must be used. An *external*

Table 10.1. Jackson Staging System for Penile Cancer

Stage	Description	Five-Year Survival Rate
0	Cancer is limited to the topmost cell layer.	Over 95%
I or A	A cancer that is confined to the glans, the foreskin, or both.	Over 95%
II or B	A cancer that involves the shaft of the penis.	85%
III or C	There are groin lymph nodes that contain cancer and can be operated on.	About 60%
IV or D	A cancer that involves adjacent structures, or the lymph nodes are inoperable, or there are distant metastases.	5%

beam or iridium-192 needles can be used. The needles are commonly placed through the penis in a procedure called *interstitial radiation*. Damage to the urethra may occur, with complications such as narrowing or formation of a *fistula*, an abnormal hole through which fluid can pass. Chronic pain or swelling can also occur. Radiation is reserved for patients with small lesions that have not spread too far below the surface. Surgery is usually required for patients who fail radiation therapy. Groin lymph nodes can be treated with external-beam radiation.

Chemotherapy

Efudex, a 5 percent 5-fluorouracil cream, can be used to treat small tumors. It must be applied twice a day for three to five weeks. There is little experience with system-wide chemotherapy for penile cancer in this country.

ANALYSIS

In this section, I will discuss the primary lesion, which is the site where the cancer first arose, and then the lymph nodes. See Appendix I for further discussion on both of these topics.

The Primary Lesion

Currently, there are differing opinions on how much healthy

tissue should be removed along with the tumor. Many urologists recommend a 2-cm margin around most tumors that have spread below the surface. Mohs micrographic surgery and other limited surgical procedures have had good results with narrower margins. As with other solid tumors, a narrow margin of excision may increase local recurrence, but there is no evidence that it decreases survival. Local recurrence can be reduced if the margins are free of tumor cells. Patients who develop local recurrence seem to have a second chance to be cured if the recurrence is promptly treated.

The Regional Lymph Nodes

The removal of lymph nodes that are not enlarged has been a topic of discussion among doctors. Some urologists support ELND.[3-5] In these studies, many patients treated without ELND returned with advanced disease in their lymph nodes. If these patients had been closely followed, their lymph nodes may have been removed before they became the cause of tumor spread. ELND in this disease is further complicated by the midline location of the penis, since cancer can spread to either the left or the right side.

The issues involved have been more thoroughly studied among patients with breast cancer and melanoma because they are more common cancers. For patients with breast cancer, the most thoroughly studied cancer, the findings are clear. ELND does not increase survival. Available data suggests that the same conclusion may be reached for cancer of the penis. At this time, it may be prudent to remove the lymph node that generally becomes involved with cancer first, called the sentinel node, on the side of the lesion and perform a complete groin lymph node removal if the sentinel node contains cancer. Lymph nodes in the pelvis only become positive for cancer after the lymph nodes in the groin are already involved.

TREATMENT ACCORDING TO STAGE

The following treatment options are recommended. Keep in mind that conservative surgery is best suited to the treatment of early cancer. Even so, I would still encourage you to ask your doctor about the most conservative options available to you in your specific case. "Standard treatment" refers to the treatment recommended as accepted medical practice.

Stage 0

At this stage, only the surface cells are involved. Patients with stage 0 lesions can be treated with 5-fluorouracil cream (Efudex), which must be applied twice a day for three to five weeks. These lesions may also be removed surgically or treated with a laser.

Stage I

At this stage, the cancer is limited to the glans and/or the foreskin. Standard treatment has been partial penectomy or radiation therapy. However, I believe that these lesions can be successfully treated with conservative surgery, such as Mohs micrographic surgery or local excision with a very narrow margin that contains no cancer cells. Margins of less than 1 cm may increase the rate of local recurrence. I believe that patients should be carefully instructed in how to examine groin lymph nodes. They should examine themselves monthly and be examined by their physician every three months. Routine ELNDs may not be necessary.

Stage II

At stage II, the tumor involves the shaft of the penis. Treatment is the same as for stage I.

Stage III

At this stage, there are operable lymph nodes in the groin. The primary tumor should be treated as described for stage I, since the presence of lymph node disease does not mean that the primary lesion needs more aggressive treatment. The patient should be treated with antibiotics and the lymph nodes examined every one to two weeks. If the swelling is due to infection, antibiotics should cause the lymph nodes to decrease in size. If they do not decrease in size, the swelling is probably caused by cancer and the lymph nodes should be removed. The traditional recommendation of waiting four to six weeks prior to evaluation may need to be shortened, since lymph nodes that contain cancer may themselves become the source of distant disease during this waiting period.

Stage IV

At this stage, other local structures either are affected by cancer, or the lymph nodes are inoperable, or the cancer has spread to distant organs. The only treatment possible is for the relief of symptoms.

FOLLOW-UP

Regular and meticulous follow-up is the most important part of conservative treatment for penile cancer. This is especially true for those who have not had an ELND. Patients should be carefully instructed in self-examination, of both the area of the primary lesion and of the groin lymph nodes. Patients should be followed every two to three months for the first two years, and then every four to six months for the next three years. Scans should be done for patients who develop symptoms. Patients who do not return regularly should be advised to have an ELND. The amount of follow-up required varies with the situation. You and your doctor will come up with a follow-up plan that is best for you.

11.

Prostate Cancer

Prostate cancer is the most common malignancy among American men and the second leading cause of cancer death among men behind lung cancer. (The incidence is nearly twice as high for African-American men, and the death rate is nearly triple. The reasons for this discrepancy are unknown.) Over 240,000 Americans are diagnosed with prostate cancer each year and over 40,000 die of the disease. Cancer deaths are few compared to the many cases because most prostate cancers grow slowly. Also, most men with prostate cancer are over sixty years of age, and they are more likely to die of other causes even if their cancer is untreated. The number of cases diagnosed is increasing due to the widespread use of the prostate-specific antigen (PSA) blood test. The real age-adjusted incidence of prostate cancer may also be increasing.

A recent autopsy study found evidence of microscopic prostate cancer in about one third of men aged twenty to fifty. A fifty-year-old man has about a 40 percent chance of developing microscopic prostate cancer during his lifetime. He has about a 10 percent chance of being diagnosed with the disease.[1] By the age of eighty, he has a 60 to 70 percent chance of having microscopic cancer cells in his prostate gland. But only about one man out of eleven, or 9 percent, will have clinically apparent prostate cancer sometime during his life, and only 3 percent of men will die of prostate cancer. Thus, there is a large gap between the number of patients with clinically diagnosed cancer and those with undetected microscopic disease. There is no other cancer with such a wide gap.

This chapter will cover the following topics: the anatomy of the prostate, the types of cancer that affect the prostate, how this cancer is graded, how this cancer spreads, what screening procedures are available, what the signs and symptoms are, how this cancer is diagnosed, how this cancer is staged, what treatments are available, my analysis of how conservative surgery can be used to treat this cancer, my recommendations for the appropriate treatment at each stage, and what sort of follow-up is needed after treatment.

ANATOMY AND PHYSIOLOGY

The prostate gland is about the size of a walnut. Divided into two lobes, it is located below the bladder and in front of the rectum. It surrounds the urethra, which carries urine from the bladder through the penis. The prostate gland produces a component of semen that contains proteins and other substances to help improve the chances of fertilization.

TYPES OF CANCER

Ninety-five percent of all prostate cancers arise from the glands that produce a component of the seminal fluid, and are called *adenocarcinomas*. Most of these cancers begin near the outside of the gland, where they may be more easily felt on rectal examination. On rare occasion, cancers arise within the ducts or connective tissue of the gland.

Doctors have tried to explain the wide gap between the large number of patients with microscopic cancer and the small number with clinically significant disease. About forty years ago, it was suggested that some prostate cancers are latent. They appear similar to more lethal cancers, but are predestined never to grow or spread. More recently, it has been suggested that so-called latent cancers are simply the smallest cancers. Researchers at Stanford University believe that cancers behave according to their size. Cancers smaller than 0.5 cc in volume (the volume of ten drops of water) do not spread, and they require years to grow.[2] About 80 percent of all prostate cancers are less than 0.5 cc in volume.

Which theory is correct? The Stanford approach is the more logical. No other cancer has been described as latent—that is, looking malignant under a microscope, but acting benignly. On the contrary, all cancers become more likely to spread as they increase in size.

TUMOR GRADE

Prostate cancer may be graded from grade 1, good prognosis, to grade 5, poor prognosis. Within one tumor there may be cells of several different grades. The *Gleason scoring system* attempts to arrive at an average score for each tumor. Pathologists simply add the two most common grades of cancer found. Gleason scores range from 2 (1+1) to 10 (5+5).

Prostate cancer can also be graded by whether it is well, moderately, or poorly differentiated. These two grading systems may be compared as follows: well differentiated, Gleason grades 2 through 4; moderately differentiated, Gleason grades 5 through 7; and poorly differentiated, Gleason grades 8 through 10.

Prostate cancer can also be assessed according to *DNA ploidy*, or the number of chromosomes within the cell. Several preliminary studies suggest that there is a strong connection between ploidy and prognosis. Diploid cells, or those with the normal twenty-three pairs of chromosomes, indicate good prognosis, while aneuploid cells, or those with an abnormal number, indicate poor prognosis.

ROUTES OF SPREAD

If a prostate cancer remains below the volume of 4 cc, or about one teaspoon, it is unlikely to spread. Some prostate cancers grow very slowly, usually requiring more than four years to double in size.[3] (In comparison, the average breast cancer doubles in size every three months.) It would require about twelve years for a 0.5-cc cancer to reach the size of 4 cc. At this size, only about 7 percent of patients will have metastases—spread to distant organs.[4]

Locally advanced disease causes the prostate to enlarge and to squeeze the urethra, which can block the flow of urine. It can penetrate through the capsule that surrounds the gland and invade the bladder or rectum. It can also spread to the nearby lymph nodes in the pelvis. Distant spread usually appears in the bones of the spine, hips, or extremities, but it can spread to almost any organ.

SCREENING

Digital rectal examination (DRE), in which the doctor feels the prostate through the rectum, has been the most common screening method. But early disease is best detected by a blood test that measures the level of prostate-specific antigen (PSA). Screening includes an annual DRE and an annual PSA determination. Patients with an abnormal PSA test may be further evaluated with transrectal ultrasound (TRUS). Ultrasound is a painless procedure in which high-frequency sound waves are passed through the body, creating pictures of the organs they bounce off of. TRUS has detected cancers as small as 0.5 cm. But it is very imprecise and misses about as many cancers as it finds.

Areas that are suspicious on either physical examination or ultrasound should be biopsied. The ultrasound can precisely guide the biopsy needle to tumors that it can find. Modern biopsy techniques have made this procedure nearly painless.

PSA Level: What is Normal?

PSA is produced by all the cells of the prostate gland, both normal and malignant. Malignant cells leak into the blood stream about ten times as much PSA as benign cells. If this blood level is elevated—greater than 4.0 nanogram (ng) per milliliter (ml) of blood—cancer may be present. If it is above 10 ng/ml without another cause, such as benign prostate disease, cancer is likely. About 75 percent of all men with prostate cancer have elevated PSA levels. Note that not all prostate cancers produce elevated PSA levels. Some cancers are too small to leak much PSA into the blood stream, while others do not produce that much PSA.

Since the prostate gland enlarges with age, PSA levels also increase with age. T. A. Stamey at Stanford University in California suggests that 95 percent of all men without cancer should fall within the following upper limits on their PSA levels:

- Forty to forty-nine years, 2.5 ng/ml.
- Fifty to fifty-nine years, 3.5 ng/ml.
- Sixty to sixty-nine years, 5.0 ng/ml.
- Seventy to seventy-nine years, 6.5 ng/ml.

Keeping these values in mind can help to eliminate unnecessary biopsies in some men over sixty. They also may help detect cancer in some men under sixty. Some urologists would rather measure PSA density—how much PSA is in each gram of prostate tissue. PSA density becomes smaller as the prostate gland enlarges. This accomplishes much the same thing as Stamey's age-adjusted rates by accounting for the effect of normal prostate growth. However, many urologists believe that a serum PSA level of 4.0 ng/ml should be used as a general guideline for biopsy in all age groups.[5] See Appendix I for additional information on PSA levels and screening.

Screening Recommendations

Both the American Cancer Society and the American Urological Association recommend screening for those men without symptoms over age forty who are African-American or who have a family history of prostate cancer, as well as for those who wish to be screened. Screening should also be considered for all men over fifty, as determined by either the doctor or the patient himself.

However, not all doctors agree on this subject. The United States Preventive Services Task Force, the International Union Against Cancer, and many European organizations have not endorsed routine screening. If all men followed the recommendations given above, the cost of screening would be high, the complications of treatment would be significant, and the benefits of early treatment remain uncertain. Prostate cancer screening has not been shown to increase the survival of patients.

Does early detection prolong life? This question can only be answered by studying large groups of men, comparing those screened to those not screened. Studies thus far have found no survival benefit from PSA screening, for either the general population or for those in special-risk groups. More accurate studies involving larger numbers of patients are underway. One study concluded that regular testing doubles the number of patients who are found to have cancer confined to the prostate gland, as opposed to finding a cancer that has already spread.[6] For this reason, men with risk factors, such as African-Americans or those with a family history of prostate cancer, should be screened. Men without risk factors will have to decide if the small benefit of regular testing is worth the time and expense.

SIGNS AND SYMPTOMS

Early prostate cancers usually have no symptoms. The first symptoms are frequent or painful urination, blood in the urine, or a decrease in the force of the urinary stream. The appearance of symptoms is usually a sign that the cancer is advanced, at least locally.

DIAGNOSIS

A tissue sample can be obtained with a *needle biopsy* through the rectum or through the area between the scrotum and the anus, called the perineum. Cancer is occasionally diagnosed while the patient is being operated on for benign prostate enlargement in an operation called a transurethral resection of the prostate (TURP).

STAGES OF DISEASE

The American Urological Association (AUA) system is most commonly used and divides prostate cancer into four stages, A through D. Unfortunately, cancers detected by ultrasound or from an elevated PSA do not have a logical place in this system. In 1992, the American Joint Commission on Cancer and the International Union Against Cancer (AJCC-UICC) devised a staging system based upon the TNM method that is explained in Chapter 5. Table 11.1 shows the AUA system and Table 11.2 shows an abbreviated version of the AJCC-UICC system.[7] In Table 11.1, approximate equivalents from the AJCC-UICC system are given in parentheses, while Table 11.2 gives AUA system equivalents. Reported five-year survival rates vary widely. Those shown in Table 11.1 are approximations.

Table 11.1. AUA Staging System for Prostate Cancer

Stage	Description	Five-Year Survival Rate
A	A cancer that cannot be felt during a DRE. It has been found via TRUS or in the tissue removed from a TURP.	
A₁	A cancer that occupies less than 5% of the tissue removed by a TURP and is of low or medium grade. Some urologists use a slightly different definition (T1$_a$, N0, M0).	Over 90%
A₂	A cancer that occupies more than 5% of the tissue removed by a TURP, or is of high grade, or additional cancer that was found after a repeat TURP (T1$_b$, N0, M0).	Over 80%
B	A cancer that can be felt during a DRE.	
B₀	A cancer that is identified by needle biopsy due to an elevated PSA level (T1$_c$).	Over 95%
B₁	A cancer that is confined to one lobe of the prostate gland, and is less than 1.5 cm in diameter (T2$_{a-b}$, N0, M0).	About 90% to 95%
B₂	A cancer that is confined to the prostate, but involves more than one lobe, or is more than 1.5 cm in diameter (T2$_c$, N0, M0).	About 85%
C	A cancer that has extended beyond the capsule that surrounds the gland (T3, N0, M0).	About 65%
D₁	A cancer that has spread to the lymph nodes (any T, N$_{1-3}$, M0).	About 40%
D₂	Distant metastases are present (any T, any N, M$_1$).	About 20%

TYPES OF TREATMENT

Surgery

Radical Prostatectomy

Radical prostatectomy is the removal of the entire prostate gland, the seminal vesicles (nearby structures which secrete and store a component of semen), and the pelvic lymph nodes. The most common side effects are incontinence induced by laughing and

Table 11.2. TNM Staging System for Prostate Cancer

Tumor Size [T]	Nodal Metastases [N]	Distant Metastases [M]
T1—Cancer cannot be felt during DRE and cannot be seen on TRUS (A)	N0—No cancer in the lymph nodes	M0—No distant metastases are present
T1$_a$—Tumor occupies less than 5% of tissue removed by TURP (A$_1$)	N1—Cancer is in a single lymph node 2 cm or smaller (D$_1$)	M1—Distant metastases are present (D$_2$)
T1$_b$—Tumor occupies more than 5% of tissue removed by TURP (A$_2$)	N2—Cancer in one or more lymph nodes 2 cm or larger with none larger than 5 cm in greatest diameter (D$_1$)	
T1$_c$—Tumor is identified by needle biopsy, generally because of elevated PSA (B$_0$)	N3—Cancer is in a lymph node greater than 5 cm in greatest diameter (D$_1$)	
T2—Tumor can be felt during DRE or seen on TRUS and is confined to prostate (B)		
T2$_a$—Tumor involves half a lobe or less (B$_1$)		
T2$_b$—Tumor involves more than half a lobe, but not both lobes (B$_1$)		
T2$_c$—Tumor involves both lobes (B$_2$)		
T3—Tumor has extended beyond capsule that surrounds gland (C)		
T4—Tumor is fixed to or invades adjacent structures (C or D)		

coughing (25 percent), complete incontinence (5 percent). Perhaps the most disturbing complication is impotence, which occurs in over 50 percent of patients. Most men who choose less aggressive treatment are trying to avoid this complication. The sensation of orgasm is preserved.

Less common complications include narrowing of the urethra (ranging from less than 1 percent up to 25 percent), blood clots (1 percent to 12 percent), wound infection (less than 1 percent to 16 percent), swelling of the legs (1 percent to 5 percent), and death (much less than 1 percent to 2 percent).[8] These numbers vary greatly, because they were taken from a number of studies.

Since the early 1980's some urologists have attempted to preserve the nerves that control erection. This has decreased impotence to about 30 percent. One study of this procedure concluded that it controlled cancer as well or better than more radical operations.[9]

Radical prostatectomy may also be used to treat patients who develop local recurrence after radiation therapy or other treatment. Unfortunately, in these cases complications increase. The number of prostatectomies increased six-fold from 1984 to 1990.

Transurethral resection of the prostate

The *transurethral resection of the prostate* (TURP) is most often used to treat benign enlargement of the prostate or benign prostatic hypertrophy (BPH). The urologist places a tube up the urethra and removes small pieces of the prostate by cutting or burning the tissue. Enough of the gland is removed to relieve the obstruction caused by the enlarged gland. Cancer has been found in 6 to 10 percent of these procedures. With the greater use of PSA testing, cancer is found less often, in 2 to 5 percent of cases. If cancer is found, some urologists will perform a repeat TURP looking for additional cancer. If more is found, additional treatment is often recommended.

TURP is also acceptable treatment for patients with an obstructed urethra due to Stage C or D cancer. TURP is not generally used to treat early prostate cancer, because it seldom removes all the tumor. However, a few urologists believe the prostate cancer can be treated with repeated aggressive transurethral resections.[10]

The complications of these operations are minimal. Most patients retain their potency, because the prostatic capsule is not removed. The rate of true, complete urinary incontinence is no more than 1 percent. Narrowing of the urethra with scar tissue or prostate regrowth is rare.

Lymph Node Sampling

In some patients, it is valuable to find out if cancer has spread to the pelvic lymph nodes prior to surgery. There is about a 10 percent chance of lymph node spread from tumors of about 5 cc in volume. This increases to about 50 percent among tumors measuring 13 cc. Most urologists agree that patients with tumors which are both low-grade and low-stage do not need lymph node sampling.

Lymph nodes can be removed through a major operation, in which the abdominal cavity is opened up, or with laparoscopic surgery. Laparoscopic lymph node sampling involves placing small tubes into the abdomen, through which the surgeon can manipulate tiny instruments to remove tissue. If the lymph nodes are positive, most urologists believe that radical surgery is not curative. Thus, urologists may perform laparoscopic lymph node sampling prior to a planned radical prostatectomy in order to avoid an unnecessary operation..

Radiation Therapy

External Beam Radiation

External beam radiation, sometimes called cobalt treatment, is more often used to treat older patients for whom surgery would be risky.[11] It is also suitable for those with advanced or incurable disease. Here, the goal is to kill as much of the tumor as possible and slow its progress. It requires about seven weeks of daily treatment, Monday through Friday, for a total of about 70 Gy.

Radiation therapy often does not eradicate the cancer. Thomas Stamey and colleagues from Stanford recently reported that radiation cures only 20 percent of patients.[12] Five years after treatment they found rapidly increasing PSA levels (indicating probable cancer) in 80 percent of patients.

Radiation therapy is also used to treat symptomatic metastases to either bones or soft tissue. About 80 percent of patients respond to this treatment, but about half of those who do respond will relapse.

Radiation therapy can cause fatigue during the period of treatment, bowel injury (10 percent) causing rectal pain or diarrhea, bladder irritation causing urinary frequency (15 percent), incontinence (4 percent) and impotence (40 percent to 60 percent).

Brachytherapy or Interstitial Radiation

Radiation can also be administered with radioactive seeds, which are inserted into the gland, using a small surgical procedure. The radiation is effective for only a short distance (about 5 millimeters) from the seeds. But, the seeds are only a short distant from the tumor cells. ("Brachy" is the Greek word for short.) This procedure is done on an outpatient basis. Most men are able to return to normal activity is less than 48 hours. Thus far, brachytherapy is producing results which are equivalent to those of surgery or external beam radiation for patients with low or intermediate grade lesions. Patients with a Gleason's score > 8 and those with T2b or T2c lesions are more likely to experience a rise in PSA , than patients treated with surgery or external beam radiation. Brachytherapy causes less radiation damage to the surrounding tissue and, thus, fewer complications than surgery or external beam radiation.

Chemotherapy

Current chemotherapeutic drugs are weakly effective against prostate cancer and are usually administered after hormonal therapy has failed. They achieve a subjective response in about 15 percent to 30 percent of patients. Patients feel better; they experience less pain, but they do not live longer. Vinblastine (Velban), estramustine (emcyt), docetaxel (Taxotere), and mitoxantrone (Novantrone) are among the drugs used.

Hormonal Therapy

The growth of prostate cancer is enhanced by male hormones called androgens. Testosterone, produced by the testicles, is the most prominent type of androgen. It represents about 95 percent of all prostate-stimulating androgens. Other androgens are produced by the adrenal glands located above the kidneys. Treatment is intended to eliminate the stimulatory effect of testosterone on prostate cancer cells. There are several ways to do this.

Removal of the testicles (orchiectomy) is the surest way to reduce testosterone. But, this has obvious disadvantages and other androgens remain active. Female estrogens, such as diethylstilbestrol, are also effective antiandrogens, but they can cause breast enlargement, blood clots, fluid retention and other complications that effect the cardiovascular system.

There are three additional types of drugs which can effectively treat prostate cancer. (These drugs are further explained in Chapter 5.) The first is a new class of drugs which cause the pituitary gland in the brain to shut off its stimulating hormonal signal to the testicles. This causes the testicles to stop making testosterone. These drugs are called releasing factor agonists. They include leuprolide (Lupron) and goserelin acetate (Zoladex). This treatment can cause hot flashes, loss of muscle and bone mass, anemia, mental changes, and men can temporarily lose their sex drive. These drugs are also expensive.

A second class of drugs work within the prostate cancer cell, blocking the effect of testosterone and other androgens. They are called antiandrogens. These drugs include flutamide (Eulexin) and bicalutamide (Casodex). The side effects include gynecomastia and hot flashes. Since impotence is uncommon, treatment with these drugs is called a nerve-sparing hormonal blockade.

The third class of drugs inhibits the conversion of testosterone to dihydrotestosterone (DHT). DHT is actually a greater stimulant to prostate cancer cells than testosterone itself. Finasteride (Proscar) is the principle drug in this class. This drug is probably the least effective against prostate cancer, but it causes the least sexual dysfunction. Men treated with Proscar are likely to preserve their potency and sex drive.

Complete Hormonal Blockade

Until recently hormonal therapy was used primarily in the treatment of advanced disease. But, in the early 1990's a few physicians began using hormonal therapy to treat patients with early prostate cancer. One form of treatment used three different drugs - one from each of the three classes mentioned above. This form of therapy has gone by several names, including complete hormonal blockade, total androgen ablation, and triple hormonal blockade. It effectively reduces the PSA level to less than 0.1 ng./ml in most patients. Patients are often treated for about a year, and then the drugs are discontinued. Normal sexual function and desire returns to most men within a few months. Some patients choose to remain on Proscar, the drug with the fewest side effects. Because of the success of this treatment, some physicians are now treating patients with only two classes of drugs. PSA levels should be carefully monitored.

There have been no scientific studies of complete hormonal blockade. But the therapy has been successfully used on hundreds of patients in Canada, California, and Europe. Scientific studies have demonstrated that hormonal blockade does prolong life in men previously treated with radical prostatectomy or radiation therapy. The treatment is thought to kill prostate cancer cells both locally and throughout the body. The evidence so far suggests that hormonal blockade is effective treatment for men with early prostate cancer.

Hormonal therapy also reduces the production of PSA by cancer cells. Thus, a very low PSA level does not guarantee the eradication of the tumor. Since reliable statistics are not yet available, you may wish to discuss this with your doctor and/or with a physician who has had experience treating patients with complete hormonal blockade.

Hormonal Therapy for Advanced Disease

When used for patients with advanced disease, there is no convincing evidence that hormonal therapy can prolong survival. Most patients (about 85 percent) respond to treatment. Responses can be subjective (the patient feels better) and/or objective (the tumor gets smaller). Hormonal therapy can decrease the rate of tumor growth, reduce pain, and increase the quality of life. These effects may persist for a period of months to years. If one form of hormonal treatment stops working, another may be tried. But each new hormone treatment is less likely to be effective. Patients whose cancer remains in the region of the prostate are much more likely to respond to hormone manipulation (84 percent) than those who develop distant disease (20 percent).[13]

Experimental Local Treatment

Microwave Thermal Therapy

A microwave heat applicator inserted into the rectum while the patient is under anesthesia. This heats the prostate gland to about 110 degrees, causing tissue destruction. This has been used primarily to treat patients with advanced disease, and can lead to a noticeable reduction of symptoms.[14]

Cryosurgery

Freezing can also destroy both malignant and benign tissue. Probes have been used to selectively freeze certain parts of the prostate gland.[15] Under anesthesia 6 to 8 probes are inserted into the prostate gland through the skin between the scrotum and the rectum. A cold liquified gas is introduced into these tubes and is used to freeze the prostate gland. TRUS and temperature probes carefully monitor the growing "iceball" in the prostate. The procedure requires about two hours of anesthesia and sometimes one day of hospitalization.

The freezing technique varies widely among urologists.[16] Some freeze the entire gland including the surrounding nerves which control erectile function. This causes impotence in nearly all patients. Some urologists, like Dr. Israel Barken in San Diego, try to avoid freezing the nearby nerves. Potency is preserved in about 70 percent of these patients. If the cancer recurs, cryosurgery can be used to treat the recurrence. The U.S. government agency which administers Medicare has determined that cryosurgery is as effective as radiation therapy - both external beam and seed implantation.

Watchful waiting

When a patient's cancer is monitored without treatment, the process is called *watchful waiting*. This approach has been used primarily with older patients with early disease and in those who refuse radical surgery and radiation therapy. Those who support watchful waiting point out that local tumor growth almost always precedes the development of distant metastases.[17]

ANALYSIS

Of the malignancies covered in this book, the behavior of prostate cancer is probably the most difficult to understand. Very few randomized trials have been performed, and these have been flawed by the small numbers of patients. Therefore, most of our information comes from retrospective studies of patients treated over the past thirty years. These studies suffer from many of the defects of retrospective trials discussed in Chapter 2 and in many studies patients were poorly treated. It is important for you to also review the information presented in Appendices I and II.

Is Age a Significant Factor ?

Men over 70 years of age may die of natural causes before their prostate cancer has even become noticeable. Because aggressive treatment (radical prostatectomy or radiation therapy) can cause significant side effects, conservative treatment may be suitable for men in this age group.

Younger men, those with a life expectancy of more than 10 to 15 years, are more likely to experience problems or even die from their prostate cancer. Aggressive treatment is often recommended for these younger men. However, there is another important consideration. The principle complication of aggressive treatment is impotence, which is more likely to bother younger men. Thus, conservative treatment may be better for them, as well. This is especially true if the tumor is well differentiated.

Lessons from Watchful Waiting

The risks of conservative treatment can also be evaluated by studying men who had no treatment at all, so-called watchful waiting. Many of these studies were done before PSA testing became available. Many of them were poorly conducted. In some studies patients did not have regular follow-up examinations. Some patients were not treated unless they developed bladder outlet obstruction. Investigators from Dartmouth reviewed 144 such poorly conducted studies.[18] Surprisingly, they found no evidence that radical surgery or radiation was superior to watchful waiting. (In these studies the "treatment" was really neglect.) The Dartmouth team tried to determine if any patients benefitted from aggressive treatment. They focused on men who were 60 years of age or younger and whose tumor had a moderate Gleason grade. These were the patients who were *most likely to benefit* from radical surgery or radiation. But even in this select group, only 3 percent of men had their lives prolonged by aggressive treatment. Despite poor treatment, the men in these 144 studies did remarkably well.

In another study 223 Swedish men with early disease were followed for 10 years. Patients who developed symptoms from locally progressing cancer were treated with hormonal therapy only.[19] These men lived about as long as men treated with radical surgery; 87 percent survived 10 years.

Additional studies are presented in Appendices I and II. The lesson here is that even men who were poorly treated did remarkably well. Many of these surprising results were obtained before PSA testing was available. They were obtained in men who were followed very poorly, and often treated inadequately even when their cancer progressed. Consider how much better these already good results could be, if these cancers were properly controlled.

Change in Attitude

Many physicians who advocate conservative treatment for prostate cancer are trying to *control* the disease. They are not trying to *cure* the disease by removing or destroying every last cancer cell. This is a change is treatment strategy and is difficult for some urologists and other physicians to accept. If this sounds risky, remember that even radiation therapy seldom eradicates every prostate cancer cell.

It is clear that the risk of tumor spread is directly related to the size of the tumor. Any procedure which can successfully reduce the size of the tumor may also reduce the chance of tumor spread during the follow-up period. According to the ideas presented in Chapter 4, patients who have survived a tumor of a specific size without developing distant spread can probably prevent the spread of cancer cells from a smaller tumor. There is no evidence concerning prostate cancer which violates this simple principle. If the tumor can be controlled locally, though not necessarily eradicated, the spread of disease can usually be prevented. Thus, conservative treatment, such as complete hormonal blockade, cryosurgery, or radiation seed implantation, becomes a reasonable option.

The Importance of Follow-up

Digital rectal examinations (DRE) and PSA testing are important parts of follow-up. Following any form of treatment the blood level may fall to near 0 ng./ml. Recurrent or progressive disease may be present, if the PSA level begins to rise. Appropriate additional treatment can be started. A goal of treatment should be to keep the PSA level as low as possible. Treatment should continue if the PSA level approaches the highest level measured prior to treatment. There is no medical evidence that prostate cancer will spread, if the tumor is well controlled.

Periodically, men will need to take a "holiday" off of hormonal treatment. This will give men a break from the unpleasant side effects of the treatment. As mentioned above, PSA levels are not reliable while men are receiving hormonal treatment. A drug holiday also permits PSA measurements which more accurately reflect the size and activity of the cancer.

TREATMENT ACCORDING TO STAGE

The following treatment options emphasize the conservative end of the treatment spectrum. "Standard treatment" refers to the treatment recommended as accepted medical practice.

Stage T1a, c

At this stage the tumor occupies less than 5 percent of the tissue removed and is of low or medium grade. Standard treatment is watchful waiting. Repeat TURP is becoming less common. But if additional cancer is found following a repeat TURP, the patient is classified stage T1b.

Stage T1b

At this stage the tumor occupies more than 5 percent of the tissue removed, or is of high-grade, or significant additional cancer was found after a repeat TURP or biopsy. Radical prostatectomy is standard treatment for patients with more than ten to fifteen years of life expectancy. External beam radiation therapy is standard treatment for patients with fewer than ten years of life expectancy. But, the benefits of aggressive therapy are so small that patient preference should play a significant role in decisions about treatment.

Patients who wish to avoid the complications of aggressive treatment, e.g., impotence and incontinence, should consider the options described above, especially complete hormonal blockade, cryosurgery, and radiation seed implantation. Some men, especially those with a low grade tumor, may choose to begin a period of watchful waiting.

Since the spread of cancer is largely determined by its size and grade, I believe that it is prudent to treat the tumor prior to a period of watchful waiting. Hormonal treatment can involve three classes of drugs discussed above. Hormonal blockade can be "customized" according to the characteristics of the tumor and patient preference. For example, some men may wish to begin treatment with an antiandrogen and finasteride (Proscar), the drugs least likely to cause impotence. Even a low fat diet may retard tumor growth.

The goal of treatment should be to reduce the PSA level to near zero for about one year or longer. Tumor growth or recurrence can be monitored with DREs and PSA tests. If the tumor returns or continues to grow, additional treatment should be pursued. Patients should understand the great importance of frequent follow-up examinations. Both the patient and the doctor should be willing to accept the risk of disease progression. Some patients with very low PSA levels may develop metastatic disease.

Stage T2

At these stages the tumor is confined to the prostate gland. The treatment options are similar to those for stage T1b disease. Some tumors lie close to the capsule of the prostate. Freezing these cancer cells risks damage to the nerves that control erection.

In patients with tumors which are large or high grade, a laparoscopic lymph node dissection may be performed. Patients with positive nodes are not candidates for radical surgery.

Stage T3

At this stage the cancer extends beyond the capsule that surrounds the gland. Radiation therapy is the primary treatment for most patients, although it is uncertain whether this treatment can increase patient survival. Patients in whom the entire tumor can be removed may consider radical prostatectomy. Hormone manipulation may also be tried. If the tumor shrinks some patients may be candidates for radical prostatectomy or radiation therapy over a smaller area. But, there is no good evidence that surgery or radiation prolongs the survival of these patients any longer than hormonal therapy alone.

Stage T4

At stage T4 the cancer has spread to lymph nodes (N1-3) or distant organs (M1). The primary therapy is hormone manipulation or castration. TURP can relieve urinary obstruction. Chemotherapy is rarely used.

FOLLOW UP

Regular and meticulous follow-up is the most important part of conservative treatment for prostate cancer. Patients should have a PSA test performed before and after surgery. They should then have a DRE and PSA test performed every six to twelve months. TRUS should also been performed as needed. Other X-rays and scans should generally be performed on patients with symptoms suggestive of recurrent disease. The amount of follow-up required varies with the situation. You and your doctor will have to decide on a follow-up schedule that's best for you.

12.

Cancer of the Rectum

Cancers of the colon and rectum affect about 138,000 Americans every year. Considered together, they are second only to lung cancer as the leading cause of cancer deaths in the United States. They affect about one out of twenty Americans, or 6 percent. Rectal cancer alone (excluding the colon) affects about 38,000 Americans annually, with almost 8,000 dying of this disease. Current research indicates that a low-fiber, high-fat diet plays a role in the development of this disease.

This chapter will cover the following topics: the anatomy of the rectum, the types of cancer that affect the rectum, how this cancer is graded, how this cancer spreads, what screening procedures are available, what the signs and symptoms are, how this cancer is diagnosed, how this cancer is staged, what treatments are available, my analysis of how conservative surgery can be used to treat this cancer, my recommendations for the appropriate treatment at each stage, and what sort of follow-up is needed after treatment.

ANATOMY AND PHYSIOLOGY

The colon and rectum make up the last 7 feet of the intestinal tract. The colon absorbs water from the bowel contents and produces formed stool. About the last 18 inches of the colon is called the *sigmoid colon*. The sigmoid colon becomes the rectum as it leaves the abdominal cavity. It is about the last 6 inches (15 cm) of the intestinal tract. The last 1 inch (2 cm) of the rectum is called the *anal canal*. The outlet at the lower end of the rectum is called the *anus*.

Three different types of cells cover this region of the body. The skin of the buttocks changes to a *mucous epithelium*—the type of moist skin that covers the lips and oral cavity—at the anus. This lines the anal canal. At the rectum proper, the cells change again to intestinal *epithelial cells*, which line the rest of the intestinal tract. All of the intestinal epithelial cells lining the rectum form a layer called the *mucosa*.

The last 2 inches (5 cm) of bowel include a complex set of muscles that control bowel movements. The rectum is suspended from a sling of muscles called the *levator ani* muscles, which are under voluntary control. The *external sphincter*, another voluntary muscle surrounds the rectum. The ridge formed by the circular muscle is called the *anal verge*. The inner muscle tube (the *internal sphincter*) lies within the wall of the rectum itself. It acts automatically, in coordination with the voluntary muscles.

TYPES OF CANCER

Most rectal cancers develop from the inside lining of the intestinal tract—the mucosa. This cell layer contains cells that produce mucus, which protects the intestinal lining from the bacteria and toxic substances in the stool, and lubricates the rectal canal. Most rectal cancers arise from these glandular cells and are called *adenocarcinomas*. These are velvety, soft tumors covered with tiny projections. Other rectal tumors include a low-level malignancy called carcinoid and lymphoma, a cancer of certain white blood cells. Malignant melanoma (see Chapter 9) can also occur in the rectum. It has been treated like melanoma elsewhere in the body, but when it occurs in the rectum it has a particularly bad prognosis.

TUMOR GRADE

Rectal cancer is usually divided into three grades, from well differentiated, grade I, to poorly differentiated, grade III. The cells in high-grade tumors are rapidly dividing and look very malignant under a microscope. As with other cancers, survival and local recurrence rates are best among patients with well-differentiated tumors.

ROUTES OF SPREAD

Rectal cancer penetrates through the various layers of the rectal wall. It starts in the mucosa and then reaches the layer underneath, the *submucosa*. At this point, it is considered invasive. It then reaches the muscular layer of the bowel, the *muscularis*, and then through and past the outside covering of the bowel, the *serosa*. As the tumor penetrates and enlarges, it can spread to the pelvic lymph nodes. Large tumors can attach to surrounding structures such as the vagina in women, the prostate in men, the bladder, or the sacrum, a bone at the bottom of the spine. This is discussed in more detail further on, since the stages of disease are defined by this spread.

Blood from most of the rectum goes first to the liver on its way to the heart, as does most of the blood from the entire gastrointestinal tract. (This allows digested nutrients to be further processed in the liver.) Thus, cancer cells from the colon and upper rectum are first carried to the liver. Occasionally, rectal cancer will spread to the lungs, brain, or elsewhere.

SCREENING

Rectal cancers arise from *polyps*. About one third of these polyps can be found on rectal examination; most are within reach of a 25-cm sigmoidoscope, a flexible scope used to view the lower part of the colon and the rectum. The American Cancer Society has made the following recommendations. Individuals over the age of forty should have an annual digital rectal examination (DRE), in which the doctor feels for the presence of growths within the rectum. After the age of fifty, individuals should have their stool tested for occult (hidden) blood annually. Prior to taking this test, the patient must follow a strict diet to reduce the chance of a false positive result. Even when carefully performed, only about 5 percent of patients with positive tests are found to have cancer. As many as 30 percent are found to have polyps. About 90 percent of patients with cancer will have a positive test. The other 10 percent have cancers that do not bleed enough to show positive.

After the age of fifty, individuals should have a sigmoidoscopic examination every three to five years. If polyps are found, they should be removed. The incidence of colon and rectal cancer can be reduced by 80 to 90 percent in patients who have regular sigmoidscopic examinations and polyp removal.[1] These tests should be performed more often in patients with ulcerative colitis, or who have a family history of colon cancer or polyps.

SIGNS AND SYMPTOMS

Rectal cancer most frequently causes a change in bowel habits, such as constipation. The shape of the stool may be narrowed by a tumor that surrounds the rectal canal. Bleeding may also occur, although bleeding can occur from other sources, such as hemorrhoids. These are all late symptoms, and pain is often a very late symptom.

DIAGNOSIS

Polyps are found by DRE or sigmoidscopic examination. A *biopsy* determines the diagnosis.

A blood test for carcinoembryonic antigen (CEA) may be elevated in some patients with this disease. This is a protein produced by some colon cancer cells. A *barium enema* X-ray examination, in which barium is introduced into the rectum to highlight the inner lining, can detect rectal tumors. An *ultrasound examination* can be performed. This test uses high-frequency sound waves to display tumor invasion and enlarged lymph nodes.

STAGES OF DISEASE

In 1932, C. E. Dukes from England described a staging system for cancer of the colon and rectum. It is based primarily on how far the tumor has invaded into the bowel wall. This system, which has been modified often, still bears his name. The TNM system, described in Chapter 5, has been accepted by the International Union Against Cancer (UICC) and the American Joint Committee for Cancer Staging and End Results (AJCC). Table 12.1 shows both systems combined. Overall staging numbers are used for ease of reference. Figure 12.1 shows the layers of the bowel.

Table 12.1 Dukes and TNM Staging Systems for Rectal Cancer

Overall Stage	Dukes	TNM	Description	Five-Year Survival Rate
0	0	T_{is}	A cancer that is limited to the topmost layer of cells, also called cancer *in situ*.	Over 95%
I	A or B_1	T_{1-2}, N_0, M_0	A cancer that is confined to the bowel wall. Penetration of the tumor into the muscle layer of the bowel is indicated by the higher designation in each system (B_1 or T_2).	Stage A—about 90%, stage B_1—about 85%
II	B_2 or B_3	T_{3-4}, N_0, M_0	A cancer that has spread through the entire bowel wall, but does not involve the lymph nodes. Involvement of adjacent structures or organs is indicated by the higher designation in each system (B_3 or T_4).	Stage B_2—about 70%, stage B_3—about 30%
III	C_{1-3}	T_{0-4}, N_{1-3}, M_0	A cancer that has invaded the lymph nodes. The numbers 1 to 3 in the Dukes system describe the extent of the primary tumor: 1, confined to the bowel; 2, outside the bowel; or 3, involving nearby structures. The numbers 1 to 3 in the TNM system describe the progression of nodal disease: 1, spread to from one to three regional lymph nodes; 2, spread to four or more regional lymph nodes; and 3, spread to a lymph node further removed along the course of a named artery.	C_1—45%, C_2—20%, C_3—15%
IV	D	T_{0-4}, N_{1-3}, M_1	Distant metastases are present.	Less than 5%

Figure 12.1 Parts of the Rectum

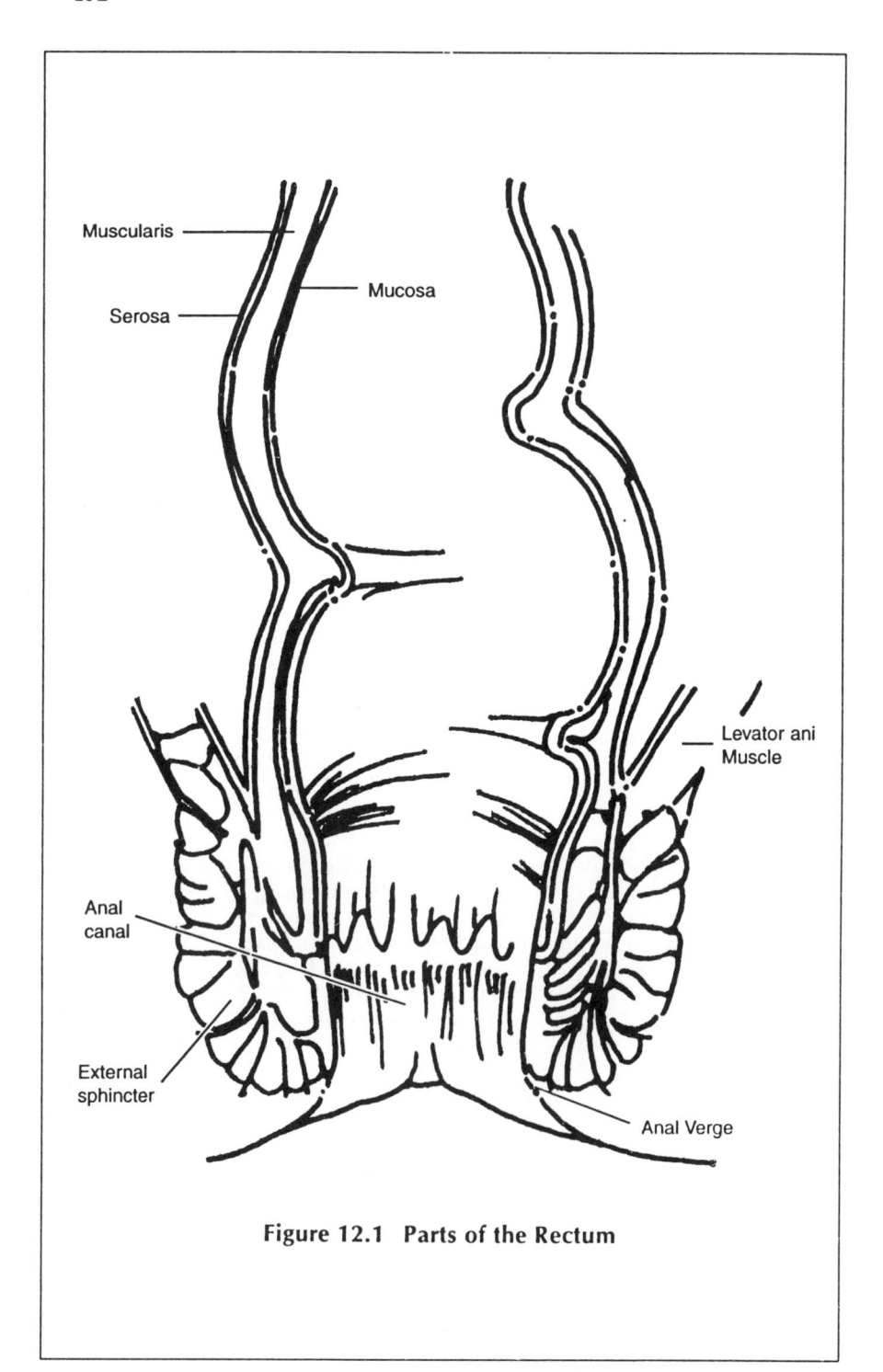

TYPES OF TREATMENT

Treatment options include surgery, radiation therapy, and chemotherapy. See Chapter 5 for more information about these treatments, including general information on the side effects associated with each treatment.

Surgery

Surgical options include the following procedures. The upper part of the rectum is accessible to the surgeon and can be easily separated from the surrounding tissue when operating within the abdomen. The lower rectum lies deep within the pelvis, where there is little room to operate.

Abdominoperineal Resection (APR)

Rectal cancer has traditionally been treated with an APR, which is performed from both the abdomen above and the rectal area below. The surgeon enters the abdominal cavity to free the colon and rectum from above. The entire rectum, the tumor, and surrounding tissue are then removed from below. This includes removal of the lymph nodes. The end of the colon is brought out through the abdominal wall in what is called a permanent *colostomy*. There is usually a large space left behind, which requires several weeks or months to heal.

Low Anterior Resection (LAR)

In this operation, the segment of intestine, both the lower colon and rectum, that includes the tumor is removed. The two open ends are then reattached. Over the past several decades, surgeons have been changing their opinion about the length of clinically healthy tissue that should be removed below the tumor, known as the margin. The goal has been to avoid injuring the sphincter mechanism, without leaving tumor cells in the patient. The margin has slowly decreased from about 5 cm down to 1 cm, a change that has allowed more patients to be treated with sphincter-saving surgery. When the margin is close—less than 2 cm—it should be examined with a *frozen section*, described in Chapter 5.

Originally, these two pieces of intestine were sewn together by hand with sutures, or stitches. In the 1970s, a stapling device was invented to help the surgeon join two segments of intestine. It works particularly well inside the pelvis. It enables surgeons to remove rectal tumors and staple the remaining colon to a short segment of remaining rectum, using a circular row of tiny metal staples. It is now in common use.

Significant leaks may occur where the segments of intestine are sewn or stapled together. This complication may occur in as many as 20 percent of patients. Therefore, a temporary colostomy is usually performed. After the two segments of bowel have healed together, the temporary colostomy is reversed and bowel movements return to normal.

Coloanal Anastomosis

In this operation, the lower colon is pulled down and sewn to the lower rectum. If the tumor has invaded near or into the sphincter muscles, these muscles may be partially removed, although they may be damaged in the process. This operation is like an LAR except that the colon is sewn to the anus and not the low rectum. This permits the removal of a tumor located very low in the rectum. The staples that are often used in the LAR are not usually used in coloanal anastomosis because the colon is being sewn to muscle, and not to another segment of intestine. Patients will still have an external sphincter to maintain continence, but they may become aware of a large volume of feces suddenly falling into the colon above the anus. This operation may require a temporary colostomy while the surgical area heals.

Pull-through Procedure

In this operation, the colon is pulled down inside and through the rectum, like one sleeve inside another. The mucosa of the rectum is stripped away so that the colon and rectum will stick together. No sutures and no colostomy are required. Incontinence and other problems with bowel habits occur in one third or more of patients.

Local Excision or Ablation

Tumors that are within 10 cm of the anus can be removed by

local excision. This works best with tumors that are less than 3 cm in diameter and involve less than a quarter of the inner circumference of the rectum. Surgeons have tried to save the rectum and avoid marring the patient with a permanent colostomy by treating these patients with local excision and/or radiation therapy. It is generally agreed that the surgeons should remove the tumor with a margin of 1 to 2 cm of visibly normal tissue. It is generally agreed that tumors excised with narrow margins should be carefully checked by the pathologist to be sure that the margins are all free of tumor cells. Different surgical incisions have been used, for example, through the anus, or through the tailbone.

Fulguration uses an electric current to burn the tumor. Afterwards, the area is allowed to heal without being closed up. The tumor can also be treated with *cryosurgery*, in which a probe freezes the tumor. Since the margins of the tumor are destroyed by these techniques, they cannot be checked by a pathologist.

Because the margins are destroyed, tumor ablation is not widely practiced. It is used primarily on patients who are medically unsuitable for extensive surgery. Patients must be examined four to six weeks for recurrence. Often two to four treatments are required to eliminate the tumor. Laser therapy has also been used, primarily in patients with advanced disease, to remove a tumor that is obstructing the intestinal tract.

Radiation Therapy

Radiation can be administered with a device placed into the rectum, a technique known as *endocavitary radiation*. Jean Papillon of Lyon, France, has great experience with this form of treatment. He administers 100 to 120 Gy of endocavitary radiation over a period of several weeks. If the tumor becomes smaller, some patients are operated on. The remaining patients are treated with *interstitial radiation*, in which radioactive needles are placed directly into the tumor.

Radiation therapy can also eradicate microscopic cells that may remain after local excision of a tumor. Usually 50 to 60 Gy is administered. Adjuvant radiation therapy, or that given in addition to surgery, can successfully reduce local recurrence rates, but it does not increase survival.

However, one study demonstrated decreased local recurrence and increased survival for patients who had low-dose radiation therapy *prior* to an APR.[2] This makes sense, since local recurrence following an APR is found deep within the pelvis. It is very difficult to detect and treat, and the recurrent disease could grow to a large size and become the source of spreading tumor cells. Thus, preoperative radiation therapy may have prevented the spread of disease in some patients. Chemotherapy can also be used to shrink tumors before surgery.

Complications that occur shortly after radiation therapy, such as rectal inflammation and bleeding, occur primarily in patients who receive over 63 Gy. Later complications include intestinal obstruction, inflammation of the intestines, and bladder contraction. The higher the dose, the higher the complication rate. Long-term complications occur in less than 5 percent of patients.

Chemotherapy

For over twenty-five years, 5-fluorouracil has been the standard drug for cancers of the colon and rectum. It can reduce the size of tumors in about 25 percent of patients. But used alone, it does not reduce local recurrence after surgery or increase survival.

Levamisole has been widely used around the world to treat worms in both humans and animals. It can stimulate the immune system. In one recent study, levamisole and 5-fluorouracil in combination increased survival in patients with stage C colon cancer.[3] This study did not include patients with rectal cancer, but the tumors are similar. Adjuvant chemotherapy has been reported in some studies to prolong the lives of some patients with advanced disease who also receive postoperative radiation,[4] although European trials have disputed this.[5]

Leucovorin is a compound that can stabilize the molecular structure of 5-fluorouracil. There is evidence that these two drugs together may prolong survival better than 5-fluorouracil alone.

ANALYSIS

Surgical procedures that spare the rectum are gaining acceptance and are available at most large medical centers. Preservation of the sphincter mechanism can be accomplished in two ways. First, a segment of intestine above and below the tumor is removed. The remaining upper segment is connected to the remaining rectum. The surgeon must remove a margin of normal-appearing intestine above and below the tumor. Second, the tumor is simply removed using a knife, electric current, cold probe, laser, or radiation. This is more appropriate for smaller tumors located close to the anus.

Many surgeons now accept a margin of 1 cm around the tumor. This represents a rapid change is surgical opinion during the past twenty years. A randomized trial conducted by the NSABP, a breast-cancer project that also did colon cancer studies, determined that a narrow margin of excision resulted in a local recurrence rate of 22 percent. When the tumor was removed with a wider margin, the local recurrence rate was only 12 percent. Despite this difference in local recurrence rates, the overall survival rate was not affected by the margin of excision. As with breast cancer, local recurrence following a limited excision did not adversely affect survival. The authors of the study concluded, "There are unmistakable parallels between the evolution of the operative strategy of carcinoma of the rectum and that of breast cancer."[6] Thus, promptly treated local recurrence does not reduce survival.

Therefore, surgeons can prudently perform one of the conservative operations I have described without compromising the patient's survival. By reading Appendix I, you should gain confidence in surgical procedures that preserve bowel continence.

TREATMENT ACCORDING TO STAGE

Conservative surgery for cancer of the rectum is widely practiced. You should have little difficulty finding a surgeon who is familiar with the operations described here. However, much of the therapy recommended here is in the developmental stages. You will want to be treated by surgeons who are familiar with these new techniques.

Keep in mind that conservative surgery is best suited to the treatment of early cancer. Even so, I would still encourage you to ask your doctor about the most conservative options available to you in your specific case. Sometimes, radiation or chemotherapy is used before surgery to help shrink a large tumor. I think this is a good use for these therapies. However, radiation therapy or chemotherapy is sometimes used after surgery to help reduce local recurrence. In addition, the use of the chemotherapy drug 5-fluorouracil is being recommended by the National Institutes of Health for otherwise healthy patients with Dukes stage B_2 and C disease. The NIH feels that this may prolong survival in some patients. These therapies are mentioned here because they are options that you may be presented with. However, I would again encourage you to talk to your doctor to find out how much these therapies can actually help to prolong your life.

Stage 0

At this stage, the cancer involves the topmost layer of cells. Local excision is the primary therapy.

Stage I

At stage I, the tumor is confined to the bowel wall. These recommendations depend on exactly where the tumor is located.

Upper 10 cm of the Rectum

Tumors that are more than about 5 cm above the anus can often be removed with a LAR. The margin must be free of tumor cells. If the margins are inadequate for the size of the tumor, consider the treatment discussed below.

Lower 5 cm of the Rectum

Small tumors can often be locally excised with a full thickness of the rectal wall. If the lesion is less than 3 cm in diameter, well or moderately differentiated, and has been completely excised, postoperative radiation therapy may not be needed.

Larger tumors may by treated with a pull-through or coloanal anastomosis. The surgeon can remove the tumor within a segment of bowel. He or she can even remove a small portion of involved muscle. Preoperative radiation therapy and/or chemotherapy may shrink the tumor enough to allow complete excision. If there are grave signs, such as high grade, or blood or lymph vessel invasion, postoperative radiation therapy may be considered.

Stage II

At this stage, the tumor has penetrated through the bowel wall. The treatments recommended depend on where the tumor is located.

Upper 10 cm of the Rectum

Treatment is the same as for stage I. Margins must be free of tumor as determined by a pathologist. Preoperative radiation therapy or chemotherapy may shrink the tumor enough to allow surgical removal of the tumor with a sphincter-preserving operation. Preoperative radiation therapy or chemotherapy may also reduce local recurrence. If the tumor invades the bladder, a partial cystectomy, or removal of part of the bladder, may be necessary.

Lower 5 cm of the Rectum

Some T_3 cancers can be excised locally or treated with a LAR or coloanal anastomosis. LAR is preferable. Preoperative chemotherapy and/or radiation therapy may allow complete excision using a coloanal anastomosis. Postoperative radiation therapy and/or chemotherapy may be considered.

Stage III

At stage III, the tumor has spread to the lymph nodes. Again, these recommendations depend on the tumor's location.

Upper 10 cm of the Rectum

Surgical excision should be considered, as described under stage II. Postoperative chemotherapy may be added, particularly for patients with more than four positive lymph nodes. It may reduce local recurrence and increase survival.

Lower 5 cm of the Rectum

Large tumors should be treated with preoperative radiation therapy and/or chemotherapy. Sphincter-saving procedures may be employed if technically possible. Large tumors that fail to respond to preoperative radiation or chemotherapy may require an APR. Postoperative chemotherapy may be added, particularly for patients with more than four positive lymph nodes. It may reduce local recurrence and increase survival.

A group of investigators has been able to increase survival somewhat by giving postoperative chemotherapy at the same time as radiation therapy. Best results have been achieved if chemotherapy was administered as a continuous intravenous infusion, running twenty-four hours a day, during the seven weeks of radiation therapy. The continuous infusion was somewhat more successful than conventional intermittent intravenous injections in prolonging overall survival.[7]

Stage IV

At stage IV, the tumor has spread to distant organs. The primary tumor should be removed locally if possible. More extensive surgery with radiation therapy is appropriate if intestinal obstruction may occur. The removal of one to three liver metastases or isolated lung or ovarian metastases may prolong suvival. Chemotherapy or biological therapy, described in Chapter 5, may be attempted.

FOLLOW-UP

Regular and meticulous follow-up is the most important part of conservative treatment for rectal cancer. Patients should be seen every three months for the first two years and every six months for the next three years. They should have a rectal examination and CEA blood test. Blood chemistry tests, chest X-rays, and ultrasound examinations of the rectal area may be performed about annually depending upon the stage of the disease. Other X-rays and scans should be performed if symptoms develop. The amount of follow-up required varies with the situation. There can be a longer interval between visits if a wide surgical margin was used, and a shorter interval if a narrower margin was used.

If the preoperative carcinoembryonic antigen (CEA) level was elevated, the test should be repeated postoperatively, and should be normal or near normal. If the CEA level is still elevated, it is likely that there still is rectal cancer somewhere in the body. If the

CEA level rises over time, it may be the first sign of an isolated local recurrence. A thorough evaluation may identify such a recurrence, which can sometimes be removed. Most elevations in CEA, though, are from distant metastases, usually detectable on X-rays or scans, or recurrences that cannot be completely removed. Recent evidence suggests that CEA follow-up tests do little to prolong life.[8]

13.

Soft Tissue Sarcoma

Soft tissue sarcomas occur in about two of every 100,000 adults. They are more common in children. This is primarily due to the high incidence of sarcomas of the skeletal muscles among children.

Soft tissue sarcomas cause about 2 percent of all adult cancer deaths. They can be caused by asbestos exposure, as in the case of mesothelioma, and radiation, as in the case of fibrosarcoma. Most sarcomas have no known environmental or hereditary cause.

This chapter will cover the following topics: the various tissues affected by this disease, the types of sarcoma that can arise, how this cancer is graded, how this cancer spreads, what screening procedures are available, what the signs and symptoms are, how this cancer is diagnosed, how this cancer is staged, what treatments are available, my analysis of how conservative surgery can be used to treat this cancer, my recommendations for the appropriate treatment at each stage, and what sort of follow-up is needed after the treatment.

ANATOMY AND PHYSIOLOGY

Sarcomas are cancers of the body tissues, as opposed to those of specific organs. They arise in bone, cartilage, muscle, fat, nerves, blood vessels, and other connective tissue. Most sarcomas arise in the extremities. But they can arise within almost any organ in the body, because all organs contain most of these types of tissue. Sarcomas are divided into those involving hard tissue, bone and cartilage, and those involving soft tissue, which includes all other tissues.

TYPES OF CANCER

There are over fifty different types of sarcomas. Within each group there are subtypes, based upon the types of cells from which the cancers arise. Each type is named for the type of cell from which it arises:

- *Angiosarcoma.* Blood vessel.
- *Liposarcoma.* Fat.
- *Fibrosarcoma.* Connective tissue.
- *Rhabdomyosarcoma.* Muscle.
- *Leiomyosarcoma.* Smooth (involuntary) muscle.
- *Neurofibrosarcoma.* Nerve covering.
- *Synovial sarcoma.* Membrane lining the joints.
- *Lymphangiosarcoma.* Lymph vessel.

Although discussion of each type of sarcoma is beyond the scope if this book, these are some of the characteristics of a few of the more common types. Liposarcoma represents about 15 percent of all cases. It is commonly found on the extremities and behind the abdominal cavity, in an area called the retroperitoneum. Liposarcomas generally occur in patients who are fifty to sixty years of age. Fibrosarcoma is another common type of soft tissue sarcoma, representing about 15 percent of all cases. It is seen in patients who are thirty to fifty-five years of age and commonly arises in the leg. Malignant fibrous histiocytoma is a highly malignant tumor that is being seen with increasing frequency, now about 20 percent of all cases. It occurs late in life, and commonly arises on an extremity or in the retroperitoneum.

TUMOR GRADE

There is some variation among soft tissue sarcomas in their overall prognosis, based on their tissue of origin. Nevertheless, prognosis is primarily determined by the grade of the tumor. Pathologists divide sarcomas into three grades, from 1, low, to 3, high. The pathologist observes the appearance of the tumor under a microscope, especially the number of cells that are dividing. The cells in high-grade tumors are rapidly dividing, rapidly growing, and very malignant in appearance. They are the most likely to spread. Low-grade tumors usually remain localized. Survival and local recurrence are related to tumor grade, tumor size, cell type, tumor location, and the presence of cancer cells in the margins when the tumor is removed.

ROUTES OF SPREAD

Soft tissue sarcomas are often surrounded by a fibrous capsule. They are much less likely to spread to regional lymph nodes than other types of cancer. Distant spread most often occurs to the lungs, brain, and bones.

SCREENING

There are no standard screening methods for this disease. They usually cause no symptoms and can arise deep within an extremity or other region of the body. Therefore, patients should see their physician promptly if they discover any new mass.

SIGNS AND SYMPTOMS

The most common complaint is the appearance of a painless mass.

DIAGNOSIS

CAT and MRI scans can show sarcomas. The scans can locate the tumor and describe the surrounding structures. A chest X-ray can detect lung metastases.

As with all tumors, a biopsy is required to make an accurate diagnosis. Many of these tumors look alike, particularly tumors that are poorly differentiated. The pathologist may need to examine many sections of each tumor to make a diagnosis. A *needle biopsy*, in which a needle is used to collect cells from the tumor, may not provide enough tissue. Therefore, an *incisional biopsy*, in which a piece is cut out of the tumor, is usually preferred. A biopsy may be done immediately prior to definitive surgery. The surgeon who prefers to do an *excisional biopsy*, in which the tumor is completely removed, should perform a definitive cancer operation. That is, he or she should take care to remove the tumor with an adequate margin of healthy tissue surrounding it.

Some sarcomas are difficult to precisely identify. They are so undifferentiated that they bear no resemblance to their cell of origin. Pathologists commonly send samples of these tumors to specialty centers.

STAGES OF DISEASE

Like other cancers, stage is determined by both tumor size and the extent of tumor spread. But among soft tissue sarcomas, tumor grade plays an very important role in determining prognosis. Prognosis is also influenced by the location of the tumor. A tumor near the body's surface has a better prognosis than one deep inside an extremity or other part of the body. There are several staging systems, including the complex TNM system, described in Chapter 5. The most commonly used system in the United States has been approved by the American Joint Committee on Cancer (AJCC). Shown in Table 13.1, it is based upon tumor grade and size.

TYPES OF TREATMENT

Treatment options include surgery, radiation therapy, and chemotherapy. See Chapter 5 for more information about these treatments, including general information on the side effects associated with each treatment.

Surgery

Traditional surgery has been amputation or wide excision including a broad margin of apparently normal tissue. When muscles have been involved, surgeons have often removed the

Table 13.1 AJCC Staging System for Soft Tissue Sarcomas

Stage	Description	Five-Year Survival Rate
IA	A grade 1 cancer that is localized and smaller than 5 cm.	85% to 95%
IB	A grade 1 cancer that is localized and larger than 5 cm.	70% to 90%
IIA	A grade 2 cancer that is localized and smaller than 5 cm.	70% to 85%
IIB	A grade 2 cancer that is localized and larger than 5 cm.	50% to 70%
IIIA	A grade 3 cancer that is localized and smaller than 5 cm.	60% to 80%
IIIB	A grade 3 cancer that is localized and larger than 5 cm.	25% to 45%
IIIC	A cancer of any grade or size with spread to the lymph nodes.	25% to 45%
IVA	A cancer of any grade, size, or lymph node status that obviously (not just microscopically) invades adjacent structures, such as major blood vessels or nerves.	20% to 40%
IVB	Distant metastases are present.	20%

entire muscle group. If the tumor has been near the shoulder or hip, the entire joint has been removed. If the tumor has involved a major blood vessel, the vessel has been removed and replaced with an artificial graft. When bone has been removed, it has often been replaced with bone graft or metal. Even after radical excision, local recurrence rates of 25 to 30 percent have been common.

Recently, more surgeons are practicing more conservative surgery, including limb-sparing techniques. Conserative surgery for soft tissue sarcomas means the removal of the tumor with a suitable margin of normal-appearing tissue. A 2-cm margin is ideal; however, this is not always possible. In some situations, the surgeon must remove only the tumor, trying to obtain a margin with no tumor cells visible under the microscope. This approach is similar to Mohs micrographic surgery, described in Chapter 5, which is practiced by some surgeons.[1]

Radiation Therapy

Postoperative radiation therapy is used to reduce local recurrence, especially after surgery that spared the limb from amputation. Doses of 60 to 70 Gy given over six to seven weeks are common. As with other malignancies, postoperative radiation therapy does not prolong survival. Radiation may also be given prior to surgery to reduce the size of a large tumor. The side effects of radiation therapy include fatigue during the period of treatment and a sunburn-like reddening of the skin. Other side effects may appear depending on where the tumor is located.

Chemotherapy

Chemotherapy has been very effective in bone sarcomas and rhabdomyosarcomas, or muscle tumors. Chemotherapy has been much less effective in other soft tissue sarcomas. Adriamycin is the most commonly used agent for these tumors. Chemotherapy in addition to surgery, or adjuvant chemotherapy, is not very effective. Patients with tumors 5 cm or smaller should not be treated with adjuvant chemotherapy.[2] Most authorities recommend that patients with large tumors or distant metastases receive treatment as participants in a clinical trial. Preoperative, or neoadjuvant, chemotherapy can be used to shrink large tumors prior to surgery.

ANALYSIS

Limb-sparing operations are gaining acceptance and are available at most large medical centers. Local recurrence following radical surgery, such as amputation, is a worrisome event, and is associated with a decreased survival rate. Local recurrence following conservative surgery has a much better prognosis. Therefore, surgeons can prudently perform a conservative operation without compromising the patient's survival.

The suggestion that local recurrence has little effect on survival would have been medical heresy not that long ago. But today, wide local excision and radiation therapy are gaining acceptance in the treatment of soft tissue sarcoma. The central question is, "What is the clinical significance of local recurrence?" Specifically, does recurrent disease cause distant metastasis or is it merely a sign of aggressive disease? If local recurrence jeopardizes patient survival, then aggressive local control measures are indicated. Current evidence overwhelmingly suggests that local recurrence is merely a sign. It can be a sign that the tumor has already spread. It can also be a sign that the tumor is very aggressive. But if local recurrence is treated promptly, there is no reliable evidence that it causes tumor spread. This observation has been confirmed by several medical centers in Europe, Japan, and the United States.

I do not believe that radiation therapy is routinely needed. If local control did affect survival, we should see this benefit among patients treated with radiation therapy. Unfortunately, this does not occur. Most authorities report that radiation therapy improves local control, but does not affect survival. The single exception to this observation is discussed in Appendix I. These observations support the present trend toward limb preservation, and should encourage both surgeons and radiation therapists to strive toward an even greater concern for the functional and cosmetic results of their therapy.

TREATMENT ACCORDING TO STAGE

The following treatment options are recommended. Keep in mind that conservative surgery is best suited to the treatment of early cancer. Even so, I would still encourage you to ask your doctor about the most conservative options available to you in your specific case. Sometimes, radiation or chemotherapy is used before surgery to help shrink a large tumor. I think this is a good use for these therapies.

Stage I

Stage I includes localized grade 1 tumors. All obvious and microscopic disease should be removed. If possible, a wide margin (2 cm) of normal tissue should also be removed. If needed to preserve important structures, the margin may be much less, as long as it does not contain tumor cells. Removal of muscle groups and wide margins greater than 2 cm of normal tissue are not necessary. Radiation therapy is not routinely necessary. It may be used if the tumor was removed with a narrow margin close to a vital structure, such as an artery or nerve.

Stage II

This stage includes localized grade 2 tumors. Treatment is the same as for stage I. Preoperative chemotherapy or radiation therapy may be used to shrink a tumor. Postoperative radiation therapy may be used more often than in stage I patients.

Stage III

Stage III includes localized grade 3 tumors. Treatment is still the same as for stage I. Preoperative chemotherapy or radiation therapy may be used to shrink a tumor. Postoperative radiation therapy may be used more often than in stage II patients. Patients with stage IIIC disease, in which the cancer has spread to the lymph nodes, should have their positive lymph nodes removed.

Stage IVA

Stage IVA includes tumors that invade nearby structures. Patients should be treated with preoperative chemotherapy and/or radiation therapy. More radical surgery is needed at this point in order to completely remove the tumor.

Stage IVB

At this stage, distant metastases are present. The primary tumor can be treated with a limited excision. If the patient has a few metastases to the lungs, these may be removed. Patients with diffuse disease—disease throughout their bodies—may wish to consider chemotherapy, but results thus far are not encouraging.

Special Considerations for Recurrent Tumors

Most authorities recommend more aggressive treatment for a tumor that recurs locally. However, two studies from Memorial Sloan-Kettering in New York indicate that promptly treated local recurrence does not jeopardize survival.[3,4] I believe that conservative surgery is suitable for recurrent tumors. However, aggressive treatment, including radiation therapy, is suitable for a patient who is anxious about the possibility of future recurrences.

FOLLOW-UP

Regular and meticulous follow-up is the most important part of conservative treatment for soft tissue sarcoma. Patients should be examined and may have chest X-rays every six months for the first two years, and then annually thereafter. Blood chemistries, scans, and other X-rays should be performed if symptoms develop. The amount of follow-up required depends on tumor size and grade. You and your doctor will come up with a follow-up plan that's best for you.

14.

Cancer of the Vagina

Cancer of the vagina accounts for only about 2 percent of all gynecologic malignancies. It is less common than cancer of the cervix. Most patients are over fifty years of age. Many cases are associated with, and perhaps caused by, the human papillomavirus (HPV). Some women whose mothers took diethylstilbestrol (DES) to prevent miscarriage during pregnancy have developed vaginal cancer.

Radiation therapy has played a prominent role in the treatment of this disease. Therefore, there has been little opportunity to use conservative surgical measures.

This chapter will cover the following topics: the anatomy of the vagina, the types of cancer that affect the vagina, how this cancer is graded, how this cancer spreads, what screening procedures are available, what the signs and symptoms are, how this cancer is diagnosed, how this cancer is staged, what treatments are available, my analysis of how conservative surgery can be used to treat this cancer, my recommendations for the appropriate treatment at each stage, and what sort of follow-up is needed after treatment.

ANATOMY AND PHYSIOLOGY

The vagina is a muscular tube that extends from the vulva to the uterus. It is about 7.5 cm long and located between the bladder and the rectum. It is lined by *squamous epithelial cells* in a layer called the *mucosa*. There are no glands in the vagina itself; lubrication comes from glands in the cervix.

TYPES OF CANCER

Over 90 percent of vaginal cancers arise from the squamous epithelial cells lining the vagina. About half of all vaginal cancers arise in the upper third of the vagina. Malignant melanoma, discussed in Chapter 9, and a variety of sarcomas, which are covered in Chapter 13, also affect the vagina. Noninvasive cancer is called *vaginal intraepithelial neoplasia* (VAIN).

TUMOR GRADE

Vaginal cancer is usually divided into three grades, from well differentiated, grade I, to poorly differentiated, grade III. This is based on how abnormal the cells appear under a microscope. As with other cancers, survival rates and local recurrence rates are best among patients with well-differentiated tumors.

ROUTES OF SPREAD

After cancer penetrates through the basement membrane—the membrane that supports the squamous epithelial cells—it is called invasive cancer. Cancer in the upper part of the vagina spreads to the lymph nodes in the pelvis, similar to cancer of the cervix (Chapter 8). About 10 to 20 percent of patients with stage I disease will develop disease in the pelvic lymph nodes. Cancers in the lower part of the vagina spread to the groin lymph nodes and later to the lymph nodes in the pelvis, similar to cancer of the vulva (Chapter 15). Cancer of the vagina can invade the surrounding tissues and structures such as the bladder and rectum.

SCREENING

The gynecologist will check for vaginal cancer at the time of the regular Pap smear.

SIGNS AND SYMPTOMS

Most vaginal cancers cause no symptoms. Abnormal bleeding or a discharge occasionally calls attention to a malignancy. Lesions in the lower vagina may cause urinary symptoms.

DIAGNOSIS

The gynecologist confirms the diagnosis by sending a biopsy to the pathologist. After a complete history and physical examination, patients may have any or all of the following tests:

- A *chest X-ray*.
- An *intravenous pyelogram*, in which an X-ray is taken of the kidneys after a dye has been introduced through a vein to produce contrast.
- A *cystoscopic examination*, in which the bladder is examined via a lighted tube.
- A *sigmoidscopic examination*, in which the rectum and colon are checked via a lighted tube.
- A *lymphangiogram*, in which the lymph vessels are examined after a dye has been introduced to produce contrast.
- A *barium enema*, in which the large intestine is examined after barium has been introduced to produce contrast.

STAGES OF DISEASE

Staging according to the International Federation of Gynecology and Obstetrics (FIGO) is shown in Table 14.1.

TYPES OF TREATMENT

Treatment of vaginal cancer is limited to surgery and radiation. Intravenous chemotherapy has a limited role in the treatment of this disease and is largely experimental. Topical chemotherapy, in the form of a lotion applied to the surface, is used for stage 0 disease. See Chapter 5 for more information about these treatments, including general information on the side effects associated with each treatment.

Surgery

Surgery ranges from local removal to *radical vaginectomy*, which includes radical hysterectomy and removal of the pelvic lymph nodes. Local removal is technically difficult, especially for lesions high in the vagina. Skin grafts are occasionally

Table 14.1 FIGO Staging System for Vaginal Cancer

Stage	Description	Five-Year Survival Rate
0	A cancer that is limited to the topmost cell layer.	Over 95%
I	A cancer that is limited to the mucous membrane.	70% to 80%
	Microinvasive cancer—There is less than 2.5 mm of invasion.	About 85%
II	A cancer that involves tissues beyond the vagina, but does not extend to the pelvic wall.	About 50%
III	A cancer that extends to the pelvic wall.	About 30%
IVa	A cancer that is growing into the lining of the bladder or rectum.	About 10%
IVb	Distant metastases are present.	Less than 10%

necessary and narrowing of the vaginal canal is a possible complication.

If a cancer of the upper vagina is managed with conservative surgery, the pelvic lymph nodes may be removed using a laparoscope, which is a tube inserted into the abdomen through which the surgeon removes tissue with tiny cutters. If the removed nodes are positive, the remaining nodes can be removed through the laparoscope. Most surgeons, though, prefer doing open abdominal surgery because they believe that the nodes can be more completely removed that way.

Cancer of the lower vagina may be treated like cancer of the vulva. The surgeon can remove the sentinel lymph nodes—those where the disease first spreads—in the groin region. This subject is more thoroughly discussed in Chapter 15.

Radiation Therapy

Radiation therapy for vaginal cancer requires dosages between 65 and 80 Gy. There are two ways to administer radiation therapy inside the vagina. In *intracavitary radiation*, radioactive cesium can be placed in a cylindrical applicator and used to treat the entire vaginal lining. In *interstitial radiation*, radioactive iridium can also be placed directly into the cancer. More advanced cancers can also be treated with *external-beam* therapy. If the cancer is in the upper vagina, the pelvic lymph nodes may need to be treated. Radiation therapy is often used when the nodes are not removed. Possible side effects include narrowing, and painful or difficult intercourse. Also, *fistulas*—abnormal passages—may form between the vagina and either the bladder or the rectum, although this is rare.

ANALYSIS

Cancer of the vagina has been managed primarily by radiation therapy. Consequently, there has been little experience with conservative surgery. Cancers in the upper vagina have been managed by hysterectomy. But the limited experience thus far is compatible with the consistent theme of this book. Promptly treated local recurrence after conservative surgery does not adversely affect survival. Therefore, local excision is a prudent option when technically possible. Pregnancy does not affect the behavior of this cancer. See Appendix I for a discussion of studies made in this area.

TREATMENT ACCORDING TO STAGE

The following treatment options are recommended. Keep in mind that conservative surgery is best suited to the treatment of early cancer. Even so, I would still encourage you to ask your doctor about the most conservative options available to you in your specific case.

Stage 0

At this stage, the cancer is limited to the topmost layer of cells. Early cancer or vaginal intraepithelial neoplasia (VAIN) is conventionally treated with laser therapy or topical application of 5-fluorouracil, a standard chemotheraputic drug. Intracavitary radiation therapy or local excision is occasionally used for this early disease.

Stage I

At stage I, the tumor is limited to the mucosa. I believe that small lesions may be treated with local removal, or local removal plus radiation therapy. This may be performed with a knife or a laser. This includes most all lesions that can be removed with a margin of normal tissue that is free of disease, as determined by a pathologist. Larger lesions may be treated with both external-beam and intracavitary radiation. If the lesion is in the upper vagina, the pelvic lymph nodes may be removed with a laparoscope. If the lesion is in the lower vagina, the sentinel groin lymph nodes may be removed. If the sentinel nodes are positive, the rest should be removed. In patients who will return regularly, the lymph nodes may be left alone. They must be examined regularly, and removed if they enlarge.

Stage II

At stage II, the tumor involves tissue beyond the vagina, but does not extend to the pelvic wall. Patients whose cancers have extended beyond the vagina are seldom candidates for any type of surgery. Radiation therapy using both external-beam and intracavitary therapy may be the best therapy.

Stage III

At this stage, the tumor extends to the pelvic wall. Radiation therapy is also the preferred therapy for advanced disease. Surgery is occasionally helpful to relieve symptoms. Chemotherapy, though experimental, may be considered.

Stage IV

At stage IV, the tumor is growing into the lining of the bladder or rectum or there are distant metastases. Radiation therapy and surgery may be used to relieve symptoms. Chemotherapy may provide a temporary response.

FOLLOW-UP

Regular and meticulous follow-up is the most important part of conservative treatment for cancer of the vagina. This is especially true for those who have not had their lymph nodes removed. Patients should be carefully instructed in self-examination. This includes both the area of the primary cancer, where possible, and the regional lymph nodes. Patients should have a physical examination, pelvic examination, and Pap smear every three to four months for the first two years, and then every six months for the next three years. Blood chemistries, chest X-rays, and scans should be done for patients who develop symptoms. The amount of follow-up required varies with the situation. There can be a longer interval between visits if a wide surgical margin was used, and a shorter interval if a narrower margin was used.

15.

Cancer of the Vulva

Cancer of the vulva is an uncommon malignancy, accounting for less than 1 percent of all cancers among women and about 4 percent of gynecologic cancers. It occurs primarily in women over fifty years of age. Many women have another malignancy, such as cancer of the cervix, and many have a history of sexually transmitted diseases. The human papillomavirus (HPV) probably plays a role in causing this disease.

This chapter will cover the following topics: the anatomy of the vulva, the types of cancer that affect the vulva, how this cancer is graded, how this cancer spreads, what screening procedures are available, what the signs and symptoms are, how this cancer is diagnosed, how this cancer is staged, what treatments are available, my analysis of how conservative surgery can be used to treat this cancer, my recommendations for the appropriate treatment at each stage, and what sort of follow-up is needed after treatment.

ANATOMY AND PHYSIOLOGY

The vulva includes the *labia majora*—the outer lips—and the tissue in between them: the *labia minora*, or inner lips, the clitoris, and the urethral opening. The vulva is lined by *squamous epithelial cells* in a layer called the *mucosa*. The area between the vulva and the anus is called the *perineum*.

TYPES OF CANCER

About 90 percent of cancers arise from the squamous epithelial cells lining the vulva. *Adenocarcinoma,* which arises from glandular tissue, and malignant melanoma, discussed in Chapter 9, account for less than 5 percent each of all vulvar cancers. Noninvasive cancer is called *vulvar intraepithelial neoplasm* (VIN).

TUMOR GRADE

Some physicians believe that tumor grade influences prognosis, from grade 1, good prognosis, to grade 3, poor prognosis. Grade is determined by examining cells under a microscope. High-grade cells are rapidly dividing.

ROUTES OF SPREAD

The cancer becomes invasive after it penetrates through the basement membrane, the structure that supports the top layer of cells. Cancer of the vulva spreads first to the groin lymph nodes. It appears first in the superficial nodes, those closest to the skin, and then in the deep lymph nodes, those beside the large blood vessels in the leg. Vulvar cancer can then spread to the pelvic lymph nodes, deep in the pelvis, in front of the tailbone. Of patients with tumors less than 2 cm in diameter, about 10 percent will have spread of disease to the groin lymph nodes. Nodal spread also depends upon the depth of invasion, ranging from 0 percent for lesions 1 mm deep to more than 25 percent for those more than 5 mm deep. Most of this is microscopic spread. That is, the lymph nodes contain cancer cells, but are not enlarged. By the time a tumor is 2 to 4 cm in diameter, about one third of patients will have spread of disease to the lymph nodes. Lesions larger than 4 cm in diameter will have spread to the groin lymph nodes in over 50 percent of patients. Spread to the pelvic lymph nodes occurs in only about 5 percent of patients. Almost all patients with pelvic spread have enlarged lymph nodes that can be easily felt in the groin. Sites of distant spread include the lungs and bones.

SCREENING

The gynecologist will check for vulvar cancer at the time of the regular Pap smear.

SIGNS AND SYMPTOMS

The most common signs include a mass or ulcer. Symptoms are burning, bleeding, a discharge, or itching associated with a mass or ulcer.

DIAGNOSIS

The gynecologist confirms the diagnosis by sending a *biopsy* to the pathologist. For patients who have no obvious evidence of tumor spread to regional lymph nodes or other organs, additional tests are not necessary.

STAGES OF DISEASE

The International Federation of Gynecology and Obstetrics (FIGO) staging system is shown in Table 15.1.

TYPES OF TREATMENT

Treatment options include surgery and radiation therapy. There is little experience with chemotherapy for this disease, although several different drugs have been tried, and patients with advanced disease may be treated preoperatively in an effort to shrink the tumor. Hyperthermia is used in some experimental programs. See Chapter 5 for more information about these treatments, including general information on the side effects associated with each treatment.

Surgery

Conservative surgical procedures are gaining acceptance in the treatment of vulvar cancer.

Radical Vulvectomy

Radical vulvectomy consists of removal of the entire vulva, together with removal of the lymph nodes in both the right and the left groin regions, performed through one large operation. In a modified radical vulvectomy, only the affected half of the vulva is removed. The lymph nodes are removed through smaller, separate incisions. Often, only the lymph nodes on the

Table 15.1 FIGO Staging System for Vulvar Cancer

Stage	Description	Five-Year Survival Rate
0	A cancer that is limited to the topmost cell layer.	Over 95%
I	A cancer that is 2 cm or less in diameter and is limited to the vulva or perineum. Microinvasive cancer—The cancer has invaded less than 5 mm below the surface with no spread of disease.	Over 90%
II	A cancer that is larger than 2 cm and is limited to the vulva or perineum. There is no spread of disease.	80% to 90%
III	A cancer that can be of any size, with spread to the urethra, vagina, or anus, or if the regional lymph nodes contain cancer.	50%
IVa	A cancer that invades the upper urethra, the pelvic bones, or the lining of the bladder or rectum; or if there are lymph nodes in the groin on both sides that contain cancer.	15%
IVb	Distant metastases are present or the cancer has spread to the pelvic lymph nodes.	5% (distant metastases) to 15% (positive pelvic lymph nodes)

affected side are removed. These modifications have already reduced the complications of vulvar surgery.

The greatest complication of radical surgery is breakdown of the vulvar and groin incisions resulting in tissue death, infection, and lymph accumulation. This can be a dreadful complication, requiring months to heal and leaving considerable scarring. Modified surgery has reduced this complication from about 50 to 85 percent to about 20 to 50 percent, depending on the study.[1] Another serious complication is constant swelling of the leg on the side of the lymph node removal (or on both sides, if the nodes were removed on both sides). Modified surgery has reduced this from as high as 69 percent to about 20 percent of patients.[2] Scarring and narrowing of the vagina, urinary incontinence, and prolapse, or falling out of position, of the vagina or uterus are less common complications. Radical vulvectomy also results in significant sexual dysfunction.[3] Decreased sexual desire, painful or difficult intercourse, inability to achieve orgasm, and embarrassment are among the common complaints, occurring in 20 to 50 percent of women. In one study, of the 9 women who were sexually active prior to radical vulvectomy, only 5 returned to sexual activity.

Local Excision

The tumor is locally removed, usually with a 2-cm margin. This can be done with either a scalpel or a laser. The pelvic lymph nodes can be removed through a laparoscope, which is a tube inserted into the abdomen through which the surgeon manipulates tiny cutters. There are a few possible complications after laparoscopic surgery. An inability to urinate may occur in about 20 percent of patients. Bowel injury is very rare. If the pelvic lymph nodes are positive, the remaining nodes can be removed through the laparoscope. Most surgeons, though, prefer doing open abdominal surgery because they believe that the nodes can be more cleanly removed that way.

Radiation Therapy

Patients who have positive lymph nodes in either the groin or the pelvis may be treated with radiation therapy. A dose of 45 to 50 Gy of *external-beam* radiation is administered to the groin on the same side as the primary tumor. The complications of radiation are similar to those of groin lymph node removal. They include swelling of the leg and death of the skin in the area of treatment in 10 to 40 percent of patients. If a large tumor has been removed with a narrow margin of excision, radiation may be used at the site of the primary tumor.

Hyperthermia

Hyperthermia involves heating the tumor in order to kill the cancer cells, since these cells are more sensitive to heat than normal cells. Possible complications include blisters and burns. These can be controlled by monitoring the patient during treatment.

ANALYSIS

The treatment of vulvar cancer has traditionally been radical vulvectomy—removal of the entire vulva together removal of the lymph nodes in both the right and left groin regions. Since about 1970, several institutions have modified this approach by removing only the affected half of the vulva and removing the lymph nodes through smaller, separate incisions, or removing only the lymph nodes on the affected side. These modifications have already reduced the complications of vulvar surgery. Local excision often leads to increased rates of local recurrence, but not always. My analysis will focus first on the primary lesion, where the tumor first arose, and then on the lymph nodes. See Appendix I for further discussion of the studies reviewed.

The Primary Lesion

Some gynecologists are removing primary lesions with a 1-cm margin. A narrower margin may increase the chance for local recurrence. To assess the effect of local recurrence on overall survival, I have combined the results of several studies. I have found 21 patients who developed local recurrence isolated to the vulva following conservative surgery, either wide local excision or simple vulvectomy. They were followed for from one to twenty-eight years. All 21 were treated with reexcision. Two developed distant disease and died. Both may have originally had advanced disease, but this was not clear from the studies. Four patients died of other causes, and the remaining 15 were alive and well when last contacted.

It is reasonable to conclude that vulvar cancer can prudently be excised with a 1-cm margin. Risk factors include tumor size, depth of invasion, amount of cancer in the margins, amount of blood and lymph vessel involvement, and tumor grade. As in the case of other early cancers, patients who develop recurrent vulvar cancer following conservative surgery seem to have a second opportunity for cure. The above results are consistent with the results of conservative surgery in other parts of the body.

The Regional Lymph Nodes

The treatment of groin lymph nodes has been changing from

routine removal of all these nodes as part of a radical vulvectomy to removal or sampling of only the most superficial lymph nodes on the side of the primary tumor. If the superficial nodes are positive, then all the nodes on that side are removed. Positive groin lymph nodes are found in about 5 percent of patients with tumor invasion of 3 mm or less, and slightly over 10 percent of patients with invasion of 5 mm or less.

Few investigators have chosen to simply observe their patients, and remove the lymph nodes if they become enlarged. Many studies have shown this to be prudent for both breast cancer and cancer of the head and neck. If these lymph nodes behave as they do in other cancers, it may soon be prudent simply observe them closely every few months. I believe this option should be offered to selected patients who can participate in a conscientious follow-up process. It is likely to become the accepted treatment policy for selected patients with early disease. Lymph nodes in the pelvis, which cannot be easily monitored, usually become positive for cancer only after the lymph nodes in the groin are already positive.

TREATMENT ACCORDING TO STAGE

The following treatment options are recommended. Keep in mind that conservative surgery is best suited to the treatment of early cancer. Even so, I would still encourage you to ask your doctor about the most conservative options available to you in your specific case. Sometimes, radiation or chemotherapy is used before surgery to help shrink a large tumor. I think this is a good use for these therapies. "Standard treatment" refers to the treatment recommended as accepted medical practice.

Stage 0

At stage 0, only the topmost layer of cells is involved. Standard treatment consists of local removal.

Stage I

At this stage, the tumor is 2 cm or less in diameter and is limited to the vulva or perineum. There is no spread of disease. Standard therapy for patients with stage I cancer with less than 1 mm of invasion is wide local excision with margins of 1 to 2 cm. For lesions with more than 2 mm of invasion, removal of the groin lymph nodes on one side is added.

I believe that most patients can be prudently treated with wide local excision, or removal, of the tumor, using 1- to 2-cm margins. I also believe that narrower margins are acceptable in selected cases, for example, to preserve the clitoris. The superficial groin lymph nodes on the side of the tumor may be removed and sent to the pathologist. If they are positive, all the groin lymph nodes on that side should be removed. If the deep nodes are positive, then the pelvic lymph nodes should be treated with surgery or radiation therapy. In selected patients with nodes that feel normal, the lymph nodes may be examined regularly by the patient and the doctor, and removed if they enlarge.

Stage II

At this stage, the tumor is larger than 2 cm and is limited to the vulva or perineum. There is no spread of disease. Standard treatment is radical vulvectomy and removal of groin lymph nodes on both sides. However, I believe that patients with stage II disease can be treated with the same strategy as that outlined for stage I.

Stage III

At stage III, the tumor can be of any size with spread to the urethra, vagina, or anus, or the regional lymph nodes are positive. Standard treatment has been radical vulvectomy and removal of the groin lymph nodes on both sides. Many investigators believe that the primary tumor and the lymph nodes should be considered separately. If the patient has stage III disease because of the size or location of the primary lesion, she may consider preoperative radiation therapy or chemotherapy. I believe that the tumor can be removed with a marrow margin of excision. This is easier if the tumor shrinks following radiation or chemotherapy. Enlarged nodes should be removed at the time the tumor itself is removed. In selected patients with nodes that feel normal, the sentinel nodes should be biopsied. If they are positive, a complete lymph node removal should be performed.

Stage IVa

At this stage, the tumor invades the upper urethra, the pelvic bones, or the lining of the bladder or rectum, or there are positive groin lymph nodes on both sides. The primary tumor should be treated as outlined for patients with stage III disease. Enlarged groin lymph nodes should be removed and the pelvic nodes treated with surgery or radiation therapy. There are experimental programs involving radiation therapy, chemotherapy, and hyperthermia. If you want to find out more about such programs, either ask your doctor or call a regional cancer center in your area.

Stage IVb

At this stage, there is spread of disease to distant organs or the pelvic lymph nodes. Local surgery or radiation therapy may be used to control symptoms. Positive groin or pelvic lymph nodes should be treated with surgery or radiation therapy. As in the case of stage IVa, there are experimental programs involving radiation, chemotherapy, and hyperthermia.

FOLLOW-UP

Regular and meticulous follow-up is the most important part of conservative treatment for vulvar cancer. This is especially true for those who have not had their lymph nodes removed. Patients should be carefully instructed in self-examination, in both the area of the primary cancer and of the regional lymph nodes. Patients should have a physical examination, pelvic examination, and Pap smear every three to four months for the first two years, and then every six months for the next three years. Blood chemistries, chest X-rays, and scans should be done for patients who develop symptoms. Patients who do not return regularly should be advised to have their lymph nodes removed. The amount of follow-up required varies with the situation. There can be a longer interval between visits if a wide surgical margin was used, and a shorter interval if a narrower margin was used.

16.

Barriers to Change

There is nothing more difficult to carry out, more perilous to conduct, or more uncertain of success than to take the lead in the introduction of a new order of things.

Niccolo Machiavelli, 1532

Now that you have made it this far, I hope you have learned many things. You have learned that the surgical treatment of cancer is in the midst of great change. For most of this century, surgeons have attempted to completely remove every cancer cell in order to achieve local control and cure. Radical surgical procedures were the "gold standard" for the treatment of most solid tumors. It now appears that more limited operations may be equally effective. You have learned that local recurrence—once a dreaded complication of surgical therapy—may be only a harbinger of distant spread, but *not* its cause. This has been clearly demonstrated for breast cancer, and preliminary evidence suggests this to be true for many other cancers. You have learned that cancer provokes a struggle within each patient—a struggle between the growing cancer and the immune defenses of the patient. I have told you the conclusions I have reached about this tumor-host conflict, conclusions that I believe explain the innocent behavior of local recurrence in so many patients.

By now, you may be forming some opinions of your own about the treatment of cancer. I hope you agree with me that many cancers can be successfully treated in a more conservative manner. Perhaps you are asking a question I've heard many times before: "If I can understand the reasoning behind conservative treatment, why don't more surgeons accept your ideas?" In this chapter, I'll try to answer that question. Please note that I am not criticizing individuals. My focus is on the system itself.

THE FORCES AT PLAY IN THE DEBATE OVER CONSERVATIVE SURGERY

To understand how we have arrived at the current system, we must understand the forces at play on doctors and patients alike.

Cultural Forces and Beliefs

Our beliefs are molded from childhood by our family, friends, educational and religious institutions, political organizations, media outlets, and fellow workers. In brief, our beliefs are influenced by our culture. Increasingly, the medical profession thinks of itself as scientific—the impartial, objective observers of the facts. But doctors are also influenced by cultural forces.

Lynn Payer, in her book, *Medicine and Culture*, examines medical practice in France, Germany, Great Britain, and the United States. Doctors in the United States are aggressive. They order more blood tests, more X-rays, scans, and other imaging procedures. They perform more coronary artery bypasses, more hysterectomies. They give more medication. Payer says, "While American doctors love to use the word 'aggressive,' the French much prefer *les médecines douces*, or 'gentle therapies.'"[1] F. M. Hull, a British general practicioner, said, "American physicians seem to regard death as the ultimate failure of their skill. British doctors . . . regard death as . . . sometimes something to be wished."[2] Americans have increasingly come to expect miracles from the health professions. Almost everyone is exposed to the power of modern medicine, its wondrous technology and miraculous results. All of this leads to a denial of death.

The hospice movement is an example of the difference in medical philosophy between Britain and the United States. The modern hospice movement began in 1968 when Cicely Saunders opened St. Christopher's Hospice in London, in a country, not coincidentally, that was devastated by two world wars. Patients with terminal cancer were treated by those who were trained to be sensitive to the needs of the patients and families. Acceptance of death is a major part of hospice care. The movement has since spread to the United States, where the emphasis is on home care.

There are also philosophical differences between France and the United States. French doctors place great faith in *le terrain*—the soil—the constitution, the natural resistance of the patient to outside insult. American doctors focus on the insult, the French on the reaction. Perhaps the current popularity of wholistic medicine, with its emphasis on the patient's resistance to disease, is a reaction to this void in traditional American medicine.

Payer attributes the aggressive nature of American medicine to the effect of the vast American frontier upon all who came to settle here. Immigrants, mostly Europeans, came to believe that anything was possible for those who could successfully conquer adversity.[3] The hypothesis presented in Chapter 4 places great faith in a patient's *terrain*. This seed-and-soil hypothesis places equal weight on both the patient *and* the disease. Conservative surgery is not very popular in the United States because Americans focus on aggressive treatment, and not the natural resistance of the patient.

Forces Influencing Doctors' Decisions

Doctors are strongly influenced by the practices of their colleagues. A traditional rule among surgeons has been, "Don't be the first in your community to adopt a new procedure, and don't be the last." If all surgeons followed this maxim, then nothing would ever change. Someone has to be the first. All professionals are expected to conform to established treatment practices—the "standard of care" practiced by other doctors. This is an ethical and legal requirement that often impedes change. In these litigious times, doctors may be held responsible for poor results, especially if more treatment could have been given.

Consider a patient with breast cancer who must decide between breast-sparing surgery and mastectomy. She may live many miles from a radiation therapy facility, may be unable to miss six weeks of work, or may be unable to find transportation. Or she may not have the financial resources to pay for radiation treatment. She and her surgeon face this statement from the National Institutes of Health Consensus Development Conference on the Treatment of Early-Stage Breast Cancer: "Although local control [of the cancer] can be obtained in some patients with local excision alone, no subgroups have been identified in which radiation therapy can be avoided."[4] What do they do?

And this is not the only official pronoucement on this matter. In 1992, four professional societies of radiologists, surgeons, pathologists, and oncologists published "Standards for Breast Conservation Treatment." Among the questions it poses is, "Are there patients for whom breast irradiation can be omitted?" No answer was given, but the implied answer was, "Today, none." None of the references in the paper's bibliography cite studies that recommend partial mastectomy alone for selected patients with early breast cancer.

In England, over one third of surgeons treat their patients with wide excision alone and no postoperative radiation therapy.[5] I believe that this experience can be repeated here, that many patients with stage I breast cancer can be spared postoperative radiation therapy. Radiation does reduce local recurrence following narrow excision, but it does not add a single day to the survival of patients. (See the NSABP lumpectomy trial discussion in Chapter 1.[6]) But the documents cited above have practically eliminated this as a treatment option for American women.

Why are doctors so reluctant to change their standards of care? Two factors are the medical journals in which the results of investigations are published and the financial considerations involved.

The Medical Journals

The well-known medical and surgical journals, such as the *New England Journal of Medicine* and the *Journal of the American Medical Association* (JAMA), receive many more papers than they can publish. Good medical journals have a review process to evaluate and screen papers. The journal's editor sends a manuscript to two or three referees. They read the paper and return it with a recommendation to publish it or reject it. Papers that challenge the prevailing ideas face an uphill battle.

They are usually reviewed by established practitioners who are defenders of the prevailing views on treatment. At a well-known journal, one negative review often leads to the rejection of the paper. This process, known as peer review, favors the repetition of accepted ideas and the suppression of innovative ones.

Recently, medical journals have begun to study the methods they use to evaluate papers submitted for publication. At an American Medical Association meeting in 1989, David Horrobin, editor of *Medical Hypotheses*, gave eighteen examples "of situations in which peer review has delayed, emasculated, or totally prevented the publication of and investigation of potentially important findings." He said, "It is my view that innovation is so rare, so valuable, and so central to the improvement of patient welfare that innovative articles should be deliberately encouraged and more readily published than conventional ones."[7] This book was written, in large part, because many of the ideas expressed here have not been adequately debated in medical and surgical journals.

Financial Considerations

Ralph Moss in his book, *The Cancer Industry*, estimated that the cost of caring for cancer in 1991 was $100 billion.[8] Patients and their families seldom consider the cost of treatment when the enemy is cancer. Treatment may be life-saving surgery, or therapy that adds only a few weeks of life. Expense is seldom a factor. Most of the participants in the health-care system make their living from the delivery of care, not by preventing disease or restraining overly aggressive treatment. There is very little incentive to conserve these health-care dollars.

For example, a young woman with breast cancer could easily spend $25,000 in treatment:

Partial mastectomy and lymph node removal	$ 2,000
Hospital (including lab, anesthesia, etc.)	$12,000
Radiation therapy	$ 6,000
Chemotherapy	$ 5,000
TOTAL	$25,000

If the patient elected to have a mastectomy and reconstruction, she could spend an additional $11,000. By eliminating the

$6,000 cost of radiation therapy, her net additional cost would be $5,000, for a total cost of $30,000.

The cost of a partial mastectomy done as an outpatient is less than $5,000. As discussed in Chapter 4, there is little evidence that the added $20,000 to $25,000 cost of more aggressive treatment adds to the quality or duration of a patient's life.

Physicians and surgeons obviously have a financial incentive to practice their specialties. There continues to be competition among specialists to treat cancer with their own particular weapons. These forces are an accepted part of a free-market economy and should ultimately lead to the best possible care for all patients. A key ingredient in this scenario is an informed consumer. Some patients continuously repeat, "Doctors are just in it for the money." These patients would be better off using their energy to learn about their disease and its treatment. An informed patient is the principle beneficiary of a health-care system that offers choice.

Forces for Patient Choice

Fortunately, women are demanding more choices and more control over the treatment for breast cancer. By 1987, seventeen states had informed-consent laws that required doctors to offer breast-sparing treatment options to their patients with breast cancer. Various organizations, such as the National Association of Breast Cancer Organizations and the National Breast Cancer Coalition, are fighting for additional breast cancer research money. I hope that such organizations will also be fighting for a more rational treatment of breast cancer.

In 1994, Jerome Kassirer, the editor-in-chief of the *New England Journal of Medicine*, stated, "When they can, patients should always participate in decisions that affect their well-being. We have always implicitly respected patients' preferences about outcomes, but in the era of formal guidelines, this may not be enough, we may need to make these assessments explicit. We already know some of the circumstances that should alert us that we are dealing with an 'ultra-sensitive decision.'"[9] Kassirer was especially concerned about treatment options that varied greatly in their complications, but only marginally in their expected benefit. He also was concerned if a patient attached unusual importance to a particular outcome or was particularly averse to taking risks. Kassirer believes that patients' opinions are often more important than that of some distant panel of experts. So do I.

CANCER TREATMENT AND THE GENERAL SURGEON

For most of this century, the general surgeon has treated most cancer patients because most cancers occur in parts of the body that are covered by general surgery. However, great changes began in the 1950s, when high-voltage radiation therapy and chemotherapy were both introduced. As we saw in Chapter 1, multidisciplinary therapy coordinated these various specialists to give the patient optimum treatment in a well-planned regimen. But multidisciplinary therapy began to suffer from the excess of treatment by committee. Disciplines that once competed to treat patients began to acquiesce to one another. The result has become a therapeutic conglomeration that may maximize treatment, often needlessly.

The specialty of general surgery has been under attack from many sides. Ear, nose, and throat specialists began calling themselves head and neck cancer specialists. Some general surgeons joined with proctologists, specialists in anal and rectal surgery, and started a specialty of colon and rectal surgery. Vascular surgeons started issuing a certificate for special training. Thus, the specialty of general surgery has no clear identity, at least in the mind of the public. By the 1990s, general surgeons were in no mood to see more erosion by surgeons calling themselves surgical oncologists. For that reason, no recognized subspecialty of cancer surgery has been established.

Forty years ago, patients saw a surgeon for an initial biopsy and advice on treatment options. Today, patients are told to see a cancer specialist, an oncologist, for up-to-date care. But medical oncologists are primarily trained to give chemotherapy. They do not perform surgery. They do not administer radiation therapy. The vast majority of their experience is with patients whose disease has already spread.

Patient care is best served by the return of a single physician to coordinate patient care. Patients will be better off if their care is managed by one caring family doctor or surgeon who understands the principles of cancer treatment outlined in this book. It may be time for the pendulum to begin swinging back the way it came. Of all the cancer specialists, the general surgeons are best able to see the broad picture. Most of the cancer cures are achieved by them. They also see patients before and after radiation and chemotherapy, and sometimes administer chemotherapy themselves. Many surgeons and family doctors are well suited to this role, because they understand to role of adjuvant therapy, that administered in addition to surgery, and they understand the value of restraint. They are learning that following surgery for cure, radiation therapy may enhance local control, but it fails to increase patient survival. They are learning that chemotherapy only rarely prolongs life for patients with solid tumors, while causing significant side effects and complications.

Surgeons will gain the respect of the medical profession if they can solve the greatest dilemma of their own specialty: why is local recurrence following limited surgery an innocent, or nonthreatening, event? Randomized, prospective trials of breast cancer, malignant melanoma, and soft tissue sarcoma have demonstrated that promptly treated local recurrence following limited surgery does not adversely affect survival.[10-12] Indeed, there are no studies that are incompatible with the conclusions of these trials. Local recurrence may be a harbinger of distant disease, but not its cause. It may reflect the size, grade, or aggressiveness of the primary tumor, but, if treated promptly, is not the cause of tumor spread. This phenomenon has not been explained, and is being ignored by many in the profession. There is not a paper in any American surgical journal that attempts to explain the innocence of local recurrence.

AT THE HEART OF THE MATTER: CHANGING BELIEFS

Throughout most of the twentieth century, cancer surgeons believed that cancer must be totally removed or eradicated to be effectively treated. Doctors and patients alike want to do "everything possible" to eradicate the cancer. Few patients with curable disease want to "take any chances" with "experimental" treatment. Cancer is such a feared disease that surgeons have been slow to challenge the wisdom of radical surgery. Proponents of more conservative operations have been soundly criticized.

I believe that we are involved in a dramatic change in our perception of locally recurrent cancer. The NSABP lumpectomy trial, discussed in Chapter 1, has forever altered our perception of local recurrence. Once a dreaded complication, locally recurrent cancer is often innocent or nonthreatening in its behavior if treated promptly. Surgeons are completely revising their understanding of cancer. This change has placed the field of cancer surgery into the midst of a change in beliefs, as defined by Thomas S. Kuhn in his book, *The Structure of Scientific Revolutions*. In it, he traces the history of several different fields of science. He concluded that progress is not a slow and steady process. Instead, it is marked by revolutionary changes, in which younger members of a profession come to view their field from a different perspective. Thinkers are forced to completely alter their point of view in response to proven observations that no longer fit into the existing way of seeing things. Examples include the change from a flat world to a round one, or from an earth-centered to a sun-centered solar system.

Kuhn concludes that advancement is not made in an orderly fashion as described in textbooks. Change is often slow and difficult. When scientists make observations that conflict with the prevailing beliefs, they must reevaluate their interpretation of nature. Kuhn points out that leaders often cling with determination to the ideas they were taught, simply because they learned them from respected mentors. Older, established scientists usually defend their cherished beliefs with passion. New observations are ignored, rejected, or forced to fit into an outdated mold. He says, "When the profession can no longer evade anomalies that subvert the existing tradition of scientific practice—then begin the extraordinary investigations that lead the profession at last to a new set of commitments.... The ones known ... as scientific revolution."[13]

The treatment of cancer has reached this state. Kuhn's chapter on the resolution of revolutions offers no easy alternative solution to this problem. He says that change occurs one professional at a time. As the famous physicist Max Planck once said, "An important scientific innovation rarely makes its way by gradually winning over and converting its opponents: it rarely happens that Saul becomes Paul. What does happen is that its opponents gradually die out and that the growing generation is familiarized with the ideas from the beginning."[14]

The innocent behavior of local recurrence following conservative surgery has been a startling discovery. It directly contradicts the beliefs of twentieth century cancer surgery. It dramatically changes the role of surgery in the treatment of cancer. No longer must the surgeon struggle to remove every last cancer cell. The surgeon now has a second chance to cure the patient if recurrent disease appears. Cancer surgery is going through a 180-degree turnaround, from the belief that the surgeon must remove every last cancer cell to the belief that a few cells left behind are not a survival hazard.

Today, surgeons in positions of influence do not wish to give up their authority. They are the principal opponents of change. Some may be willing to change, but at their own pace, a pace that may be too slow to help you. The presentation of new ideas in medical schools, journals, and meetings is regulated by many who have earned their positions of authority supporting the principles of radical surgery. They are able to accept or reject ideas that challenge their beliefs. This system has fostered the repetition of erroneous ideas, and has suppressed those who challenge them.

I believe that resistance to change is not motivated primarily by self-interest. The great majority of practicing surgeons are following the advice of their leaders, and all are caught up in a process they may be unable to control. Resistance to change may be inevitable, the result of our inability to alter long-held, cherished beliefs.

17.

Conclusion and Ten Questions to Ask Your Doctor

You have now had a chance to consider a great deal of information about cancer. I hope that you have not found it too difficult. Some patients may feel that their decision about a particular form of treatment is a life-and-death matter. This is usually not true. At the time of treatment distant metastases have either been established or prevented. The type of initial surgery or radiation therapy does not alter this fact. Regrettably, there are no blood tests and no imaging studies that can detect whether microscopic disease has spread. Thus, patients must live with this unknown–an uncertainty that may be difficult to live with. It is tempting to try to reduce anxiety by accepting aggressive initial treatment. But his is not advisable. The advantage of aggressive initial therapy is its ability to reduce the chance that cancer will recur at the site of initial treatment, known as reducing the rate of local recurrence. Aggressive initial therapy cannot cure disease that may have silently spread to other parts of the body.

If you have read other books on the treatment of cancer, you may have noticed that they seldom present a range of treatment options. For each stage of each cancer there is usually a single treatment recommended. Occasionally there is a choice between surgery and radiation, such as for prostate cancer and cancer of the cervix. But the types of options suggested in this book are seldom encouraged.

You may need to make a decision about treatment for yourself or someone you care about. If so, here are some suggestions. Don't rush into treatment. Make an appointment to see your doctor, usually a surgeon. If the diagnosis was made by your family doctor, he or she will refer you to a surgeon. Then take a few days to study and understand the issues. Tumors become more likely to spread as they grow, so you should not waste time, but a few days won't hurt. If the tumor has already been removed, you have plenty of time to consider additional treatment. Get emotional support from a friend, or find a support group for patients with your particular illness (see Appendix II). Go to your surgeon or family doctor and tell her or him that you want to bring this book. Here are some questions you may want to ask your doctor. I have included my answers and chapter references for more information.

1. HOW MUCH SURGERY DO I NEED?

For most of this century, radical surgery has been the cornerstone of cancer treatment. Surgeons tried to remove the visible tumor, cells that may become malignant, and a generous safety margin of normal tissue. The trend lately has been away from radical surgery, for example, lumpectomy for breast cancer instead of mastectomy. Other cancers are now being studied to learn whether conservative surgery is effective. Definitive results for many of these cancers will not be available for many years. I believe that biological principles learned from breast cancer, the most thoroughly studied so far, can be applied to other malignancies. Most cancers can be prudently treated by removal of the cancer along with a margin of normal tissue confirmed by a pathologist to be free of cancer. An added 1 to 2 cm of apparently healthy tissue may also be removed to help reduce the chance of local recurrence. These ideas are reviewed in the Preface, Chapter 1, and Chapter 4.

2. HAS THE CANCER SPREAD?
CAN THE SURGEON GET IT ALL?

At the time of surgery, cancer cells may have already spread to other parts of the body. Small colonies the size of mustard seeds may be growing in nearby lymph nodes or distant organs. There are no tests that can reliably detect the early spread of cancer. CAT scans, MRIs, and X-rays are generally of little help for patients with early disease. Tumors must be about 1 cm in diameter to be seen by most imaging techniques. Some blood tests, such as that for prostate-specific antigen, can detect the early appearance of cancer or the reappearance of disease following treatment. But such tests do not yet exist for most cancers in their earliest stages.

The conservative treatment recommended in this book requires regular check-ups with your doctor after treatment. Recurrent cancer after a conservative operation must be promptly treated. Chapter 2 discusses how cancer spreads.

3. WHAT HAPPENS TO TUMOR CELLS THAT REMAIN AFTER SURGERY?

The fate of cancer cells in the area of surgery is quite controversial. For most of this century, surgeons have seen the grave consequences of locally recurrent cancer. Indeed, local recurrence after radical surgery is usually a sign that distant spread has already occurred. However, after conservative surgery, local recurrence is not such a bad sign. Promptly treated recurrences can be removed without threatening patient survival. Surgeons who believe they have a second chance to remove tumor cells are less prone to perform radical surgery at the first operation. This is one of the most surprising conclusions of modern cancer studies. It is discussed in Chapters 3 and 4.

4. WHAT IF THE CANCER HAS SPREAD TO THE LYMPH NODES?

If the surgeon can feel enlarged lymph nodes and concludes they may contain cancer, he will remove them. Occasionally, the surgeon will remove the lymph nodes just to test for the presence of cancer, even if they are not enlarged. He can learn if the cancer is early and localized or has spread to the nodes. The more spread has occured, the worse the prognosis. Some doctors recommend chemotherapy for patients whose disease has spread to the lymph nodes. The answer to this question varies, depending in part upon the success of chemotherapy in each type of cancer. See question 7 below and refer to Chapter 5.

5. WHAT PROBLEMS SHOULD I EXPECT FROM SURGERY?

Permanent disability is related to the amount of normal tissue removed to completely excise the tumor. If surgery may cause significant functional or cosmetic complications, the surgeon should thoroughly explain the anticipated disability or deformity. He should also strive to reduce the amount of healthy tissue removed. This may be helped by asking a pathologist to check the borders around the tumor until all microscopic evidence of cancer has been eliminated, and removing only that amount of tissue. Only your doctor can clearly explain how his suggested treatment is likely to affect you. Refer to Chapter 5 and the chapters about each cancer, Chapters 6 through 15, for more information.

6. DO I NEED RADIATION (X-RAY) THERAPY?

If your doctor is concerned that cancer cells may remain in the surgical field or nearby lymph nodes, radiation can often kill these cancer cells. Radiation kills cancer cells in those specific areas of the body where the X-ray beam is pointed. Adjuvant radiation therapy, or radiation following complete removal of the tumor, reduces local recurrence, but rarely, if ever, increases patient survival. Cancer can still return in areas of the body already treated with radiation.

Radiation can cause a temporary burn of the skin, like a sunburn. Most patients feel fatigued during the several weeks of therapy, and nausea is a side effect. Radiation therapy may also slightly increase your chances of developing a second malignancy, including leukemia. Refer to Chapter 5 for more information on radiation therapy. Refer to Chapter 4 to learn why killing cancer cells locally has little effect on survival.

7. WHAT ABOUT CHEMOTHERAPY?

Chemotherapy is often recommended for patients following surgery. If the surgery removed all visible cancer, such treatment is called adjuvant chemotherapy. A few patients with breast and colon cancer may have their lives prolonged slightly, but virtually none are cured because of chemotherapy. Almost all patients experience the side effects of chemotherapy, such as vomiting and hair loss. Since the benefit of chemotherapy may be so minimal and does vary among tumors, you will want to ask your doctor specifically, "How many added months of survival are gained by the average patient with my stage of disease?" Refer to Chapter 5.

8. ARE YOU SYMPATHETIC TOWARD THE CONSERVATIVE TREATMENT OF CANCER?

Here are some characteristics of general surgeons who are sympathetic toward conservative surgery. Generally, they began treating patients with breast-sparing surgery during the mid-1980s. Surgeons who waited until later were trained to respect the principles of radical surgery, and may have more difficulty parting with those principles. Most patients with operable breast cancer can be prudently treated with breast-sparing surgery. If your surgeon still performs mastectomy on many of his patients, even the "modified" mastectomy, he may be less than sympathetic to conservative surgery.

If you are consulting a gynecologist or urologist, you should ask if he or she is sympathetic toward conservative treatment. Surgeons who are committed to radical surgery may be clearly hostile toward lesser treatment. Surgeons who treat cancer should be aware of the results of the NSABP lumpectomy trial, discussed in Chapter 1, since it is one of the most thorough studies on the surgical treatment of cancer. Ask your surgeon if he believes that the biological principles learned from that study apply to your disease as well.

Most surgeons will reveal by their attitude their opinion about conservative surgery. This is discussed in Chapters 1 and 16.

9. CAN YOU REFER ME TO SOMEONE WHO ADVOCATES A POSITION THAT IS DIFFERENT FROM YOURS?

Many authorities stress the importance of a second opinion, but this does little good when both opinions come from the same school of thought. In the 1970s, a patient with breast cancer could have sought two opinions or two dozen and still have been treated with a mastectomy. Today, patients with other malignancies are in that same situation. If you are concerned about the functional or cosmetic consequences of surgery, get a second opinion from an advocate of conservative treatment. If there is a large hospital in your area, see if they have a doctor referral service. Also, contact a couple of the organizations listed in Appendix II, since talking to other people with cancer might lead you to a suitable doctor.

You might wish to call ahead and ask if the doctor is willing to discuss the treatment recommendations presented in this book. If you find a surgeon who is sympathetic to the general ideas expressed here, you will be on the right track for one of your opinions. This book simplifies some very complex issues and cannot consider all the factors that lead to a final treatment decision. Only you and your surgeon can do that.

I have supported partial mastectomy without radiation therapy since the late 1970s. Nevertheless, I have always suggested that patients obtain the opinion of physicians whose views differ from my own. I encourage all patients to learn both sides of this debate directly from physicians who *advocate* opposing views. (You wouldn't ask a Ford salesperson about a Honda.) Your surgeon should be willing to direct you to a colleague who advocates a different mode of treatment.

10. WHY DO PATIENTS WHO DEVELOP LOCALLY RECURRENT CANCER FOLLOWING CONSERVATIVE SURGERY DO SO WELL?

The innocent or nonthreatening behavior of locally recurrent cancer remains a real mystery. Some doctors have given it only passing thought. My own impression is that it should profoundly affect a surgeon's attitude about how much normal tissue he should remove. My explanation of this mystery is found in Chapter 4. If you have the time and patience, become familiar with these ideas. I hope Chapter 4 will give you some peace of mind regarding the recommendations presented in this book.

IN CONCLUSION

In order to summarize important principles of cancer treatment in this book, I have had to simplify many complicated and controversial areas. The answers offered here may need to be modified for each individual case, but the questions are valid for all cases. Doctors are under some pressure to recommend aggressive treatment. You will want to find a doctor who makes you feel comfortable and is willing to consider the conservative recommendations presented here. Visit your doctor with a companion to provide emotional support. He or she may also help you remember questions you need to ask, ask questions of the surgeon while you collect your thoughts, and, later, help you remember the overall discussion as you consider your options. Also, carry a notepad along. If you encounter a specialist who is unwilling to consider your concerns, you may need to get the opinion of another doctor.

To participate effectively in the decisions regarding your treatment, you will need to work, study, and prepare. Many patients spend more time considering the purchase of an appliance than they do studying treatment options for cancer. Don't be satisfied with the simple answers offered above. Read this book and others until you are confident that you understand the issues. The many unknowns in cancer serve as a great equalizer between doctors and their patients. See Chapter 2.

Here are some general principles for conservative cancer treatment. Remember, they are general: Cancers small enough for surgical excision often can be removed with a 1- to 2-cm margin of normal tissue. (Two cm is about the diameter of a nickel.) If narrower margins are necessary to preserve an important part of the body, a pathologist should confirm that there is no cancer at the edge of the tissue removed. Radiation therapy may be considered if the tumor is attached to a nerve, the vocal cords, or another important structure. But additional radiation after surgery "just to be sure" seldom, if ever, prolongs life. Seek the advice of someone who does not feel constrained by legal requirements to recommend only standard treatment. Include a visit to your family doctor or, if you can, to a doctor who has made similar decisions for himself or a family member.

You have already taken the first step if you have gotten this far. Conservative treatment will often be associated with a higher risk of locally recurrent cancer, but the appearance of local recurrence does not mean that the choice of conservative treatment was wrong. However, as patients exercise their right to choose treatment, they must also accept the risks associated with each choice.

HEART TO HEART

Patients who wish to receive conservative therapy will face many barriers. Aided by the information presented in these pages, however, you should be able to find treatment that preserves bodily form and function without compromising your opportunity for cure. The goal of the physician and surgeon is to do everything possible to make their patients' lives happier and healthier, longer if possible, and more comfortable to bear. The physician should help the patient accept that there are things that are outside the control of science and medicine. In short, patients and doctors alike can all benefit from these well-known words:

> God, give us grace to accept with serenity the things that cannot be changed,
> Courage to change the things which should be changed,
> And the wisdom to distinguish the one from the other.
>
> Reinhold Niebur, The Serenity Prayer, 1942

Appendix I

Selected Studies in Conservative Surgery

This Appendix includes a history of treatment for various cancers, as well as a summary of studies in which conservative surgery has been used. I have attempted to include all the relevant information for each cancer. I have not intentionally excluded any study that may have not supported the thesis of this book. For example, in the section on soft tissue sarcomas, I include a study which claims that local recurrence does adversely affect survival. I also include a rebuttal to this conclusion.

The information addressed in this book falls within three different surgical specialties: general surgery, gynecology, and urology. Each of these specialties requires at least five years of residency training after the completion of medical school. No one book can encompass the information of a single training program, much less three. A single book cannot adequately deal with a single cancer, much less ten. But this is an exhaustive review of the available information on the subject of conservative surgery for each cancer discussed.

If you made it this far, you are probably smart and intensely interested in learning. This book does not prepare you to debate with your doctor. But it should prepare you to understand the issues. The following studies should serve as benchmarks for you own decisions. In case it's not clear by now, I hope you will seek out a surgeon who is genuinely sympathetic to conservative treatment for at least one opinion. See Appendix II for research studies published from 1995 to 2001.

CHAPTER 6: BLADDER CANCER

The first cystectomy for bladder cancer was probably performed in Cologne, Germany, in 1887 by B. Bardenheuer.[1] F. H. Martin performed the first cystectomy in the United States in 1899. Most surgeons avoided the procedure because so many patients died or had serious complications. For example, Hugh Young of Johns Hopkins in Baltimore, known as the father of urology, never performed the operation.

The earliest cystoscope was invented in 1877. It was improved during the 1880s, an improvement due in part to Edison's incandescent light bulb. The cystoscope allowed bladder tumors to be removed or cauterized (burned away) without major surgery by going through the urethra in an operation known as transurethral resection, or TUR.

Radium was first used to treat bladder tumors in 1903. A variety of techniques were used to place radon seeds or other sources of radiation directly inside the bladder. The development of high-voltage radiation therapy during the 1950s increased the use of external-beam radiation.

Antibiotics were available by the 1940s, by which time advances had been made in anesthesia. This made surgery easier, and the radical cystectomy was again favored by some urologists. Unfortunately, the survival results remained discouraging. By the 1950s, some urologists returned to TUR.

In 1956, J. A. Nichols and V. F. Marshall of New York Hospital reviewed their experience from 1932 to 1948 with 112 patients using local removal and fulguration, or the use of electric current to destroy a tumor.[2] They concluded that patients with bladder tumors of a low grade and low stage could be successfully treated with bladder-sparing surgery. Patients with high-grade or high-stage lesions did not do so well and, they suggested, needed more aggressive surgery.

In 1987, H. W. Herr of Memorial Sloan-Kettering Hospital in New York reviewed the treatment of 45 patients with muscle-infiltrating bladder cancer using TUR.[3] Patients were followed for three to seven years. Thirty-two patients, or 71 percent, developed further bladder cancer. Twenty-one of these were retreated with TUR, and were doing well when last evaluated. Eleven patients developed new bladder cancers—not recurrences—that were treated by cystectomy. Four of these patients died of bladder cancer. Four patients developed metastatic disease; two had no disease in the bladder. The overall survival of patients free of disease was 82 percent. There is no evidence that any deaths were due to the limited initial surgery.

Five years later, Herr reviewed the experience of other urologists who treated bladder cancer with TUR.[4] He concluded that TUR was as effective as radical surgery. For patients with cancer that deeply invaded the bladder muscle, the five-year survival rate for TUR was 57 percent; for radical cystectomy, it was 60 percent. These figures are not statistically different. Herr concluded, "From this review, transurethral resection does not appear to cause metastasis or jeopardize surgical cure."

In 1992, P. Sweeney and associates from Case Western Reserve University in Cleveland summarized the experience from over ten hospitals with partial cystectomy.[5] They found 532 patients who had been treated with partial cystectomy. Local recurrence developed in about 60 percent—38 percent to 78 percent, covering a wide range of surgical techniques, tumor grades, and so forth—of patients. But only 8 percent of patients treated with partial cystectomy required surgical treatment later. The majority were treated with repeat TUR or fulguration. Patient survival was determined by both the grade of the tumor and the stage of the disease. The type of treatment did not affect survival.

Consider the survival of patients whose recurrences were treated with cystectomy. M. H. Faysal and T. S. Freiha from Stanford University in California treated 117 patients with partial cystectomy.[6] They reviewed these cases in 1979. Recurrences developed in 78 percent of patients. About half of these patients developed recurrences that were of a higher stage than their first cancer. About 40 percent developed recurrences that were of a higher grade than their first cancer. However, the authors do not mention their follow-up schedule and state that information was obtained from the California Tumor Registry. Patients may not have been seen every three months, as many urologists now recommend. About 49 percent of these patients lived for five years following treatment of their recurrence. The survival rate was higher for patients who were ultimately treated with cystectomy, but these patients may have had less advanced recurrences. Those who had no cystectomy may have had advanced disease, and were thus inoperable.

In other studies, investigators from the Cleveland Clinic and the University of Iowa have reported favorable experience with bladder-sparing surgery.[7,8] Investigators at Massachusetts General Hospital have designed a treatment plan that combines TUR, systemic chemotherapy, and external-beam radiation.[9]

CHAPTER 7: BREAST CANCER

Chapter 1 covers much of the history of breast cancer treatment. Beginning with the radical mastectomy of Halsted, it reviews the studies that have led some surgeons to practice tumor removal plus postoperative radiation therapy. However, during the late 1980s, 55 to 90 percent of all patients with stage I disease elected to have a mastectomy.[10,11] Some patients did not wish to undergo several weeks of radiation treatment, or they found that radiation facilities were not easily available.[12] Others chose mastectomy because they feared local recurrence. This is the reason that most surgeons recommend the routine use of postoperative radiation therapy following any form of breast-sparing surgery. In Chapter 4, I tried to reassure you that local recurrence following conservative surgery is not a grave event. Removing a second, recurrent cancer at the same site does not impair survival. In this Appendix, I would like to examine the role that radiation therapy plays in breast-sparing surgery, and encourage selected patients to avoid radiation altogether.

In the United States, the lumpectomy trial conducted by the NSABP, a breast cancer project, is largely responsible for the increasing popularity of breast-conserving surgery.[13] This study proved that lumpectomy or lumpectomy plus radiation therapy can achieve survival rates equal to mastectomy survival rates for patients with stages I and II breast cancer. (Stage I cancers are 2 cm or less with no lymph node spread, while stage II cancers are 2 cm to 5 cm, or with spread to the nodes in the armpit.) The study also showed that patients treated with lumpectomy alone had a very high rate of local recurrence. These results are summarized in Table A.1.

Most breast cancers send out strands of tumor cells in many directions. In the NSABP trial, most patients had a tumor removed with a margin that was within 1 cm. Although the primary mass was removed, in many patients some cancer cells remained along these strands. There were so few cells that they could easily be missed, even by a careful surgeon and pathologist. Thus, lumpectomy alone, without radiation therapy, resulted in a high rate of local recurrence. I believe that the secret to successful surgery is a wide margin of excision. Excision of a 1- to 2-cm margin of tissue can remove most or all of the cancer cells along strands of tissue radiating from a tumor.

Partial Mastectomy Versus Lumpectomy and Radiation Therapy

There is no doubt that radiation therapy killed tumor cells in most of the patients treated by lumpectomy and radiation. It reduced local recurrence from 43 to 12 percent. That is dramatic. But can these cells be eliminated by surgery alone?

I believe that, based on recent experience, surgeons who perform a careful wide excision, a real partial mastectomy, can achieve results equal to those achieved by lumpectomy and radiation therapy. In this section, I will focus on the experience of those surgeons who have treated patients with breast-sparing surgery alone. I have included the results of the NSABP study primarily for comparison.

Appendix I

Table A.1. NSABP Lumpectomy Trial Results

Treatment	Local Recurrence	Survival Rate After 8 Years
Mastectomy	8%	82%
Lumpectomy alone	43%	83%
Lumpectomy with radiation	12%	84%

In 1939, Vera Peters of Princess Margaret Hospital in Toronto began to treat patients with tumor excision both with and without radiation therapy.[14] By 1974, she had treated 184 patients with excision and postoperative radiation therapy, and 19 patients with excision alone. Only 1 of the 19 patients developed "progressive disease." The survival rates in these two groups were the same. (More recent results from this institution are presented in Table A.2.)

George Crile, Jr., of the Cleveland Clinic began treating patients with partial mastectomy in 1955. About 20 percent of his patients, those with more advanced disease, received postoperative radiation therapy.[15] In 1990, he reviewed his experience with 291 patients treated through 1975, the year Dr. Crile stopped performing surgery.[16] Thirty-two patients, or 11 percent, developed local recurrence in the breast. This includes patients from both groups, those who were treated with surgery alone and those who also received radiation therapy.

In 1993, the Cleveland Clinic reported its experience in treating 328 patients—in addition to the patients Crile studied—with cancers 2 cm or less in diameter. Following partial mastectomy, about 11 percent of stage I patients developed local recurrence after five years. Of these patients, 14 percent developed local recurrence after ten years. The importance of wide margins is demonstrated in the results from the Cleveland Clinic, where margins of 1 to 2 cm are standard.[17]

In 1971, Robin Tagart of Newmarket General Hospital in England began to treat the first of 37 patients with partial mastectomy without postoperative radiation. He ended his study in 1978, when he learned that 37 percent of them had developed local recurrence in the treated breast,[18] although he did continue to perform wide excision with radiation therapy. But Tagart concluded that the initial treatment used did not affect survival, even when limited to partial mastectomy alone.

Several other institutions have recently reported their experience with breast-conserving surgery without radiation therapy.[19,20] All agree that survival is not adversely affected by the omission of radiation therapy.

Table A.2. Local Recurrence Rates in Patients with Tumors of 2 cm or Less

Trial	Number of Patients	Margins	Pathologically Positive Axillary Nodes (%)	Rate of Recurrence
Royal Marsden[21]	81	≥ 2.5 cm	None*	11%**
Uppsala-Örebro[22]	381	~ 1 cm	None	18%+
Cleveland, 1957–1975[23,24]	152	≥ 2 cm	12%	11%
Cleveland, 1975–1988[25]	328	≥ 2 cm	None	11%
Roswell Park[26]	8	1 to 2 cm	22%	13%
Miami[27]	59	≥ 1 cm	22%	10%
NSABP[28]	298	<1 cm	None	27%
Princess Margaret[29]	207 (low risk)++	0.5 to 1 cm	None	14% (low risk)
Milan, Italy[30]	280	2 to 3 cm	33%	9%

* Clinical staging (see Chapter 5).
** Includes axillary (armpit) lymph node recurrences.
\+ Includes updated information from a 1994 study.
++Tumors of 2 cm or less in patients fifty years of age or older.

Partial Mastectomy and Smaller Tumors

I will now focus on patients with tumors 2 cm or less in diameter. Table A.2[31] presents the experience of several institutions in treating patients with such tumors. Most breast cancer patients in the United States are now treated with tumors of this size. Larger tumors are more difficult to adequately treat using surgery alone and are much more likely to result in local recurrence.

These studies show that patients whose tumors can be removed with a 1- to 2-cm margin of tissue can often be spared postoperative radiation therapy. Local recurrence rates of 11 percent or less can be achieved in most patients with tumors of 2 cm or less. In 1990, the Uppsala-Örebro Breast Cancer Study Group reported a local recurrence rate of 10.2 percent. However, in 1994, the same group reported an unexpected and markedly higher local recurrence rate among patients treated without radiation therapy of 18.4 percent.[32] They speculated that as more hospitals and doctors were added to the study, the criteria for inclusion in the study were less strictly followed. They concluded that some patients may have had "overlooked multifocality [numerous areas of cancer] on preoperative mammograms, margins of surgical excision that were too narrow, and less extensive pathological examination of the specimen [tissue removed at surgery] that resulted in incomplete removal of mutifocal lesions."

Physicians at the Royal Marsden Hospital, Uppsala-Örebro Hospital, the Cleveland Clinic, the Roswell Park Memorial Institute, and the University of Miami believe that radiation therapy can be safely eliminated in selected patients. Princess Margaret and the National Cancer Institute in Milan, Italy, use radiation routinely. There is agreement that before she can forgo radiation therapy, a patient should have lymph nodes that are free of disease, and that there should be little or no evidence of surrounding cancer.

Recurrence is less common among older patients. Thus, investigators at the Royal Marsden Hospital in England recommend that patients less than fifty years of age be treated with radiation therapy. Investigators at Roswell Park Memorial Institute in Buffalo recommend radiation therapy for patients less than seventy years of age. Surgeons from the University of Miami use postoperative radiation therapy if the tumor invades into nerves, lymph vessels, or blood vessels.

There are several factors that influence recurrence rates after surgery: the size of the primary tumor, the width and pathological status of the margin, lymph node status, patient age, the presence of cancer in the cells lining the milk ducts, tumor grade, DNA analysis, and invasion of tumor into blood vessels, nerves, or lymphatic vessels. If patients are carefully selected based upon these factors, satisfactory local control can be achieved with surgery alone.

CHAPTER 8: CANCER OF THE CERVIX

In the early 1800s, cancer of the cervix was treated with removal of the cervix. By the 1890s, Emil Ries of Chicago and John Clark of Baltimore had both described the radical hysterectomy, including pelvic lymph node removal. The procedure was popularized in Europe by Ernst Wertheim of Austria. By 1911, he had treated 500 patients and published a clear anatomical description of both the way this disease spread and of his operative technique. This operation still bears his name.

Radiation therapy was also used to treat cervical cancer. Johns Hopkins Hospital in Baltimore was a leader in this field under Howard Kelly, the first professor of gynecology, in the 1890s. In 1933, Joseph Meigs of Massachusetts General Hospital began to use surgery to treat patients who failed radiation therapy. His extended radical hysterectomy, which included pelvic lymph node removal, gained in popularity after World War II.

In 1948, Alexander Brunschwig of Memorial Hospital in New York introduced radical pelvic exenteration for recurring cervical cancer.

All the pelvic organs were removed. This required a permanent diversion of both the urinary and digestive tracts to openings in the abdominal wall. This operation is seldom used today.

By the 1950s, the limits of radical surgery had been reached. As with many other cancers, surgeons began to consider more conservative measures. For cancer of the cervix, most of this work has been done in Europe. From 1958 to 1988, Erich Burghardt and colleagues at the University of Graz in Austria performed conization—removal of a cone-shaped section of the cervix—on 26 patients with stage Ia$_2$ cervical cancer, or cancer limited to the cervix.[33] Five-year results are available on 18 patients. Three developed local recurrence. All were treated with radical hysterectomy and/or radiation therapy. One of these patients missed her follow-up appointment for three years and returned with stage II$_b$ disease, or cancer that has spread beyond the cervix. She died three years after radical hysterectomy and radiation therapy. The other two patients were free of disease after treatment of the recurrence. One had radical hysterectomy, the other had radiation therapy. Another 93 patients with stage Ia$_1$ disease were treated with conization. None developed local recurrence.

In 1978, K. J. Lohe of the University of Munich and colleagues from the Universities of Erlangen, Freiburg, Heidelberg, and Cologne published their experience with 134 patients with microscopic cancer (stage Ia$_2$).[34] They treated 118 of these patients with hysterectomy. About 20 percent also received radiation therapy. Sixteen were treated with conization. Of these, 9 also had radiation therapy. After five years, 94 percent were living; after ten years, 85 percent were living. None of the patients treated with conization developed a recurrence or died of cervical cancer. The authors concluded, "If proof is given that the microcarcinoma [microscopic cancer] was totally removed with the conization, further operative measures, in general, may become unnecessary."

E. Holzer and colleagues from Austria treated 61 patients with conization alone—53 with stage Ia$_1$ disease and 8 with stage Ia$_2$ disease.[35] All patients whose tumors were completely excised were alive and well after three years.

Per Kolstad of Norwegian Radium Hospital in Oslo treated 48 patients with stage Ia disease with conization (15 of them were at stage Ia$_2$).[36] During the three- to seventeen-year follow-up, 4 of the 48 developed local recurrence. All were treated with additional surgery or radiation therapy. None of the 48 developed distant metastases or died of cancer.

K. Ebeling from the University of Berlin and colleagues from six other hospitals in the former East Germany reported on 530 patients with stage Ia cervical cancer.[37] Of these, 496 were treated with hysterectomy and 34 were treated with conization. Following hysterectomy, 17 patients, or 3 percent, developed local recurrence. Following conization, 2 patients, or 6 percent, developed local recurrence. There was no significant difference in the fatality rates between the limited surgery (1.1 percent) and radical surgery (2.8 percent). The authors noted that following limited surgery "as a rule the recurrences can be easily treated with secondary treatment [another operation] to avoid fatality."

M. Morris and others from M. D. Anderson Hospital in Houston reported on 14 patients with microinvasive cancer—3 mm or less—treated with conization.[38] The average depth of invasion was 1.6 mm and the average follow-up was 26.5 months. No patient developed a recurrent cancer.

Since 1987, D. Dargent of Hopital E. Harriot in Lyon, France, has treated 9 patients by removing most of the cervix in an operation called a trachelectomy.[39] He reported in 1992 on these patients, who had stage Ia$_2$ through IIa disease. On follow-up examination, one patient was found to have a 2-cm cancer of the inner lining of the cervix. This recurrence had been missed on an earlier follow-up. It was removed, but she died after a large mass of undifferentiated cancer was found in the bone of her right hip eighteen months later. A second patient developed a cervical intraepithelial neoplasia related to the human papillomavirus. This was treated by laser therapy. One patient was treated for cervical narrowing. One was treated for failure to menstruate. Thus, 8 of the 9 women were alive and well when last contacted, and 4 had children.

Benjamin Greer and others from the University of Washington Medical Center in Seattle performed a conization biopsy on 50 patients with stage Ia$_2$ cancer.[40] Thirty-three, or 66 percent, had positive margins and 17, or 33 percent, had negative margins. All were treated with hysterectomies, and the uterus of each patient was examined. Four of the 17 patients with negative margins, or 24 percent, were found to have residual disease in the uterus. Wider margins of excision and careful examination of the cone specimen should significantly reduce the number of patients with residual disease.

S. Rutledge and colleagues from the University of Western Ontario treated 47 patients who developed recurrent cervical cancer following radiation therapy.[41] Although radical pelvic exenteration has been commonly practiced for this condition, the authors concluded that conservative surgery—in these advanced cases, radical hysterectomy—could be prudently performed in selected patients.

Cancer During Pregnancy

In 1993, V. Sivanesaratnam and associates from the University Hospital of Kuala Lumpur in Malaysia reported on 14 patients who developed cervical cancer during pregnancy.[42] All were treated with a hysterectomy. If the pregnancy was in the last trimester, the baby was delivered. Surgery was delayed to improve fetal viability—the ability of the fetus to live outside of the mother—in two patients. One of these patients developed a local recurrence, which was successfully removed. She was alive and well when last contacted. These patients did as well as similar cervical cancer patients who were not pregnant. This suggests that pregnancy itself does not adversely affect the course of this disease.

B. J. Monk and F. J. Montz from the UCLA School of Medicine in Los Angeles reported on 13 patients treated between 1955 and 1991.[43] Following a cone biopsy, seven of these patients delayed their delivery and treatment until fetal maturation, one from the first trimester, and three each from the second and third trimesters. All patients eventually delivered their children and received standard therapy. The only death occurred in a patient who had a large, deeply invasive lesion, diagnosed 35 weeks into her pregnancy. With an average follow-up of twenty months (ranging from 2 to 228 months), all the remaining patients are alive and free of disease.

B. Duggan and associates from the University of Southern California delayed therapy in 8 pregnant patients.[44] Four of them were less than twenty weeks pregnant. All 8 patients had definitive therapy after delivery. They were all free of disease when last seen.

CHAPTER 9: MALIGNANT MELANOMA

Studies of malignant melanoma fall into two catagories: those that look at treatment of the primary lesion, and those that look at treatment of the lymph nodes.

The Primary Lesion

In 1908, Sampson Handley delivered the famous Hunterian Lectures on malignant melanoma to the Royal College of Surgeons of England.[45] By his own admission, Handley had never treated or seen a case of primary malignant melanoma, basing all of his recommendations upon a single autopsy of a patient who had died of widespread melanoma. Nevertheless, his recommendations became the standard of treatment for most of this century. Handley suggested removing a 1-inch circumference of skin and a 2-inch margin of tissue underneath the skin all around the melanoma. That recommendation was later expanded to 5 cm, and even 15 cm in selected cases.[46,47]

Several investigators supported this trend by reporting premalig-

changes in the skin within several centimeters of the primary lesion.[48-50] As recently as 1990, D. L. Morton of Los Angeles recommended margins of 3 cm for melanomas of intermediate thickness.[51]

Researchers with the World Health Organization evaluated the records of 593 patients.[52] They concluded that when lesions were removed with a margin of 2 cm or more, the local recurrence rate was about 5 percent. If the margin of excision was reduced to 1 or 2 cm, the local recurrence rate increased to about 12 percent. Surprisingly, the increased rate of local recurrence did not cause a reduction of patient survival.

In 1983, C. Schmoeckel and associates from the University of Munich analyzed 577 cases of localized malignant melanoma seen at that institution.[53] Only 3 patients, or 2.9 percent, treated with margins of greater than 3 cm developed local recurrence, while 36, or 10 percent, treated with narrower margins developed locally recurrent disease. The increased rate of local recurrence did not adversely affect survival. Mathematical analysis demonstrated that local recurrence was an indicator of a poor prognosis, but not its cause.

In 1985, P. J. Heenan and associates from the University of Western Australia reported on 189 patients with localized malignant melanoma. Of these, 74 patients had lesions thicker than 1.5 mm, and 71 percent of the 189 were treated with a skin graft or flap.[54] They concluded, "Wide excision as the standard treatment of malignant melanoma is not justified." In 1992, Heenan and colleagues presented additional information on 530 patients.[55] Surgical margins of less than 1 cm were used on 35 percent of these patients. Neither local recurrence nor survival was adversely affected by narrow margins of excision.

In 1977, T.T.E. Pitt from Preston and Northcote Community Hospital in Victoria, Australia, reviewed the literature on margins of excision for melanoma and stated, "There is no evidence ... to show that wide excision confers greater protection than narrow excision in the treatment of malignant melanoma."[56] In 1983, A. B. Ackerman and A. M. Sheiner from the New York University School of Medicine performed a similar review, which also included information from the WHO study.[57] They concluded, "In short, surgery for a primary cutaneous [skin] melanoma should be no different from surgery for any other malignant neoplasm [cancer] that is primary to the skin. Excision of additional centimeters of normal skin does not enhance survival." D. E. Elder and colleagues from the University of Pennsylvania studied 105 patients with malignant melanoma and concluded, "Our data suggest that the extent of local surgery does not influence patient survival."[58]

I have found only two studies suggesting that narrow margins of excision and suvival rates are linked. In 1983, D. R. Aitken and colleagues from Ohio State University concluded that "patients with deeper lesions excised with a margin of less than 2 cm had a significantly greater risk of dying."[59] The following year, they reversed this position.[60] In 1966, J. A. Lehman reported a difference in the five-year survival rates of 42 patients treated with either simple closure (33 percent) or skin graft (52 percent).[61] This suggested that patients lived longer following wide excision and skin grafting. This conclusion is probably incorrect. (It should be noted that this study was done before Clark's levels or Breslow's depths of invasion were measured, when melanomas were classified as either superficial spreading or nodular.) It is likely that skin grafts were used primarily on patients who had thin melanomas—lesions that simply spread out over a wide area, often 2 to 3 cm in width. Other lesions were nodular in appearance—not as wide, but thicker. The thicker lesions were probably removed with a narrow excision and simple closure. The difference in survival figures was probably due to the difference in the types of patients being treated, not the effectiveness of the surgery.

In 1993, M.G.E. O'Rourke and colleagues from Mater Misericordiae Adult Public Hospital in Queensland, Australia, provided additional data that supports conservative surgery for malignant melanoma.[62] They studied 187 patients, 22 percent of whom had lesions that invaded to Clark's level IV or deeper (see Figure 9.1). Of these, 86 had their lesions removed with a margin of less than 1.5 cm, while the remaining patients were treated with surgical margins of greater than 1.5 cm. There was no significant difference in the recurrence rates for these two groups. The researchers recommended margins of 1.0 cm to 1.5 cm for localized disease. In the editorial that accompanied this article, H. F. Seigler of Duke University in North Carolina recommends a 2-cm margin.[63] M. Brown and L. A. Goldsmith recommend narrow margins free of tumor cells in cosmetically sensitive areas such as the face and hands.[64]

Many studies have demonstrated that patients treated with a narrow margin, less than 1 to 2 cm, have an increased chance of developing local recurrence. If your surgery would leave a disfiguring scar, you will want to consider the evidence that supports narrow margins of excision. There has never been a paper published demonstrating that narrow margins of excision reduce survival. There has never been a study demonstrating that wide margins improve survival.

The Regional Lymph Nodes

For decades, surgeons in the United States have debated the value of removing regional lymph nodes, even if the nodes were not enlarged. This has been called an elective lymph node dissection (ELND). It is well known that 30 to 60 percent of patients with lesions of 1.0 to 4.0 mm have microscopically positive lymph nodes, or nodes with cancer cells in them. Some surgeons have wanted to remove these melanoma cells before they spread to distant organs. Some arguments for and against this procedure have been summarized.[65-67]

It is now agreed that patients with either thin lesions or thick lesions are unlikely to benefit from ELND. Patients with thin lesions (less than 1 mm) are unlikely to have melanoma cells in their regional lymph nodes. Patients with lesions greater than 4.0 mm are likely to have melanoma cells already spread to distant sites. In either case, an ELND has little chance of improving survival. The debate now centers on patients with lesions of intermediate thickness.

Among the best-known studies that support ELND are those by C. M. Balch and associates. In 1981, they studied 1,786 patients treated between 1955 and 1980 at the University of Alabama in Birmingham (UAB) and the Sydney Melanoma Unit (SMU) in Sydney, Australia. They concluded that ELND benefited patients with lesions between 1.5 and 4.0 mm.[68] They reported a ten-year survival rate of 70 percent among patients treated with ELND. Patients treated with wide excision alone were less likely to survive ten years: 15 percent at the UAB and 45 percent at the SMU.

Contrary evidence has come from the World Health Organization, which conducted a randomized, prospective trial in Europe. The trial studied patients treated by wide excision with or without ELND.[69] These investigators concluded that ELND offers no survival advantage over wide excision alone. They reported a 55 percent to 60 percent ten-year survival rate among patients with 2.0- to 4.0-mm lesions treated with wide excision with or without ELND. The Mayo Clinic in Rochester, Minnesota, also performed a randomized, prospective trial and reached a similar conclusion.[70]

I believe that this debate hinges on one very important factor: how carefully was each patient followed after surgery? The UAB started a melanoma registry in 1975. Information for their study was obtained from "patient records and by telephone interviews with the patients, their families and their primary physicians."[71] Many UAB patients treated with wide excision alone developed easily palpable nodes, that is, the nodes could easily be felt. Indeed, 31 percent of patients who returned with melanoma in their lymph nodes had five or more positive nodes.[72] The survival of these patients was no greater than that of patients who had palpable nodes when they were first seen at UAB. Thus, the follow-up procedures at UAB were of no advantage over patient self-evaluation and referral.

The SMU began evaluating patients prospectively in 1964. Patients were seen every two to four months during the first two years.[73] I believe that the threefold difference in ten-year survival rates between UAB and SMU—15 percent versus 45 percent—may be due to the extent of nodal disease in the two studies. Patients treated by wide excision alone at the UAB may have had a lower survival rate because they were followed less frequently and developed sizeable disease in their nodes. The tumor burden of extensive nodal disease may have been responsible for some deaths at the UAB that were prevented by earlier node removal at SMU. Thus, the real issue may not be whether an ELND is needed, but at precisely what size do positive lymph nodes become an added survival risk.

By contrast, patients in the WHO trial were all followed prospectively, every one to three months, and treated promptly if nodal disease appeared.[74] These patients had a 50 percent five-year survival rate. This was equivalent to the survival of patients who had positive lymph nodes after an ELND. In other words, consider those patients with microscopic cancer in their lymph nodes. One group has an ELND. The other group has surgery several months later, after the lymph nodes have become barely palpable. The WHO trial concluded that the survival of both groups of patients is the same. This experience differs from that reported by Balch, where disease in the nodes was allowed to grow, not to the tumor burden—the cells being shed into the blood stream—of early disease, but to the readily palpable tumor burden of clinical stage III disease.

There may also be a few individuals with thin lesions who develop disease in the nodes and die as a result of the tumor burden of the nodes. In the WHO trial, among patients with primary lesions of 1.0 to 1.9 mm, 14 percent had positive lymph nodes, regardless of treatment. The ten-year survival rates of these patients were 85 percent for immediate removal, and 66 percent for delayed removal. This study suggests that patients with thin lesions live longer if they are treated with ELND at the same time their melanomas are removed. This conclusion is contrary to currently accepted practice, but there were not enough patients in this study to reach a firm conclusion.

There might be an actual difference in survival if the tumor burden of the recurrence in the nodes exceeds both the tumor burden of the primary lesion and the defense threshold of the patient. Some patients who survive a thin primary lesion may be unable to survive their nodal disease. I believe the records of individual patients should be reviewed to see if excessive deaths have occurred among patients whose nodal disease exceeded the volume of the primary lesion. Such a study could easily be performed at any large cancer hospital.

It is also possible that in a few other patients, melanoma within regional lymph nodes may metastasize to distant organs before it becomes apparent. The WHO trial dealt in averages. There are no

Appendix I 259

tests to identify these patients. There are two studies currently in progress that address this matter, the NCI Intergroup Melanoma Committee in the United States and the WHO Melanoma study in Europe. I would suggest that these investigators make an effort to carefully measure the volume of cancer in the lymph nodes. This is difficult to do. But it is important for surgeons to learn the volume of tumor that the average patient can tolerate before the tumor spreads. This tumor volume should be compared to the volume of the primary tumor for each patient. Future studies should also include an immunological evaluation of each patient. Chapter 4 explains the battle between the tumor and the patient.

In conclusion, some retrospective studies may have exaggerated the benefit of ELND, because some patients treated with delayed lymph node removal developed sizable recurrence in their nodes. They died because of the volume of the recurrent disease. Malignant melanoma is a highly aggressive malignancy that can spread from a small primary or regional lymph node. This is unlike breast cancer, the most thoroughly studied cancer, which can usually be felt before it spreads. For this reason, ELND makes more sense for malignant melanoma than it does for breast cancer. Hopefully, the studies now in progress will answer some of these questions.

CHAPTER 10: CANCER OF THE PENIS

The following material covers two topics: the primary lesion and disease of the lymph nodes.

The Primary Lesion

In 1886, W. McCormick recommended total amputation of the penis together with removal of the lymph nodes in the groin on both sides. This approach was also recommended by Hugh Young of Johns Hopkins in Baltimore. Since 1936, Frederick Mohs and his associates from the University of Wisconsin have treated patients with penile cancer using Mohs micrographic surgery,[75] described in Chapter 5. In 1992, they reviewed their experience with penile cancer patients. The five-year survival rates for these patients were as follows:

- Stage I, cancer confined to glans or foreskin—18 survivors out of 21, or 86 percent.
- Stage II, cancer involving the shaft of the penis—5 survivors out of 8, or 62 percent.
- Stage III, cancer involving the lymph nodes—0 survivors out of 2, or 0 percent.

Among these 23 survivors, there were two local recurrences: both patients had considerable disease along the urethra. Surgeons in Japan and Spain have also had experience with this technique and recommend it.[76,77] R. S. Malek of the Mayo Clinic in Rochester, Minnesota, advocates the use of laser surgery for superficially invasive cancers.[78]

Simon Horenblas and associates from the Netherlands Cancer Institute have treated patients with penis-conserving surgery since 1956.[79] Their techniques have included local excision, radiation therapy, and laser therapy. In 1992, they reported on 51 patients. Local recurrence rates were as follows:

- T_1, cancer invades connective tissue—3 out of 30, or 10 percent.
- T_2, cancer invades the body of the penis—6 out of 19, or 32 percent.
- T_3, cancer invades the urethra or prostate—2 out of 2, or 100 percent.

These stage designations are part of the complicated TNM system, described in Chapter 5, which is often used in research studies.

Consider the fate of the patients in this study who developed recurrent disease. The three patients with T_1 tumors had local recurrence isolated to the penis, that is, there was no cancer in the lymph nodes or elsewhere. They were retreated, and none died of penile cancer. Four of the patients with T_2 disease had local recurrence isolated to the penis. They were retreated, and none of these patients died of penile cancer. Two of the patients with T_2 lesions developed recurrent cancer on the penis and positive lymph nodes in the groin at about the same time. After retreatment, one of these patients died of penile cancer and the other was alive and well when last seen. The patients with T_3 tumors died of penile cancer. Simply stated, patient outcome was decided by the original stage of their disease, not by the extent of their original surgery, and not even by the recurrence of disease on the penis. Promptly treated recurrent disease did not reduce survival.

Those who argue against conservative surgery commonly point to the high rates of local recurrence following conservative surgery. P. F. Schellhammer and others in *Campbell's Urology*, an important textbook in this specialty, cited recurrence rates of 32 and 50 percent from two different studies following local excision or circumcision as primary treatment.[80]

Consider these studies. W. S. McDougal and others studied 65 patients seen at the Vanderbilt University School of Medicine in Nashville between 1960 and 1980.[81] A total of 19 patients were treated with local excision or circumcision and 6, 32 percent, developed local recurrence. There were only 19 patients with stage I disease. The authors do not say if these were the same 19 patients as those treated conservatively, but presumably the groups were identical or nearly so. None of the stage I patients died of penile cancer. Thus, none or very few of the patients treated conservatively appear to have died of cancer. This paper appears to support the thesis of this book, but the authors have failed to completely report this information.

Consider the second study cited in *Campbell's Urology*. A. S. Narayana and others reported on a group of 219 patients treated at the University of Iowa.[82] Most of them were referred to the university after initial treatment elsewhere. More than half of the patients waited more than six months to consult a physician. There are two good reasons for these patients to have poor results. First, patients who do well do not need to be referred to a university medical center for additional care. Second, most of these patients delayed in seeking treatment. Ten of the 20 patients, 50 percent, treated by circumcision developed local recurrence and were treated by partial amputation. This is a very high local recurrence rate. It suggests that this paper concerns patients with advanced disease. The survival of patients who developed local recurrence was not reported. Again, the authors did not consider the effect of local recurrence on survival.

In both of the above cases, *Campbell's Urology* exaggerated the risk of local recurrence following limited surgery. The textbook also failed to report the data suggesting that local recurrence following conservative surgery poses little, if any, risk to survival.

In another study, M. S. Jensen reviewed 511 cases treated in Denmark from 1942 to 1962.[83] If patients with T_1 and T_2 tumors are considered together, local recurrence rates were 27 percent for circumcision or excision, 5 percent for partial amputation, and 1.3 percent for total amputation. About 16 percent of patients in each group died of penile cancer. Here again, initial treatment and local recurrence had no apparent impact on survival. Current evidence is compatible with the suggestion that promptly treated local recurrence is not an added risk to survival.

The Regional Lymph Nodes

The removal of lymph nodes that are not enlarged has been debated. The issues involved have been more thoroughly studied among patients with breast cancer and melanoma, because they are more common cancers. For patients with breast cancer, the findings are clear. This operation does not increase survival. For patients with malignant melanoma, there is still debate. But it appears that patients who are treated promptly following the development of disease in the lymph nodes do as well as those who had normal-feeling nodes that contained cancer removed as part of their original surgery.

Ramon Cabanas of Victory Memorial Hospital in Brooklyn has recommended that surgeons biopsy a single lymph node in the groin area, called the sentinel node.[84] This is the lymph node where penile cancers usually first spread. Whether this node should be removed on the right or left side is determined after dye is injected into the lymph vessels near the tumor and its flow followed by X-ray. Cabanas recommends a complete node removal if the sentinel node is positive. However, some authors have found tumor cells in the groin lymph nodes of patients with negative sentinel nodes.

In 1993, Murali Kamat and colleagues of Tata Memorial Hospital in Bombay, India followed 16 patients with lymph nodes that felt normal or were microscopically free of cancer after skinny needle biopsy.[85] All 16 developed disease in the nodes. In 4 patients, the disease was so advanced that the nodes could not be removed. These patients died of their disease. The other 12 had surgery. Signs of advanced disease were found in 10. Eight of these 12 patients were alive and well 2.2 years after removal of their lymph nodes. The other 4 patients had died of their disease. The primary problem here was a failure to promptly remove enlarging nodes.

R. Ravi reported the experience of the Cancer Institute of Madras, India, in treating 423 patients with invasive penile cancer.[86] He concluded that neither lymph node removal nor biopsy of nodes in the groin were routinely indicated.

Some urologists support ELND.[87-89] In these studies, many patients treated without ELND returned with advanced nodal disease. If these patients had been closely followed, their lymph nodes may have been removed before becoming the cause of tumor spread. Current evidence is compatible with the suggestion that promptly treated regional lymph node recurrence is not an added risk to survival. Therefore, normal-feeling lymph nodes do not need to be routinely removed.

CHAPTER 11: PROSTATE CANCER

During the late 1880s, several surgeons performed a variety of operations to remove all or part of the prostate and occasionally part of the bladder. In 1904, Hugh Young at Johns Hopkins Hospital in Baltimore, assisted by William Halsted, performed a

Appendix I

radical prostatectomy. The incision was made between the anus and the scrotum, in an area called the perinum. The seminal vesicles, nearby structures that screte a component of semen, were also removed. But, unlike Halsted's radical mastectomy for breast cancer, Young's radical prostatectomy did not remove the regional lymph nodes. Most patients had disease that was too advanced for surgery, and few urologists mastered this operation. It was never widely performed.

By 1925, urologists at the Mayo Clinic in Rochester, Minnesota, began to recognize the pelvic lymph nodes as the earliest site of tumor spread. But urologists seldom tried to remove these nodes surgically, because patients with lymph nodes that contained cancer were not considered curable. By 1937, Young reported a 50 percent five-year survival rate following radical perineal prostatectomy. In the mid-1930s, transurethral resection (removal of tissue through the urethra) became accepted in the treatment of cancer that obstructed the flow of urine. In 1941, Charles Huggins reported that prostate cancer grew in response to male hormones. Castration and female hormones became accepted treatment for patients with advanced disease.

In 1945, another prostatectomy technique was introduced. An incision was made through the lower abdomen, and the prostate was approached from behind the pubic bone. Urologists used this incision to operate on the bladder, so they were familiar with this approach. The retropubic prostatectomy became a popular operation for prostate cancer.

Radiation therapy was used with mixed results in the early part of this century. By the 1950s, megavoltage irradiation was able to deliver sufficiently high doses of radiation to effectively treat most stages of the disease.

Of all the malignancies covered in this book, prostate cancer is probably the most difficult to understand. Few randomized trials, involving only small numbers of patients, have been performed. Therefore, most of our current information comes from retrospective studies of patients treated over the past twenty years.

Determining PSA Screening Levels

Tests for prostate-specific antigen (PSA) can be useful in following the progress of a specific cancer patient, as discussed in Chapter 11. But doctors are still trying to determine how PSA levels should be used in screening, that is, at what PSA level a man without any symptoms should undergo biopsy.

Investigators at the Washington University School of Medicine measured PSA levels in over 10,000 men.[90] The levels were between 4 and 10 ng/ml in 694 men. Of these, 652 patients had abnormal digital rectal examination (DRE) or transrectal ultrasound (TRUS) results. These 652 men were biopsied, and 27 percent tested positive. Another 208 men had PSA levels greater than 10 ng/ml. All of them were biopsied and 59 percent tested positive.

Some researchers prefer to judge the value of PSA screening by considering only patients with normal DRE results, since an abnormal DRE is likely to lead to a biopsy anyway. In a study of 6,630 men, the DRE results were normal in 484 men with abnormal PSA levels.[91] A total of 401 men had PSA values from 4 to 10 ng/ml, and 21 percent of them had positive biopsies. The other 83 men had PSA values of 10 or greater, and 42 percent of them had positive biopsies. The percentages of positive biopsies were lower in this study because men with abnormal DRE results were excluded from the figures. Among men with a normal PSA value, less than 4 ng/ml, an abnormal DRE result led to a positive biopsy in 16 of 233, or 7 percent, of patients. Abnormalities in both DRE and TRUS led to a positive biopsy in 32 of 232, or 14 percent, of patients with a normal PSA reading.

Questions Regarding Treatment

Between 1984 and 1990, the rate of radical prostatectomy increased nearly sixfold in the United States.[92] This has occurred for several reasons. First, the incidence of prostate cancer has been increasing. Second, PSA testing has increased the detection of prostate cancer. Third, nerve-sparing surgery has reduced the incidence of impotence following radical prostatectomy. Fourth, a randomized trial suggested that radical prostatectomy is more effective that radiation therapy in treating cancer confined to the prostate.[93] Nevertheless, the number of patients in this trial was too small to arrive at firm conclusions.

It is difficult to evaluate prostate cancer treatment. Patients may not have their entire prostate or even their entire tumor removed. Tumor growth or recurrence may not be detected. In other parts of the body, by contrast, conservative treatment almost always involves complete removal of the cancer, which can then be precisely measured. Recurrent cancer is also easier to detect and measure in most other organs.

Thus, important questions remain unanswered after a prostate operation. How large was the tumor? Was it entirely removed? When did it recur? What happened to patients whose recurrences were promptly treated? Without this information, it is difficult for urologists to accurately evaluate treatment results.

Appendix I

An example of this difficulty is reported by H. Matzkin and colleagues from the University of Miami.[94] In 1994, they reviewed nine papers dealing with untreated stage A1 disease. This is the earliest stage. They reported progression of the cancer, either locally or distantly, in 2 to 50 percent of patients. These wide-ranging results illustrate the difficulty of dependable information about this disease.

There is an additional problem with current statistics on prostate cancer. DRE, TRUS, and PSA tests are the primary tools used to measure the disease. Most of the clinical studies urologists now rely on were done prior to the widespread use of the PSA test and TRUS. Urologists had difficulty evaluating the progression of prostate cancer using only the DRE. In some cases, surgical treatment was withheld until urinary obstruction developed.

The Importance of Follow-up

Let us consider the practical significance of all this. Most patients today are diagnosed with early prostate cancer. They have an elevated PSA or cancer is found during an operation called transurethral resection of the prostate (TURP), which is performed on patients with benign prostate enlargement. These patients may wish to consider no further treatment, just watchful waiting. What is a urologist likely to recommend?

Urologists from Johns Hopkins Medical School recently said, "[Fifteen] to 20 percent of patients with untreated A1 disease develop metastatic [spreading] disease with an average follow-up of ten years."[95] This statistic is sufficient to encourage the most stouthearted to pursue aggressive treatment. But let us consider the source of these numbers.

The figure of 20 percent comes from a 1986 Mayo Clinic study reported in 1986.[96] Fifteen men with stage A1 disease were followed for ten years. Three of these patients, or 20 percent, developed metastatic disease, and all three were alive when the study ended. In spite of this high rate of tumor spread, the Mayo doctors suggested that "careful ongoing surveillance of young men with stage A1 prostatic cancer seems mandatory." However, there is no evidence in this study that these patients had regular follow-up examinations. The PSA and ultrasound tests were not generally available and were not mentioned in the study.

I have reviewed over a dozen studies concerning men with stage A1 prostate cancer. Many failed to distinguish between local and distant progression of disease—often a life-or-death distinction. Few studies have clearly described a regular follow-up program. Patients with early prostate cancer may have developed metastatic disease because they were not carefully followed. Growing cancer was not promptly detected and removed.

The success of careful follow-up evaluation is clear. Several urologists have treated their patients who have stage A_1 disease with a second TURP. Between 1975 and 1989, M. Ziegler and colleagues from the University of Saarlandes, Homburg/Saar, Germany, performed a second TURP on 120 patients with stage A_1 disease.[97] Of these patients, 26 percent had residual tumors, or tumors that were found during the second procedure, and 74 percent had none. The tumor-free patients were followed closely. None developed prostate cancer by the end of the study and none died. Patients with residual tumor were treated according to their age and physical condition.

In contrast, about 80 percent of stage A_1 patients who have radical prostatectomies will be found to have residual tumors after surgery.[98] Some of them will have both a higher stage and a higher grade of disease. This suggests that patients who are treated with a second TURP do not have all of their cancer removed by the second operation.

A Major Study Analyzes Watchful Waiting

A thorough study of prostate cancer was conducted by the Prostate Patient Outcomes Research Team (PPORT), a multi-institutional, multispeciality group based at Dartmouth Medical School in New Hampshire.[99,100] This group considered the entire English-language medical literature on prostate cancer from 1966 through 1991, and selected 144 articles for review. The PPORT study found only one study out of 144 that fulfilled its five standards of quality. All the other papers had substantial flaws. Even in this often-quoted study, the frequency of follow-up examinations was not considered among the five standards of quality. The authors compared the treatment efficiency of aggressive treatment (radical prostatectomy or radiation therapy) versus watchful waiting.

This study found no definitive evidence that aggressive therapy was superior to watchful waiting for most patients with stage A or B cancer (cancer confined to the prostate), those with well-differentiated tumors, and those over seventy-five years of age. They concluded that if the benefits of radical surgery or radiation therapy could be obtained with a simple pill, it is likely that the Food and Drug Administration would not approve the sale of the drug, because it would be considered ineffective. (This is even more remarkable when you consider that the FDA's position would be negative even for a theoretical drug with no side effects.) The PPORT researchers concluded that all men with well-differentiated tumors and all men over seventy-five years of age were unlikely to benefit from aggressive therapy.

The men most likely to benefit from aggressive treatment are those age sixty years and younger with moderately differentiated cancer, or Gleason grades 5 through 7. If these patients are followed for ten years, about 2 percent of those treated aggressively will die of cancer or its treatment, and about 5 percent of those followed with watchful waiting will die of prostate cancer. Thus, of all these younger patients with prostate cancer, only 3 percent may have their lives prolonged by aggressive treatment. The PPORT points out that some informed patients may be reluctant to trade several years of good quality life in the near future for a 3 percent survival advantage in the distant future. They agree that this choice rightly belongs to the patient.

This study has been criticized by Washington University urologist William Catalona and others, because it focuses on potent men under sixty years of age, the very patients most likely to have complications.[101] Catalona also believes that too many patients with early disease were used to predict the progression of cancer in all patients. Patrick Walsh of Johns Hopkins also believes that the PPORT study was flawed. He thinks it underestimated the rate at which prostate cancer spreads.[102] Walsh and others believe that the survival benefits of radical prostatectomy may be two to three times as great as those calculated by the PPORT study team.

If you are still inclined to do everything possible to eradicate the cancer, consider one more aspect of the PPORT report. The authors stated, "We assumed that patients received no treatment for local progression of disease unless symptoms or findings of bladder outlet obstruction occurred." These patients apparently received little if any follow-up evaluation, not even a yearly DRE. This treatment was called "watchful waiting," but it was not particularly watchful. If these patients had been carefully followed with DREs, PSA blood tests, and TRUS, progressive disease could have been detected and treated much sooner. The entire theme of this book concerns the importance of the early detection and removal of progressive or recurrent disease. The success of conservative treatment relies upon regular follow-up examinations. The availability of TRUS and the PSA blood test can only improve the results of watchful waiting and other conservative measures. The 3 percent survival advantage of aggressive treatment—which may be two to three times greater, if Walsh and others are correct—may decline to 1 percent or less, as patients take advantage of modern detection procedures. Patients must understand, however, that these tests are not perfect. In very rare cases, prostate cancer may spread in patients with a normal DRE, a normal PSA, and a normal TRUS.

Studies From Other Institutions

Doctors at the Karolinska Institute in Finland and Memorial Sloan-Kettering Cancer Center in New York reviewed the medical literature since 1980 regarding the treatment of prostate cancer. They compared the results of radical prostatectomy, external radiation, and deferred treatment—waiting, though not necessarily watchful.[103] Ten years after the initial diagnosis, the survival rates were 93 percent for radical prostatectomy, 74 percent for external radiation, and 84 percent for deferred treatment. These rates do not include deaths from other causes. These results are not from randomized studies and could be biased for the reasons discussed in Chapter 2. Patients with the smallest tumors may have been treated with radical prostatectomy. There was no uniform way to compare the patients for tumor grade and stage. Radiation has usually been used on patients with more advanced disease. Furthermore, the frequency of follow-up examinations was not determined. The differences in survival may reflect tumor growth among untreated patients.

Surgeons from Memorial Sloan-Kettering treated 75 patients with stage B prostate cancer from 1946 to 1986 and followed them for fifteen years.[104] Initially, patients had a DRE every three months. Twenty-three patients developed evidence of progressive disease and were treated with TURP. The fifteen-year survival of these patients was equal to or better than the expected survival of men without cancer of similar age. The authors claimed that "no deliberate selection was evident." However, the study was not a review of the hospital's entire experience.

This treatment was very similar to that recommended in this book. But these impressive results were obtained without reduction of the initial tumor volume, without any treatment during the first year after diagnosis, and without the aid of PSA or TRUS. I believe that the careful follow-up of these patients contributed to these good results. Only 5 of the 75 patients developed distant metastases without first demonstrating local progression of disease. This further suggests that the tumor is unlikely to spread if the size of the cancer in the prostate can be kept under control.

Men with prostate cancer are much more likely to die from other causes. Of men who are diagnosed with prostate cancer at age sixty, about 25 percent are likely to die from other causes within ten years. This increases with age; about 60 percent of those age seventy-five are likely to die from other causes. In other words, the potential benefit of aggressive treatment decreases with age. Therefore, the patients who are most likely to benefit from aggressive treatment are younger, less than sixty-five years of age, with moderately or poorly differentiated tumors.

Unfortunately, some studies have suggested that patients with poorly differentiated cancer also do poorly following aggressive treatment. In 1980, when Hugh Jewett reviewed the experience of Johns Hopkins Hospital in Baltimore with 447 patients treated with radical prostatectomy, none of his patients with poorly differentiated tumors survived fifteen years free of disease.[105] However, recent experience with similar patients suggests that these results can be improved upon. In 1994, urologists at Johns Hopkins reviewed their experience with 63 similar patients treated in the prior ten years.[106] Distant metastases only developed in the seven patients with positive pelvic lymph nodes. They concluded that many patients with poorly differentiated tumors may benefit from an attempt at cure. A review article in the *New England Journal of Medicine* concluded that men with grades 1 and 2 cancer may receive a small survival benefit from aggressive treatment, but "the relative benefit of aggressive treatment for grade 3 cancer is less clear."[107]

Treatment Options: A Middle Ground

Many articles portray the options as aggressive therapy, on one hand, and watchful waiting, on the other. I believe that patients should consider some of the choices between these two extremes. L. P. Sonda from the Univeristy of Michigan said, "Some urologists believe that prostate cancer can be cured by repeated aggressive resection [TURP]."[108] Unfortunately, it is often difficult to determine the precise location of some prostate cancers, even with TRUS. Furthermore, a cancer located on the periphery of the gland would be difficult to reach with a TURP scope. Therefore, few urologists agree with this statement.

At one time, urologists felt that TURP might cause prostate cancer to spread. This is another reason that TURP has never been considered a suitable operation for patients with prostate cancer. In 1947, it was shown that much of the fluid used to wash out the small chips of tissue made its way into the blood stream. It was feared that the surgeon who cut through cancer may also wash some cancer cells into the blood stream and increase the spread of prostate cancer.

Furthermore, patients treated with radiation therapy seemed to do worse if they were diagnosed with a TURP as opposed to a rectal biopsy. It was suggested that TURP caused the dissemination of cancer cells. This supported an attitude that inadequate initial therapy may do more harm than good. Several studies have failed to confirm this association. Doctors at the Baylor College of Medicine in Houston showed that those patients who were first treated with

TURP had done poorly because many had more advanced disease in the first place. Many of them had required a TURP because their cancer was so large that it obstructed urine flow. Doctors at Memorial Hospital in New York also concluded that TURP did not adversely affect patients with prostate cancer.[109] Today, there is general agreement that patients with stage A or B disease are not harmed by a TURP prior to radiation therapy—that TURP does not cause prostate cancer cells to spread.[110] A TURP may make a subsequent prostatectomy technically more difficult. But it does not increase the complication rate of a later radical prostatectomy.[111]

If prostate cancer is diagnosed from a TURP, some urologists recommend a second TURP or TRUS-guided biopsy. A follow-up TURP usually finds additional prostate cancer in about 30 percent of patients. But a follow-up radical prostatectomy usually finds additional cancer in about 60 percent of patients. This suggests that 30 percent of patients may have their prostate cancer missed by a second TURP. Some urologists have been concerned by this finding. This may not be surprising, though. The initial TURP was not intended to cure the cancer. Furthermore, recall the high incidence of microscopic prostate cancer found at autopsy in men of all ages mentioned at the beginning of Chapter 11.

In 1995, urologists at Baylor reported on 40 patients who developed recurrent cancer after radiation therapy.[112] They were all treated with radical prostatectomy. Many patients developed surgical complications, but the survival results were excellent. The best results were obtained in the 18 patients whose disease was confined to the prostate gland or the tissue immediately surrounding it. After five years, the disease had not progressed in 82 percent of these 18 patients. Among all patients, the survival rate—counting only those who died of their cancer, and not other causes—was 95 percent at five years and 87 percent at eight years. These results are similar to those following standard radical prostatectomy in patients who did not receive radiation therapy. This study suggests that radical prostatectomy after a recurrence may also be effective for patients who were initially treated with some form of incomplete prostatectomy.

In summary, most prostate cancer is out of the reach of the TURP scope. But some patients can still be treated with a TURP. They may wish to consider having additional tumor removed prior to a period of wachful waiting.

Other treatment options include one of the incomplete prostatectomies described in Chapter 11, cryosurgery, and microwave thermal therapy. I believe that the spread of prostate cancer is largely determined by its size, and that additional ways should be found to reduce the bulk of a prostate cancer prior to a period of watchful waiting.

Appendix I

Even if countless studies affirm a policy of watchful waiting, it will always carry a degree of risk. A patient may experience local tumor growth and later develop distant tumor spread. He will always wonder, "What would have happened if . . .?" As the patient and the doctor embark on this uncertain voyage, they must remain in regular contact. New information, procedures, and diagnostic tests should be promptly incorporated into the follow-up plan. Ian Thompson, a noted researcher in this field, has said that each patient has a "window of curability."[113] Reliable information suggests this to be true for prostate cancer and other solid tumors. The patient and the doctor must be willing to share the responsibility for vigorous follow-up care and for the outcome of their treatment decision.

CHAPTER 12: CANCER OF THE RECTUM

Ernest Miles developed the abdominoperineal resection (APR) in 1908, in the same period when radical surgical procedures where developing for cancer of the breast, head and neck, and cervix. In 1960, surgeons at St. Mark's Hospital in London tried to improve patient survival by increasing the number of lymph nodes they removed.[114] Their operation was extended significantly to remove lymph nodes throughout the abdomen. They found no survival advantage for extended surgery.

Procedures Developed to Spare the Rectum

Surgeons have devised several techniques to attach the colon to the sphincter mechanism after tumor removal. In 1939, C. F. Dixon of the Mayo Clinic in Rochester, Minnesota, introduced the low anterior resection (LAR). In the early 1940s, H. E. Bacon of Temple University School of Medicine in Philadelphia began to use the pull-through procedure, a technique first described in the late 1880s.

For most of this century, surgeons have tried to remove at least 5 cm of normal rectum below the tumor. In the 1970s and 1980s, more surgeons tried to preserve normal bowel function. Margins of 2 cm were tried and became accepted. Some surgeons now accept a margin of 1 cm below the tumor, if absolutely necessary to save the rectum.[115] In 1975, surgical stapling devices were introduced to staple together the two ends of intestine. Thus, this technically difficult procedure became much easier.

In 1974, M. W. Sterns from Memorial Sloan-Kettering Hospital in New York compared LAR to APR for patients with mid-rectal cancers. He reported no differences in local recurrence and survival rates between the two forms of treatment.[116] These results have been confirmed by many surgeons, including results from a randomized, prospective trial.

Well into the 1970s, surgeons believed that they had to preserve the last 3 to 7 cm of the rectum to maintain continence. However, surgeons have observed that sphincter competence can remain after the colon was sewn to the lower 1 to 2 cm of the rectum.[117] Surgeons became able to treat both larger tumors and lower tumors with sphincter-saving procedures. Preoperative radiation therapy of 50 Gy and excision of the entire rectum have been performed on patients with tumors that averaged 4 cm in diameter. Memorial Sloan-Kettering and Jefferson University in Philadelphia have both reported excellent results.[118] Chemotherapy has been added before or after surgery, and may offer a slight survival benefit.[119]

In 1992, surgeons from M. D. Anderson Hospital in Houston reported their experience with ten patients with large tumors of the lower (sigmoid) colon and rectum.[120] The patients required extensive operations, including removal of the bladder, to remove the tumors. No one required a permanent colostomy and all survivors had normal bowel function. Their local recurrence and survival results were comparable to those following APR.

The Use of Local Excision and Radiation Therapy

For most of this century, local excision has been used to treat small, superficial lesions. George Binkley of Memorial Hospital in New York used radium needles or excision to treat early cancers in the 1920s. Electrocoagulation or fulguration was first described as primary treatment is 1935. Low-energy radiation therapy was used in the 1930s and 1940s to treat small tumors of the rectum, but the complications usually exceeded the benefit.

The modern experience with local excision can be traced to the work of R. J. Jackman and C. E. Culp of the Mayo Clinic.[121] In 1973, they reported local recurrence in only 4 of 25 patients treated with local excision. Surgeons at St. Mark's Hospital increased their experience with local excision from 1 to 9 percent of cases between 1948 and 1972, and recommended this treatment for patients with tumors of a favorable grade. They performed an excision of the full thickness of the rectal wall, and insisted on margins that were free of tumor cells.

Between 1954 and 1982, surgeons at Memorial Sloan-Kettering treated 57 patients with local excision.[122] This represented only about 4 percent of all their patients with invasive rectal cancer. Twenty-seven patients had no adverse prognostic factors, and none of them died of rectal cancer. Thirty patients had adverse prognostic factors; 9 of these patients were treated with APR for recurrent disease and 3 died of rectal cancer. Twenty-one of these 30 patients had no further surgery, and 3 died of rectal cancer.

In 1990, R. A. Graham and colleagues from the Dana Farber Cancer Institute in Boston reviewed sixteen studies of patients treated with local excision alone.[123] The overall local recurrence rate was 19 percent, and 42 percent of these patients were treated with additional surgery. Patients with favorable disease had recurrence rates that varied from 6 to 11 percent. Favorable criteria included Dukes's stage A disease, a well or moderately differentiated tumor, and margins free of tumor cells.

J. Papillon of the Centre Leon Bernard in Lyon, France, was one of the first to use endocavitary radiation therapy as the primary treatment of rectal cancer, beginning in 1951. His treatment was limited to very early tumors.[124] Endocavitary radiation is used in the United States primarily to reduce local recurrence following local excision or in patients with incurably advanced disease. By 1985, surgeons at the Mayo Clinic were recommending local excision for patients with grade 1 tumors less than 3 cm in diameter.[125] Experience from several institutions suggests that local excision and postoperative radiation therapy for selected stage I lesions (cancer confined to the bowel wall) produce local recurrence and survival results that are equivalent to those of more aggressive surgery.[126]

Surgeons at Memorial Sloan-Kettering believe that local excision may be suitable for some patients with larger lesions. They treated 14 patients with local excision and postoperative radiation therapy. The lesions averaged 4.4 cm. Three patients had local recurrences, which were treated with APR. The patients were followed for an average of twenty-eight months. One patient died of cancer. Thirteen patients had no evidence of disease in the pelvis when last seen. The overall survival rate at three years was 88 percent.[127]

Two Kinds of Local Recurrence

Following APR, local recurrence is associated with markedly decreased survival, usually leading to death within fifteen to eighteen months.[128] Surgeons from the Free Hospital in Amsterdam reported their experience with cryosurgery to treat patients with recurrent rectal cancer.[129] They began their paper: "Locally recurrent rectal cancer is, in most cases, unresectable [not treatable by surgery] and incurable." Tumors with characteristics that favor local recurrence are also most likely to spread. Risky tumors are large, high grade, and mucus-producing, among other factors. Once these aggressive tumors are removed, there is little more that can be done to hinder their deadly course. The outcome in these patients is not influenced by the scope of the original surgery. This topic is more fully discussed in Chapters 2 and 4.

Local recurrence following conservative surgery has a markedly different prognosis. Surgeons at the Royal Melbourne Hospital in Australia treated 28 patients with local excision.[130] Six of these patients developed local recurrence and required additional surgery. All 6 were followed for an average of fifty months after their second operation; all 6 were free of all local and distant disease.

Surgeons from the Roswell Park Cancer Institute in Buffalo studied 50 patients who developed local recurrence following surgical removal of cancer in the colon or rectum. These local recurrences developed at the site where the two segments of intestine were sewn together. Forty-five of these patients developed cancer elsewhere and survived an additional sixteen months. All 5 patients with cancer isolated to the site of surgery were alive with no evidence of cancer an average of thirty-seven months following the recurrence. Three patients were still alive more than five years following the second operation.[131]

Surgeons from the Lahey Clinic in Boston treated 40 patients with cancer of the rectum using local excision on 7 patients and electrocoagulation on 33 patients.[132] Overall, 30 patients, or 75 percent, survived five years free of disease or were free of disease when they died of other causes. Thirteen patients had recurrent cancer isolated to the rectum. Eight of the 13 patients—62 percent—were free of disease an average of 5.6 years following additional treatment.

In 1986, the NSABP, a breast cancer project that also included colon cancer research, reported the results of its study comparing APR to LAR in patients with lesions in the middle and upper rectum.[133] Both operations were equally effective. Patients treated with LAR lived as long as those treated with APR. About one fourth of the patients were treated with a lower margin of less than 2 cm. Twenty-two percent of these patients developed local recurrence. Patients treated with a margin of greater than 3 cm experienced a 12 percent local recurrence rate. Thus, a narrow margin of excision almost doubled the local recurrence rate—22 percent versus 12 percent. This did not reduce survival. The authors concluded, "There are unmistakable parallels between the evolution of the operative strategy of carcinoma of the rectum and that of breast cancer." Promptly treated local recurrence does not reduce survival. Techniques of this sort allow surgeons to remove tumors that are within 5 cm of the anus.

In 1994, surgeons at Memorial Sloan-Kettering published their experience treating 130 patients with LAR and coloanal anastamosis.[134] Five patients, or 4 percent, developed isolated local recurrence. From their data it appears that 2 of these patients were alive and well, 2 were living with disease, and 1 was dead of disease. The death occurred in a patient with advanced disease. These results are remarkably good and suggest that promptly treated local recurrence is not a risk to survival for patients with this disease.

CHAPTER 13: SOFT TISSUE SARCOMA

Many soft tissue sarcomas are surrounded by a thick capsule. In the early part of this century, some surgeons would simply extract the tumor out of the capsule. Since tumor cells were present in the capsule, this operation resulted in a high rate of local recurrence. In 1936, Shields Warren and George Sommer of Harvard Medical School in Massachusetts reported 150 cases of fibrosarcoma treated with operations ranging from local excision to radical excision. Sixty-four patients, or 43 percent, developed local recurrence.[135] As with other cancers, local recurrence was recognized as a grave sign. This encouraged more aggressive surgery.

By the middle of the century, surgeons at most major hospitals were performing amputations or very wide local excisions. In 1948, Arthur Stout analyzed 144 cases of fibrosarcoma seen at Presbyterian Hospital in New York from 1907 to 1946.[136] The type of treatment used varied over this long period, but was generally local excision. Of these 144 patients, 64 (60 percent) developed local recurrence, and 86 (80 percent) were alive at last follow-up. Stout concluded that this was a remarkably good survival rate among patients who developed local recurrences so frequently. Nevertheless, he did recommend the removal of an extra margin of tissue in order to achieve local control.

During the 1950s, the treatment of soft tissue sarcomas was very aggressive. In 1957, Zelig Lieberman and Lauren Ackerman reviewed 100 cases seen at Washington University in Saint Louis and concluded, "The worst thing that can happen is local recurrence."[137] Many authors have presented data supporting this conclusion, but most have failed to consider the size and grade of the tumors.[138-140] In many studies, surgical margins were not considered in assessing local recurrence as an independent risk factor. Patients with obvious residual tumor did have a decreased survival, a reflection of tumor size.

Conservative Treatment, Local Recurrence, and Survival

By the early 1960s, surgeons began to change their ideas about local recurrence. In 1963, L. Atkinson at St. Vincent's Hospital Tumor Clinic in Sydney, Australia, became an early proponent of conservative management of soft tissue sarcomas.[141] He concluded, "An observation-only policy is advocated for those patients without local recurrence following enucleation or other similarly inadequate procedures."

Limb-sparing surgery was initiated in the United States by H. D. Suit at M. D. Anderson Hospital in Houston in 1963. Researchers at Anderson reported on 300 patients treated with conservative surgery and postoperative radiation therapy between 1963 and 1977. Of the 40 patients, 32, or 80 percent, who developed extremity recurrences were controlled by further surgery.[142] This study carefully noted the effect of tumor grade and size on both local recurrence and survival. It concluded, "The incidence of distant metastases was not increased in patients who have had a local recurrence after this conservative approach."

Later, at Massachusetts General Hospital, Suit analyzed 170 patients treated from 1971 to 1982 with conservative surgery and radiation therapy.[143] Of the 19 patients with local recurrence, 12 were suitable for repeat surgery. Nine (75 percent) of these were alive and 7 (56 percent) had no evidence of any disease from 1.0 to 3.5 years after the repeat procedure. In 1988, Suit reported that 6 of these patients had been disease-free for more than five years.[144]

The many difficulties associated with retrospective studies can be reduced by a mathematical technique called *multivariate analysis*. This allows the effects of tumor size and grade to be statistically isolated so that the possible effect of local recurrence on survival can be studied. It is known that large, high-grade tumors often cause both local recurrence and distant metastases. Some doctors have concluded that local recurrence causes distant metastasis. This conclusion is incorrect. Multivariate analysis helps to clarify this puzzle.

S. A. Leibel reviewed 81 patients with soft tissue sarcomas of the extremity seen at the University of California—San Francisco from 1960 to 1978.[145] The development of distant metastases was not related to the type of initial surgery performed or whether radiation therapy was given. By the mid-1980s, the American College of Surgeons[146] and the National Cancer Institute (NCI) had concluded that local recurrence did not adversely affect survival.

The NCI study, done in 1985 by D. A. Potter and associates, analyzed 358 patients with high-grade soft tissue sarcomas of the extremities treated with surgery and high-dose radiation therapy at the NCI between 1975 and 1982.[147] Local excision resulted in local recurrence in 12 of 128 patients. There were no local recurrences in patients treated with amputation. Nevertheless, there was no survival difference between the two groups. The authors concluded, "The significant salvage [cure via a second surgery] of patients with isolated, locally recurrent disease indicates that local failure is not necessarily a poor prognostic factor."

B. Rööser of University Hospital in Lund, Sweden, treated 325 patients with sarcomas of the extremities from 1964 to 1983.[148] He considered the effects of surgical margins, tumor grade, tumor size, and tumor necrosis (the burden on the patient created by the death of tumor cells) on local recurrence and survival. He said, "Local recurrence after surgery with a wide or radical margin is in many cases probably only a predictor of a grave prognosis and not the reason for metastasis." Rööser concluded, "However, for most patients prognosis seems to be determined already at the time of diagnosis of the primary tumor." Investigators from Lund also measured the interval from initial diagnosis to the time of metastasis, comparing patients with and without local recurrence.[149] Again, local recurrence did not appear to cause any additional metastases and was not an added threat to survival.

T. Ueda and associates from Osaka University Medical School treated 163 patients with soft tissue sarcomas.[150] Patients were initially treated with narrow excision or wide excision. There was a 73-percent local recurrence rate in the narrow excision group and a 10-percent recurrence rate among patients treated with wide excision. Radical surgery was used in 25 of the 66 patients who developed recurrent disease. This included patients from both incision groups. Using multivariate analysis, the researchers determined that initial surgical treatment did not influence ultimate survival. Ueda said his data supported the conclusion of others "that local recurrence was not necessarily a poor prognostic sign in patients with localized [soft tissue sarcoma]."

In 1985, M. Brennan and colleagues from Memorial Sloan-Kettering Cancer Center in New York concluded, "Local recurrence did not appear to be a major determinant in survival. Current emphasis on local control may be much less important to survival than thought."[151] They analyzed 451 patients with soft tissue sarcomas of the extremity treated from 1982 to 1987.[152] Multivariate analysis demonstrated that local recurrence did not affect survival. They also performed the first randomized, prospective trial of wide local excision and radiation therapy. They reported that radiation therapy enhanced the local control of soft tissue sarcomas, but failed to improve survival.[153]

In 1987, C. Collin reviewed the experience of Memorial Sloan-Kettering with 423 adults who had extremity sarcomas from 1968 to 1978.[154] Operations involving patients who had margins that were free of tumor cells but close to the tumor were classified as "marginal" operations. When compared to patients with adequate margins, there was no survival difference. The study said, "Therefore, as long as the microscopic margins were negative, survival did not appear to be affected by increasing the soft tissue margins about the tumor."

If local control of the tumor helps to enhance survival, we should see this benefit among patients treated with radiation therapy. Unfortunately, this relationship does not occur. Most authorities report that radiation therapy improves local control, but does not affect survival.[155]

An Opposing View is Expressed

A. T. Stotter and associates from the Royal Marsden Hospital in London concluded that local recurrence was a significant risk to survival.[156] They considered local recurrence as a "time-dependent" factor and reported that patients who developed local recurrence had 4.54 times the risk of developing distant metastases as those who did not. This analysis is similar to that of B. Fisher and colleagues, who demonstrated in a breast cancer project called the NSABP that local recurrence after lumpectomy for breast cancer is associated with a 3.41 greater risk of distant disease.

R. G. Margolese, also of the NSABP, found two types of local recurrence in the lumpectomy trial for breast cancer described in Chapters 1 and 7: "persistence of residual disease," and the "local manifestation of disseminated disease."[157] Fisher made an important distinction, that local recurrence "is a marker of risk for, not a cause of, distant metastasis."[158]

In similar fashion, the local recurrence of soft tissue sarcoma may occur in two forms: the persistence of residual disease and the return of tumor cells from a distant metastasis to the site of the original tumor. Of the patients in the Royal Marsden study, 60 percent had high-grade tumors, and local recurrences appeared in 42 percent of these patients. Many of these recurrences were in patients who had already developed distant metastases. Stotter's findings do not contradict those summarized above. These two forms of local recurrence are more thoroughly discussed in Chapter 4.

The suggestion that local recurrence has little effect on survival would have been heresy just a few years ago. But today, wide local excision and radiation therapy are gaining acceptance in the treatment of soft tissue sarcoma. The central question is, "What is the clinical significance of local recurrence?" Specifically, does recurrent disease cause distant metastasis or is it merely a sign of aggressive disease? If local recurrence jeopardizes patient survival, then aggressive local control measures are indicated. Current evidence overwhelmingly suggests that local recurrence is merely a sign. It can be a sign that the tumor has already spread.

It can also be a sign that the tumor is very aggressive. But if local recurrence is treated promptly, there is no reliable evidence that it causes the tumor to spread. This observation supports the present trend toward limb preservation and should encourage surgeons and radiation therapists to strive toward an even greater concern for the functional and cosmetic results of their work.

CHAPTER 14: CANCER OF THE VAGINA

Cancer of the vagina has been managed primarily by radiation therapy. Consequently, there has been little experience with conservative surgery. Cancers in the upper vagina have been managed by hysterectomy. In 1970, it was discovered that many women whose mothers took diethylstilbestrol during pregnancy to prevent miscarriage developed vaginal cancer, primarily clear cell adenocarcinoma. Pregnancy does not affect the behavior of this cancer.

The Registry for Research on Hormonal Transplacental Carcinogenesis in Chicago found 219 patients with stage I disease, or cancer limited to the mucous membrane.[159] Most were treated with vaginectomy and radical hysterectomy, but 17 underwent local excision alone. Two of these patients developed distant metastases, and died of their disease. Five patients had recurrences in the vagina, and were treated locally. Four of these were alive and well 13.7 to 18.7 years after their original diagnosis. One patient was living with disease. Including those patients who received radiation therapy, there were 43 who had some form of local therapy. The ten-year survival of patients treated conventionally was the same was for those treated by local excision—90 percent versus 88 percent. This occurred in spite of a higher ten-year recurrence rate among the locally treated patients—17 percent versus 27 percent. This is compatible with the consistent theme of this book. Promptly treated local recurrence after conservative surgery does not adversely affect survival.

M. S. Hoffman and associates from the University of South Florida treated 9 patients with invasive cancer using upper vaginectomy.[160] Four patients had tumor invasion of 3.5 mm or more and they received supplemental radiation therapy. The other 5 had invasion of less than 2 mm. Two of the 9 patients developed local recurrence and one died. The other 7 had no evidence of disease from four to fifty-four months after upper vaginectomy.

CHAPTER 15: CANCER OF THE VULVA

I will deal with two aspects of vulvar cancer: treatment of the primary lesion and treatment of the regional lymph nodes.

The Primary Lesion

N. F. Hacker and J. Van der Velden of the Royal Hospital for Women in Paddington, Australia, reviewed the experience of eleven hospitals that treated patients with small cancers of 2 cm or less.[161] They considered 165 patients treated with a "radical local excision," which consisted of 1- to 2-cm margins of excision, and 365 patients treated with a radical vulvectomy. Local recurrence appeared in 12 of the 165 (7.2 percent) patients treated with local excision and in 23 of the 365 (6.3 percent) treated with radical vulvectomy. This difference is not statistically significant. For most patients with early disease, these authors recommended a "radical local excision" plus removal of the groin lymph nodes on one side. They removed the nodes on both sides if the tumor invasion was greater than 1 mm. For patients with stage II cancer, which is cancer confined to the vulva or perineum, and an otherwise normal vulva, the authors also recommended a radical local excision plus removal of the nodes on both sides.

Most encouraging for the advocates of conservative treatment was the 1990 report from J. M. Heaps and colleagues from the UCLA School of Medicine in Los Angeles.[162] They reported no local recurrences among 91 patients whose tumors were excised with a margin of more than 1 cm. Their study included patients with all stages of disease.

To assess the effect of local recurrence on overall survival, I have combined the results of several studies. I have found 21 patients who developed local recurrence isolated to the vulva following conservative surgery—wide local excision or simple vulvectomy. They were followed for from one to twenty-eight years. The studies are summarized in Table A.3. All 21 were treated with reexcision. Two developed distant disease and died. Both may have originally had advanced disease, but this is not clear from the papers. Four patients died of other causes, and the remaining 15 were alive and well when last contacted.

Included in Table A.3 is a report from C. Dipasquale and associates of the University of Padua in Italy. They reported their experience with three young patients treated with local excision.[163] The first patient delivered two children, but developed recurrent cancer in the pelvic lymph nodes ten years after her surgery. This was treated with radical surgery. She lived an additional thirteen years, dying of her cancer twenty-three years following her original operation. (This patient is not included in Table A.3 because her recurrence was in the lymph nodes, not the vulva.) The other two patients developed local recurrences, which were excised. They were alive and well about eight and fifteen years after their original surgeries. Both delivered children.

Table A.3 Local Recurrence and Survival After Conservative Surgery

Year	Author of Study	Vulvar Recurrences	Cancer Deaths
1990	Burke[164]	1	0
1990	Heaps[165]	8	1
1990	Hopkins[166]	5	1
1991	Dipasquale[167]	2	0
1992	Berman[168]	5	0
Totals		21	2

K. C. Podratz and colleagues from the Mayo Clinic in Rochester, Minnesota, reported on 224 patients treated for invasive cancer from 1957 to 1975.[169] Twenty-seven patients were treated with wide excision alone. Among stage I patients, local recurrence developed in 16 percent. Of the patients who developed local recurrence isolated to the vulva following all types of treatment, 50 percent lived five years after their primary treatment. B. Piura and associates from Queen Elizabeth Hospital in Gateshead, England, treated 73 patients for recurrent cancer.[170] Patients with recurrences limited to the vulva had "acceptable" survival results, but the figure was not provided by the authors. The authors also concluded that the distribution of the recurrences and the survival outcomes of the patients were only minimally influenced by the type of initial surgery.

M. P. Hopkins and associates from Northeastern Ohio University College of Medicine have observed that patients who developed local recurrence localized to the vulva following limited excision can be successfully treated with repeat surgical excision.[171]

Malignant melanoma, discussed in Chapter 9, that occurs on the vulva is usually treated by gynecologists. K. O. Rogo and associates from University Hospital of Umea, Sweden, and T. Davidson and colleagues from the Royal Marsden Hospital in London compared their experience with both radical excision and local excision.[172,173] Both groups have supported local excision for this dread disease. Rogo treated a patient who had at least five excisions of local recurrences over a period of eight years. She finally died of unrelated causes. Patients and surgeons alike cringe at the sight of recurrent cancer. However, this patient is another example of the principle that promptly treated local recurrence following conservative surgery is not a risk to survival.

It is reasonable to conclude from the above studies that vulvar cancer can prudently be excised with a 1-cm margin. Risk factors include tumor size and depth of invasion. As with other early cancers, patients who develop recurrent vulvar cancer following conservative surgery usually have a second opportunity for cure.

The above results are consistent with the results of conservative surgery in other parts of the body. I have been disappointed to find in the gynecology literature so few patients treated by local excision. Even more surprising have been the large number of investigators who have failed to report the outcome of patients so treated. Gynecologists who wish to understand the role of conservative surgery should report their results in a manner that allows the reader to determine the percentage of patients who develop local recurrence. The survival rates of these patients should also be reported.

The Regional Lymph Nodes

The treatment of lymph nodes in the groin has been changing from routine excision of all these nodes as part of a radical vulvectomy to removal or sampling of only the most superficial lymph nodes on the side of the primary tumor. If the superficial nodes are positive for cancer, then a complete one-sided lymph node removal is performed. Positive groin lymph nodes are found in about 5 percent of patients with invasion of 3 mm or less, and slightly over 10 percent of patients with invasion of 5 mm or less.

In 1992, J. Y. Lin and associates from George Washington University Hospital in Washington, D.C., analyzed their experience with 82 patients.[174] They compared this to the results of eleven other institutions. There were three categories of surgery: radical vulvectomy and two-sided node removal, modified vulvar excision (several types) with separate groin incisions, and modified vulvar excision with one-sided node removal. They discovered that reducing the scope of both the vulvar excision and the number of lymph nodes removed did not increase the risk of local recurrence at either the site of the tumor or the groin lymph nodes. They had some concerns about patients who had node removals on one side and then developed cancer in the opposite groin. But this occurred in less than 4 percent of patients, and in only 0.4 percent of those with stage I tumors.

From 1970 to 1979, P. J. DiSaia and colleagues from the University of California–Irvine Medical Center treated 20 patients with a policy that used the most superficial groin lymph nodes as sentinel nodes.[175] If they were positive, a complete two-sided groin node removal was done. The pelvic lymph nodes, which are harder to reach, were only removed on the side of the positive sentinel node. Eighteen of the patients with negative groin lymph nodes had no evidence of recurrence from seven to seventy-four months after surgery. All 18 patients had complete preservation of sexual function.

Appendix I

Neither of the patients with positive groin nodes had disease in the pelvic lymph nodes, and neither had additional recurrence. Both patients, however, reported significantly adverse changes in sexual responsiveness.

Few investigators have chosen to simply observe their patients, and perform a delayed lymph node removal if the nodes become enlarged. Many studies have shown this to be prudent for both breast cancer and small cancers of the head and neck. If the nodes in the groin behave as they do in other cancers, it may soon be prudent to simply observe them closely every few months. I believe this will be the ultimate conclusion, and it should be investigated. But since a superficial lymph node removal has few complications, it may be prudent at this time to learn the status of the sentinel nodes on the side of the cancer.

Lymph nodes in the pelvis only become positive after the lymph nodes in the groin are already involved with cancer. Gynecologists have debated whether the pelvic lymph nodes should be removed surgically or treated with radiation therapy. There has been a multi-institutional study of patients with positive groin lymph nodes following radical vulvectomy and two-sided groin lymph node removal.[176] About half the patients were treated with radiation therapy to both groins and to the pelvic lymph nodes. The other half had surgical removal of the pelvic lymph nodes on the side of the disease. The study concluded that patients with two or more positive nodes in the groin lived longer if they were treated with radiation.

I found several problems with the study. First, patients treated with surgery had more advanced disease. Second, 24 percent of patients treated with surgery had recurrent disease in the groin lymph nodes, a high rate of recurrence. Radiation therapy reduced groin recurrences to 5 percent. Third, patients treated by surgery had fewer recurrences in the pelvis than patients treated with radiation. This study does not demonstrate that radiation is better therapy for patients with positive groin nodes. These results suggest that patients treated with surgery started with more advanced disease. Surgery may control cancer in the pelvic lymph nodes better than radiation therapy.

Appendix II

Selected Studies in Conservative Surgery (1995-2001)

Since 1995, hundreds of additional research studies have been published about the cancers discussed in this book. All of the research evidence supports the principles outlined in this book. I have found no studies which conflict with the principles of conservative surgery described here. Your confidence in conservative surgery will increase as you read how successful it has been in a wide variety of cancers.

Each section concludes with the Texas Cancer Center Treatment Analysis for each cancer. These comments are intended to supplement the Analysis section that appears near the end of each chapter in Part II.

CHAPTER 6: BLADDER CANCER

Since 1995, bladder-sparing treatment has become available at several major cancer centers. Treatment usually involves transurethral resection (TUR) of the bladder, radiation therapy and chemotherapy. Survival following conservative treatment appears comparable to that of radical surgery (cystectomy). But, I am aware of no scientific trials that have confirmed this. Overall 5-year survival rates of about 50 to 60 percent have been reported.

Combination treatment is complex and expensive. It usually requires more than 6 months to complete. The side effects of chemotherapy can be severe. In two prominent studies 4 percent of patients died from the chemotherapy. Advances in reconstructive surgery have improved the quality of life for patients who elect to have their bladder removed. Radical cystectomy is still the standard treatment for patients with invasive bladder cancer.

Limited Surgery Alone

Regrettably, the study of bladder-sparing treatment has not progressed in the orderly fashion that occurred in the study of breast cancer. (See Chapter 1) Conservative surgery alone has received little attention. M. Laufer of Johns Hopkins Oncology Center in Baltimore has pointed out that surgery alone (without radiation or chemotherapy) has been "incompletely evaluated" due to the small number of patients studied. However, he concluded that the outcome of treatment as measured by preservation of the bladder and overall survival is "not dissimilar to" the results of radical surgery.[1] In 2001, H.W. Herr and associates of Memorial Sloan-Kettering Cancer Center reported their experience with 99 patients whose initial treatment was aggressive TUR alone.[2] After 10 years, Herr concluded that surgery alone was successful in patients whose tumor could be completely removed by surgery. This is an opinion which Herr has maintained for many years. (See Appendix I.)

Studies of Combination Treatment

Since 1995, many articles have been written on bladder-sparing treatment. Most of these studies have involved the combined use of surgery, radiation therapy, and chemotherapy. In 2000, H. L. Kim and G.D. Steinberg of the University of Chicago published a good review of combination therapy for bladder cancer.[3]

C. N. Sternberg and associates from the San Raffaele Scientific Institute in Rome treated 87 patients with preoperative chemotherapy.[4] Fifty-five of these patients responded to chemotherapy and were then treated with bladder-sparing surgery. The five-year survival rate of these patients was 71 percent. The authors support bladder-sparing surgery for patients who respond to chemotherapy and recommend additional scientific study.

H. W. Herr and associates from the Memorial Sloan-Kettering Cancer Center treated 111 patients with preoperative chemotherapy.[5] Sixty patients had no evidence of cancer after the treatment; nevertheless, 17 of them decided to have a cystectomy. The remaining 43 patients underwent bladder-sparing surgery. Twenty-four of these patients (56 percent) were treated for recurrent cancer in the bladder. Ten years after treatment 32 patients (74 percent) were alive and 25 had a functioning bladder. Among the 17 patients who elected to have a cystectomy, 11 (65 percent) were alive at ten years. In this study patients who were treated with bladder-sparing surgery appeared to live longer than those treated with cystectomy. Compare the ten-year survival rates of 74 percent (bladder-sparing surgery)

Appendix II 287

vs. 65 percent (cystectomy).

J. E. Montie of the University of Michigan, Ann Arbor, reviewed the literature on bladder-sparing surgery.[6] He said that about 50 percent of patients developed recurrent cancer in the bladder and that about half of these recurrences invaded the muscle of the bladder. Montie went on to call these recurrences "an additional source of metastatic disease and death." He supported this conclusion by referring to the study by Herr above - a study which found no additional deaths among patients treated conservatively.

Montie also referred to a paper by William Tester and associates from the Albert Einstein Cancer Center in Philadelphia.[7] They treated 91 patients with invasive bladder cancer using preoperative chemotherapy and radiation. The authors concluded that, ". . . bladder preservation can be achieved in the majority of patients, and that overall survival is similar to that reported with aggressive surgical approaches."

Montie found no evidence of improved survival among patients treated with cystectomy. Nevertheless, he concluded that cystectomy was "optimal therapy" for bladder cancer. Montie presented no scientific evidence which suggested that conservative surgery was a threat to survival. His negative opinion of conservative surgery was based, in part, on 2 studies which, in fact, supported conservative surgery. Montie's findings support the views presented here.

Texas Cancer Center Treatment Analysis

I believe that conservative treatment will become more popular and that the side effects of bladder preservation will decline as doctors refine, reduce or eliminate their use of radiation and chemotherapy. For no other cancer has organ-sparing treatment involved such an aggressive use of adjuvant radiation and chemotherapy.

All available medical evidence continues to support the increased use of bladder-sparing treatment. I believe that many urologists continue to have a bias against bladder-sparing treatment, just as breast cancer surgeons had a bias against breast-sparing treatment. Bladder cancer has a very high rate of local recurrence and there continues to be no evidence that local recurrence is a threat to overall survival. The Texas Cancer Center supports the position of the NSABP that local recurrence is a marker for distant metastasis, not its cause. Promptly-treated local recurrence does not spread.

CHAPTER 7: BREAST CANCER

The most significant research on conservative surgery for invasive breast cancer was published prior to 1995. It proved that conservative surgery and radiation therapy is safe and effective treatment. In 1990, the National Institutes of Health recommended that all patients treated with lumpectomy should have postoperative radiation. This remains standard practice in the U.S. Today doctors are trying to determine if postoperative radiation therapy prolongs the lives of any patients. If it does, precisely which patients benefit? As I have repeatedly stated, there is no evidence that adjuvant radiation therapy prolongs the lives of women with early breast cancer.

The Effects of Radiation Therapy

In 2000, a group of British physicians reviewed 40 different scientific studies to determine the risks and benefits of radiation therapy.[8] They reviewed the treatment of 20,000 women treated with either mastectomy or breast-sparing surgery. They found that radiation reduced local recurrence at 10 years from about 30 percent to about 10 percent. But, radiation therapy had little effect on overall survival. After 20 years the "survival was 37.1 % with radiotherapy versus 35.9%" without. The investigators explained that the radiation techniques used decades ago caused damage to the heart. They concluded that modern radiation techniques should increase the overall survival rate at 20 years by 2 - 4 percent.

The effect of radiotherapy on survival is very controversial and very complex. A slight survival benefit of radiation therapy has been reported in some patients with stage II and III breast cancer. For many years I have suggested that radiation therapists should attempt to precisely show how their treatment effects survival. Do some unirradiated patients develop local recurrences which are difficult to find, e.g., high in the arm pit or under the breast bone? Do some recurrences grow to a large size? Could the spread of tumor cells from these recurrences have been prevented by better surgery - either initially or later? C.D. Atkins of New York correctly observed that radiation therapy was of little survival benefit to patients who had adequate surgical treatment.[9] And the British investigators agreed with Atkins.

It is generally recognized, that despite the large mass of information available, many important questions remain to be answered. Thus far, the mass of information is compatible with the principle thesis of the Texas Cancer Center: Locally recurrent cancer does not become a threat to survival unless it exceeds the volume of the primary tumor.

Appendix II 289

Partial Mastectomy Without Radiation

This topic was covered in Appendix I. Since 1995, additional studies have supported the selective elimination of radiotherapy following breast-sparing surgery. J. de Csepel and associates of Mount Sinai Medical Center in New York studied 43 patients who did not receive radiotherapy.[10] They concluded that some elderly patients, those with other diseases and those with metastatic cancer could decline radiotherapy. Investigators in Austria and Australia have recently eliminated radiation therapy from the treatment of selected, elderly patients.[11,12] They agree that breast-sparing surgery and tamoxifen are sufficient for some patients.

Ductal Carcinoma In Situ (DCIS)

Most of the recent significant progress in breast cancer research has occurred among patients with ductal carcinoma in situ (DCIS). DCIS is an initial step in a process that leads to invasive breast cancer. Until recently, mastectomy was the most common form of treatment. But, lumpectomy with radiation therapy has become an accepted alternative. As stated on page 138, radiation therapy reduces the rate of local recurrence without increasing survival. This important principle applies to both invasive breast cancer and DCIS, as well. Some surgeons are now eliminating radiation from the treatment of selected patients. The selection of these patients is largely determined by three important prognostic criteria: 1) tumor size, 2) tumor grade, and 3) the margin of excision. These criteria have been combined into the Van Nuys Prognostic Index (VNPI). Consider these important factors as you read the studies below.

In 1998, B.F. Fisher and the NSABP investigators published the 8-year results of their B-17 trial.[13] About 400 women with DCIS were treated with lumpectomy only. Most of the tumors were smaller than 2 cm. When pathologists examined the cut edges of the tissue removed by the surgeons, they found no tumor cells. But, as in the earlier NSABP lumpectomy trial for invasive breast cancer (B-06), the margins of excision were narrow. (The significance of margins is discussed in Appendix I.) Within eight years after treatment two types of recurrences developed. Some patients (about 12 percent) developed additional DCIS; some patients (also about 12 percent) developed *invasive* breast cancer.

A second group of about 400 patients was randomly assigned to receive lumpectomy followed by radiation therapy. Radiation had its greatest effect in reducing *invasive* recurrences - from about 12 percent to about 4 percent. Radiation also reduced the number of *noninvasive* recurrences (DCIS) from about 12 percent to about 8 percent. Again, radiation therapy did not improve survival.

Now consider some more precise numbers. Of 403 women treated with lumpectomy alone, there were 53 invasive recurrences and 51 noninvasive recurrences. Only one of these women died of breast cancer. That is 1 death, that might have been prevented by radiation, out of 403 women treated with lumpectomy alone. (The 3 other deaths in this group could not have been prevented by radiation, since these 3 women did not develop a local recurrence.) Of the 411 women treated with lumpectomy and radiation, two patients died following a local recurrence - twice the number as in the radiation-free group.

Among the entire group of 814 women, most of the breast cancer deaths (8 of 14) occurred in women who developed metastatic disease without having a recurrence in the breast. Two patients died from cancer in the opposite breast. Only 3 patients died following a recurrence in the treated breast.

Among the patients who received no radiation there were four deaths attributable to breast cancer. Among those who received radiation there were 10 deaths attributable to breast cancer - a 2 1/2 fold difference. According to my calculations this difference comes within 1 percent of being statistically significant. Yet, the NSABP investigators did not call attention to these results. It is clear that radiation therapy did not improve the survival of patients in this study. In fact, the results suggest that more patients may have died of breast cancer if they received radiation.

Another NSABP trial (B-24), demonstrated that among patients treated with lumpectomy and radiation, the addition of tamoxifen reduces the incidence of all breast cancer recurrences from 13.4 percent to 8.4 percent, but there was no survival benefit.[14] M.J. Silverstein and associates from the University of Southern California studied 133 patients whose DCIS had been excised with a margin of 1 cm or more.[15] They concluded that these patients did not need postoperative radiation therapy. In April, 1999, the Consensus Conference on the Treatment of In Situ Ductal Carcinoma of the Breast was held in Philadelphia.[16] This group concluded that invasive carcinoma of the breast develops each year in about 1 percent or less of patients treated with local excision - with or without radiation. There was no general agreement on the optimal form of treatment, but many panelist considered wide excision alone (1 cm margin or greater) to be acceptable. Some participants said that even patients with high grade lesions can be treated in this manner.

Appendix II

Erroneous Conclusions about Radiation Therapy

Most radiation therapists support the routine use of radiation after breast-sparing procedures. Recently, they have written over a dozen articles evaluating the threat of locally recurrent breast cancer.

These articles follow a similar pattern. Investigators follow patients who were treated with breast-sparing surgery. They divide these patients into two groups - those who develop recurrent cancer in the treated breast and those who do not. The investigators observe that patients who remain free of local recurrence live longer than those who develop local recurrence. This is correct. They conclude that patients die from distant metastases caused by the recurrence. This is not correct. Even in the well-known NSABP lumpectomy trial, patients treated with lumpectomy alone, who then developed local recurrence, were 4.6 times as likely to develop distant metastases as those who remained free of local recurrence. But, the NSABP investigators concluded, correctly, that local recurrence was the indicator of a poor prognosis, but not its cause.

Beginning on page 73, I try to explain these perplexing observations. In brief, there are two types of recurrence. Traditional local recurrence is a sign that the tumor has already spread. But, the persistence of tumor cells following conservative surgery (local persistence) is not a grave sign. Combining these two forms of recurrence leads to the confusing observations above. Following lumpectomy alone some patients developed traditional local recurrence. It was almost exclusively these patients, who developed distant metastases. (I also try to explain this confusing matter here in Appendix II. See Malignant Melanoma, Erroneous Conclusions.)

B. Haffty and associates from Yale reported their experience with 973 patients treated with conservative surgery and radiation therapy.[17] They concluded, "Whether early breast tumor relapse is a marker for or cause of distant metastases remains a controversial and unresolved issue."

Radiation therapists from the Hotel-Dieu de Quebec Hospital, Universite Laval reviewed the charts of 2,030 patients treated with breast-sparing surgery between 1969 and 1991.[18] At 10 years 13 percent of patients had developed local recurrence. Only 55 percent of these patients survived 10 years. Of patients who remained free of local disease, 75 percent survived ten years. The authors reported that the risk of distant metastasis was 5.1 times higher among patients with local recurrence. (As mentioned above, in the NSABP lumpectomy trial this figure was 4.6 times.) They concluded that local recurrence was the source of new distant metastases and the cause of death in some patients. This conclusion is incorrect.

These investigators measured the size of the local recurrences. They found 27 patients had recurrences less than 1.5 cm in diameter; these patients had a 10-year survival of 72 percent. There were 94 patients who developed recurrences larger than 1.5 cm; they had a 10-year survival of 32 percent. Compare the 10-year survival of patients with small recurrences (72 percent) to that of patients with no recurrence (75 percent). This supports the many other studies which have proven that promptly-treated local recurrence does not spread. It also support my 1980 statement, "For instance, a patient who survives a carcinoma of 2 to 3 cm in diameter without developing distant metastases may be expected to survive a similar volume of tumor in adjacent breast or lymphatic tissue." [19]

Of course, locally recurrent cancer can spread if it grows too large. Even today we do not know what "too large" means, because few investigators have measured the size of recurrences. For many years I have suggested that investigators should compare the size of each recurrence to the size of the primary (original) tumor. I believe that "too large" is any size which exceeds the size of the primary lesion.

Texas Cancer Center Treatment Analysis

Some radiation therapists would like to demonstrate that their treatment prolongs lives of patients and may exaggerate the benefits of radiotherapy. The Texas Cancer Center supports the increased use of breast-sparing surgery for both invasive and in situ breast cancer (DCIS). It is clear that radiation therapy does not prolong survival for patients with early disease. The Texas Cancer Center also supports the position of the NSABP that local recurrence is a marker for distant metastasis, not its cause. Promptly-treated local recurrence does not spread. (See chapter 7 and Appendix 1.)

CHAPTER 8: CERVICAL CANCER

The leader in fertility-sparing surgery is Daniel Dargent of Hopital Edouard Herriot in Lyon, France.[20] Between 1987 and 1995, he treated 47 women with radical trachelectomy and laparoscopic pelvic lymph node dissection. Twenty-nine patients were stage Ib or higher and seven patients had tumors which were 2 cm in diameter or larger. After a mean follow up of 52 months, 1 patient developed a local recurrence, 1 developed a distant metastasis, and a third died of progressive disease. Of the 16 patients who tried to become pregnant, 10 delivered a normal child.

M. Roy and M. Plante of Quebec City, Canada treated 30 patients with radical trachelectomy and laparoscopic pelvic lymph node dissection between 1991 and 1998.[21] Two years after surgery, 29 patients were alive and free of cancer. One patient developed an intraabdominal recurrence and died of advanced disease. Of the 6 patients who tried to become pregnant, 4 delivered healthy babies by caesarean section and 2 were pregnant when the paper was written. The authors updated their experience in May, 2000.[22]

A. Covens and associates of Toronto, Ontario, Canada, treated 32 patients with radical trachelectomy and laparoscopic pelvic lymph node dissection between 1994 and 1998.[23] After two years the recurrence free survival rate was 95%. One patient developed an intraabdominal recurrence and died of advanced disease. Of the 13 patients who tried to become pregnant, 4 were successful, 3 delivered healthy children by caesarean section. The authors called their procedure "an acceptable alternative" to radical hysterectomy for patients with early stage I disease.

Surgeons in England, Germany and Italy are also beginning to use this fertility-sparing approach to cervical cancer. A group of surgeons at Tohoku University in Japan has begun to use conization for selected patients who have lesions with 3 to 5 mm of invasion.[24]

Texas Cancer Center Treatment Analysis

The Texas Cancer Center supports the increased use of trachelectomy for selected patients with invasive cancer of the cervix. The Texas Cancer Center also supports the position of the NSABP that local recurrence is a marker for distant metastasis, not its cause. Promptly-treated local recurrence does not spread.

CHAPTER 9: MALIGNANT MELANOMA

Studies of malignant melanoma fall into two categories: those that look at treatment of the primary lesion, and those that look at treatment of the lymph nodes.

The Primary Lesion

Since 1995, conservative treatment for melanoma has increased. Mohs micrographic surgery has become accepted treatment in several academic medical centers. J.A. Zitelli and colleagues of Shadyside Medical Center in Pittsburgh conducted a prospective study of 535 patients treated for melanoma using the Mohs technique.[25] Eighty-three percent of lesions were successfully excised with a 6 mm margin; a 1.2 cm margin was required to remove 97 percent of all lesions. They achieved 5-year survival rates which were equivalent to patients treated by standard wide-margin surgery. Local recurrences from inadequate excision of the primary tumor were very rare (0.5 percent). The authors recommend Mohs micrographic surgery when narrow margins are desired.

S.N. Snow and associates of the Mohs Surgery Clinic in Madison, Wisconsin, treated 179 patients with melanoma from 1981 to 1991.[26] They concluded that the Mohs technique was effective treatment for patients with melanomas of thin and intermediate thickness. For deeper lesions the number of cases was insufficient to evaluate.

By 1998, K. M. Keaton and associates at the UT M. D. Anderson Cancer Center studied 278 patients with thick melanomas, i.e., deeper than 4 mm.[27] The median tumor thickness for their patients was 6 mm. After a median follow-up of over 21 years, the local recurrence rate was 27%. These investigators found that local recurrence did not significantly affect overall survival. They concluded that a 2 cm margin of excision was adequate for patients with thick lesions (> 4 mm).

D.A. Hudson and associates of the University of Cape Town, South Africa, treated 106 patients with stage I melanoma of the face.[28] Margins of excision ranged from less than 1 cm to greater than 2 cm. Seven patients developed local recurrences, but these were not influenced by the size of the excision margin. The authors concluded that stage I melanoma of the face should be treated with a complete excision, microscopically confirmed by a pathologist. They found that this could be achieved with margins of excisions of less than 1 cm.

Erroneous Conclusions

Many studies have now proven that a narrow margin of excision - and the local recurrence which may follow - does not adversely affect survival. This conflicts with the prevailing paradigm and some investigators are now resorting to faulty research techniques to support their erroneous beliefs.

X. D. Dong and associates of Duke University Medical Center studied 648 patients who developed local recurrence following the removal of the original melanoma.[29] The Duke investigators reported that 48.5% of these patients died within five years of their local recurrence. (They did not compare this mortality rate to that of patients who remained free of local recurrence.) They concluded that this mortality rate was high and that local recurrence caused the melanoma to spread. They suggested that patients may benefit from more aggressive local therapy, e.g., wider margins of excision.

This study is seriously flawed, because there are at least two types of local recurrence. First, cancer cells may have already spread to a distant organ (metastasis), before the original melanoma was removed. As the metastasis grows it may shed additional cancer cells into the blood stream, where they eventually make there way back to the site of surgery. (Experimental research has shown that cancer cells are attracted to tissue, which has been injured by surgery.) This first type of local recurrence (traditional local recurrence) has a very bad prognosis, because the cancer has already spread. Modern scans and other tests may not detect the distant metastasis until it is almost an inch in size. The metastasis may not be detected until months after the local recurrence is first seen. The distant metastasis may appear to follow - and thus be caused by - the local recurrence. But, this is incorrect. Actually, it's the other way around.

The second type of recurrence involves cancer cells left behind in the skin following the removal of the original melanoma. I prefer to call this "local persistence." Local persistence is not a threat to patient survival. Patients who are able to prevent the spread of disease from their original melanoma, are able to prevent the spread of disease from a recurrent - or persistent - melanoma. This is precisely the way breast cancer behaves.

Any group of patients who have developed local recurrence will include those with both types of recurrence. The inclusion of patients with traditional local recurrence will adversely affect the calculated survival of the whole group. The inclusion of patients with "local persistence" will not affect the group's survival. Even in the well-known NSABP lumpectomy trial, patients who developed local recurrence were 4.6 times as likely to develop distant metastases as those who remained free of local recurrence. But, the NSABP investigators concluded correctly that local recurrence was the indicator of a poor prognosis, but not its cause.

X. D. Dong and associates of Duke University combined patients with two types of local recurrence in their study. It is not surprising that these patients had a poor prognosis. Many of them already had distant metastases and developed traditional local recurrence from the distant disease. Some of the patients had local persistence and their survival was not affected. But, they were lost in this faulty study. Contrary to the study from Duke, aggressive local therapy has no affect on patient survival.

The Regional Lymph Nodes

Sentinel Lymph Node Biopsy

Sentinel lymph node biopsy is a new technique which removes only those few lymph nodes which are close to the melanoma - those nodes where the melanoma is most likely to spread. Before surgery a dye is injected into the skin around the melanoma. The dye flows into the nearest (sentinel) lymph node(s) and a scan identifies the node(s) in question. The is called lymphatic mapping. A blue colored dye allows the surgeon to see the sentinel lymph node while performing the biopsy. (Dyes can also be used which highlight positive lymph nodes on X-rays.) By removing very few lymph nodes the surgeon can usually determine the status of all the nodes in the region. If cancer cells are found in the sentinel node, the surgeon usually removes most of the remaining regional nodes. This technique causes few side effects and can be performed on any patient about whom there is any question of lymph node spread. For most patients this technique has largely eliminated the decades long debate about the value of elective lymph node dissection in patients with melanoma. There is much we can learn from this debate and, regrettably, these lessons are likely to be ignored. (This is what happened in the 1970's when breast cancer surgeons learned the removal of the lymph nodes under the arm did not improve survival. They continued to perform the surgery in order to see how far the cancer had spread, and to determine which patients might benefit from chemotherapy.)

Surprising New Information about Elective Lymph Node Dissection (ELND)

In 1996, Intergroup Melanoma Trial published the results of a randomized trial of 740 patients with localized melanoma, 1.0 to 4.0 mm thick.[30] Half of the patients received an elective lymph node dissection (ELND), when the melanoma was removed. The other patients had their lymph nodes left intact. If the lymph nodes later became enlarged with cancer cells, they were removed. The primary patients to benefit from an ELND were those with thin lesions, 1.0 - 2.0 mm. This was surprising, because these patients were the *least* likely to have positive regional lymph nodes. Why did ELND benefit those patients least likely to have positive lymph nodes? The authors of this study offered no explanation for their surprising results. My explanation, published in 1995, can be found on page 258. My explanation has been repeatedly published in the medical literature.[31,32,33,34,35,36,37] It remains the only explanation of this surprising observation. It has never been refuted. (It is also published on our web site, www.texascancercenter.com, under the section: Treatment Options/Melanoma/Medical Mysteries.)

Texas Cancer Center Treatment Analysis

The Texas Cancer Center continues to support the use of limited surgery for malignant melanoma, especially in cosmetically sensitive areas. Sentinel lymph node biopsy is appropriate for many patients with intermediate level lesions.

CANCER OF THE PENIS

Studies of cancer of the penis fall into two categories: those that consider treatment of the primary lesion, and those that consider treatment of the lymph nodes.

The Primary Lesion

Since 1995 several institutions have reported good results with therapy which preserves the penis. From 1973 to 1993, J. C. Soria and associates from the Institute Gustave-Roussy in Villejuif, France treated 102 patients with invasive cancer of the penis.[38] Conservative treatment was feasible in 72 patients. Treatment included interstitial brachytherapy either alone or with limited surgery. Penile integrity was maintained in 49 (68 percent) of these patients. The five-year survival rate of the entire group of 102 patients was 63 percent.

A. J. Chaudhary and colleagues of the Tate Memorial Hospital in Mumbai, India treated 23 patients with interstitial brachytherapy from 1988 to 1996.[39] Five patients developed recurrences either locally or in the lymph nodes. Four of these patients were successfully treated with additional surgery and were free of disease on their last hospital visit. The authors concluded that brachytherapy offers "excellent local control rates."

R. Sarin and associates from the Royal Marsden Hospital in England treated most of their 101 patients with external beam radiation therapy.[40] Others were treated with surgery or brachytherapy. Recurrent disease eventually appeared in 36 patients, 26 of whom were successfully controlled with additional treatment.

D. N. Tietjen and R.S. Malek of the Mayo Clinic in Rochester, Minnesota, treated 52 men with laser surgery.[41] They concluded that with the exception of deeply invasive (T2) lesions, local control was similar to that achieved by more conventional therapies. T. Windahl and S. Hellsten of Orebro Medical Center in Sweden treated 32 men with laser therapy.[42] Thirty-one months after treatment all men were free of disease.

D. Gotsadze and associates from the Oncological Research Center in

Tbilisi, Georgia reported their experience with 223 patients who were conservatively treated between 1959 and 1996.[43] Most were treated with radiotherapy. Local control was initially achieved in 135 (60.5 percent) of 223 patients. Local recurrence developed in 24 patients (17.7 percent) and ten patients (4.5 percent) developed positive regional lymph nodes. The 5-year survival rate was 83 percent. The authors concluded that organ-sparing treatment of penile cancer is justified. Local failure can be surgically corrected by surgery without compromising survival.

The Regional Lymph Nodes

D. Theodorescu and colleagues from Memorial Sloan-Kettering Cancer Center in New York reported on their experience with 42 patients treated between 1980 and 1994.[44] The patients all had clinically negative inguinal lymph nodes. All patients with grade 2 and 3 lesions developed positive inguinal lymph nodes, requiring surgical removal. These authors concluded that patients with grade 1 tumors do not need an elective lymph node dissection (ELND). That has also been supported by other studies.

Although sentinel lymph node biopsy has gained acceptance for several types of cancer, Pettaway and associates from the UT M. D. Anderson Cancer Center had unfavorable results with this technique between 1985 and 1994.[45] Twenty patients were treated with an extended sentinel lymph node dissections. All were negative for metastases, but 5 patients developed inguinal metastases an average of 10 months later. The author concluded that sentinel node dissection was not reliable for patients with penile cancer. As with other new techniques, it is likely that results will improve as surgeons gain experience with the procedure. Since malignant cells may spread to both the right and left sides of the body, it is usually necessary to examine both sides. (See the section on cancer of the vulva in this appendix for more information about sentinel node biopsies.)

Texas Cancer Center Treatment Analysis

The Texas Cancer Center continues to support the use of conservative treatment for cancer of the penis.

CHAPTER 10: PROSTATE CANCER

Fowler and associates of the Massachusetts General Hospital studied the treatment recommendations of cancer specialists and concluded, "... while urologists and radiation oncologists do agree on a variety of issues regarding detection and treatment of prostate cancer, specialists overwhelmingly recommend the therapy that they themselves deliver."[46]

Screening Recommendations

F. Labrie and associates of Laval University in Quebec City, Canada, began a randomized trial of prostate cancer screening in 1988.[47] By 1997, 46,193 men had entered the study - 38,056 were screened and 8,136 were not. There were only 5 prostate cancer deaths among the men who were screened. But, among those who were not screened, 137 men had died of prostate cancer. This represents a 69 percent decrease in prostate cancer deaths among men who were screened and promptly treated. It is clear from this study that prostate cancer screening can save lives. Also, the type of treatment is not nearly as important as the importance of early detection.

Brachytherapy or Interstitial Radiation

The Northwest Tumor Institute in Seattle has a very large experience with this technique. H. Ragde and L. Korb reported 10-year results of 152 patients with T1 to T3, low to high grade prostate cancer.[48] All patients received Iodine-125 brachytherapy with or without external beam radiation. Only 3 patients died of prostate cancer, and 66 percent of patients were free of disease after 10 years. The authors concluded that their results were comparable to those of radical prostatectomy.

J. Sharkey and colleagues of the Urology Health Center in New Port Richey, Florida have used brachytherapy to treat 1,048 patients since 1991.[49] After five to nine years, over 90 percent of their patients have stable PSA levels of less than 1.5 ng./ml. This result has been confirmed by a negative biopsy rate of 90 percent in 600 men. Incontinence occurs in less than 1 percent of patients, and impotence occurs in about 10 percent.

In the May 13, 1996, issue of Fortune magazine, Andy Grove, then chairman of Intel, explained his choice of interstitial radiation to treat his stage B prostate cancer. P.C. Walsh, a urologist at Johns Hopkins in Baltimore wrote an editorial which was critical of Groves' decision.[50] Walsh stated,"It is now clear that most patients who received digitally directed interstitial radiotherapy under that protocol are dying of the disease." My letter-to-the-editor was published in the Journal of Urology.[51] I pointed out that Walsh referred to a study conducted between 1970 and 1985 of men with advance disease - 72 percent had tumors larger than 2 cm. Local failure occurred in 48 percent of men, and only 18 percent of these men had additional hormonal treatment. It is not surprising that this group of men did poorly. Today most men are treated with early disease. Local recurrence is promptly detected and treated. Walsh's editorial reflected his strong bias favoring radical surgery and was of little help to men wrestling with the complex decision.

Complete Hormonal Blockade

Urologists in the U.S., Canada and Europe are investigating the use of hormonal treatment for early prostate cancer. As early as 1977, the South Sweden Prostate Cancer Study Group treated men with localized disease using either immediate estrogen therapy or delayed treatment.[52] By 1993, there was no difference in overall survival between the groups, but the risk of dying of prostate cancer was higher in the deferred treatment group. Between 1985 and 1993, the Medical Research Council in England treated 934 men with localized prostate cancer. Men were randomly assigned to immediate hormonal blockade or deferred treatment - treatment which was delayed until symptoms developed.[53] Overall survival was longer in men who received immediate treatment, and there was a 21 percent reduction is deaths due to prostate cancer.

Since 1989, S.B. Strum and associates of the Prostate Cancer Research Institute in Los Angeles have used hormonal blockade - an antiandrogen and a LHRH agonist.[54] They have treated 255 men and achieved undetectable PSA levels in 216. Some men who maintained an undetectable PSA level for more than one year elected to discontinue hormonal blockade. PSA levels remained low for an average of about 3 years. Only one patient developed a prostate cancer recurrence which was not responsive to further hormonal treatment.

Combination Treatment

N.N. Stone and R.G. Stock of Mount Sinai Medical Center in New York reported that hormonal therapy given before and after brachytherapy can reduce the size of the prostate and improve local control.[55] Patients with high risk disease had results that were similar to those of men with low risk cancer. Two years after treatment, 62 men agreed to have prostate biopsies; 60 (97 percent) were negative for tumor. Hormonal therapy given prior to radiation also prolongs overall survival.[56]

A. D'Amico and associates from the Joint Center for Radiation Therapy in Boston treated 1,586 men with 3-dimensional conformal external beam radiation.[57] Hormonal blockade was provided to 276 men for six months surrounding the radiotherapy. Men with intermediate and high risk cancer were much less likely to fail if they were treated with hormonal blockade.

When given prior to radical prostatectomy, endocrine treatment reduces the incidence of positive surgical margins, but it does not improve survival.

Cryosurgery

J.K. Cohen and associates of the Medical College of Pennsylvania in Pittsburgh treated 383 patients with cryosurgery. Five years later 71 percent had a negative biopsy and 60 percent of patients had a PSA of < 1 ng./ml.[58]

Watchful Waiting

The results of pure watchful waiting are not good and few men now choose this option. As discussed above, there are now good alternatives to aggressive surgery and radiation.

Sweden and Denmark have reliable cancer registries. They have found a high rate of prostate cancer deaths among men who postpone treatment. Men below the age of 75, who are diagnosed with nonmetastatic prostate cancer, have a greater than 50 percent chance of dying of prostate cancer if they do not receive immediate treatment.[59] Furthermore, as mentioned above, the screening study from Quebec City found a 69 percent reduction in prostate cancer deaths among men who were screened and immediately treated.

Texas Cancer Center Treatment Analysis

The Texas Cancer Center supports the increased use of conservative treatment for cancer of the prostate. Men should chose the type of treatment they prefer, since there is no evidence that overall survival is affected by this decision.

CHAPTER 7: RECTAL CANCER

Sphincter-sparing surgery is now widely practiced in U.S. medical centers. Since 1995, dozens of articles have been written on this subject - most all of them favorable. Most patients with rectal cancer should have no trouble finding a surgeon who practices conservative surgery. This progress can be attributed, in part, to the surgical subspeciality of colon and rectal surgery. These surgeons had an incentive to distinguish themselves from their more traditional colleagues, the general surgeons.

In 1997, A. K. Ng and associates from Harvard Medical School reviewed the worldwide experience with sphincter-sparing treatment for rectal cancer.[60] They found 4 studies dealing with nonsurgical therapy, e.g., cryosurgery, electrocoagulation, and endocavitary radiation. There were 14 studies dealing with local excision alone - without radiation or chemotherapy. There were 11 studies dealing with local excision and radiation - with or without chemotherapy.

Ng and associates found that local recurrence rates varied among the different studies. About 50 percent of patients were successfully salvaged with additional surgery. This resulted in overall local control rates and survival rates similar to that for abdominoperineal resection. The authors concluded that patients with small, favorable T1 tumors should be treated with local excision alone, if negative margins could be achieved. Patients with T2 lesions or T1 lesions with "unfavorable" clinical or pathological characteristics should receive both radiation and chemotherapy. Patients with T3 lesion should be treated with radiation and/or chemotherapy either before or after surgery. Recently, the trend has been toward preoperative treatment.

V. Valentini and colleagues from Rome treated 81 patients with T3 rectal cancer using preoperative radiation and chemotherapy.[61] In 46 patients the tumor decreased in size and 63 patients were able to have a sphincter-sparing procedure. R. A. Graham and associates of the New England Medical Center in Boston treated five patients with T3 lesions using local excision, and postoperative radiation therapy, 5-FU and leucovorin.[62] After these patients were followed for 56 months, there had been no local or regional failures. Two patients had died of distant disease. The authors support the use of this treatment for selected patients with T3 tumors.

M. Mohiuddin and colleagues of the University of Kentucky treated 70 patients who had tumors located in the last 2 cm of the rectum.[63] This area is difficult to treat, because it is so close to the sphincter muscles. Patients received high-dose radiation therapy before surgery. An average of 4 years later, 9 patients (13 percent) developed local recurrence. The statistical 5-year survival rate was 84 percent.

N.A. Janjan and associates of the UT M.D. Anderson Cancer Center treated 45 patients with aggressive preoperative radiation and chemotherapy.[64] The tumor decreased in size in 86 percent of patients and sphincter preservation was possible in 79 percent of patients who had surgery.

A word of caution was reported by D. Shibata and colleagues of Memorial Sloan-Kettering Cancer Center.[65] They surveyed patients who had received sphincter-sparing treatment for locally advanced rectal cancer.

Appendix II

The majority of patients (56 percent) reported unfavorable bowel function. The author suggested that some patients with advanced disease may do better with a permanent colostomy.

The Influence of Local Recurrence

J. Garcia-Aguilar and associates of University of Minnesota issued another "word of caution."[66] They reviewed 82 patients treated with excision only. All tumors were removed with negative margins and had favorable pathologic characteristics. Ten of 55 patients with T1 tumors (18 percent) and 10 of 27 with T2 tumors (37 percent) developed local recurrence. Seventeen of the 20 underwent surgery to remove the recurrence. They warned that these recurrences rates were higher than those reported among patients treated with adjuvant therapy. After 54 months (4.5 years) of follow-up, 77 percent of T1 patients and 55 percent of T2 patients were alive and free of disease. The authors noted that these survival rates were equivalent to those of patients treated with radical surgery. This study demonstrates again that local recurrence does not adversely affect survival.

Texas Cancer Center Treatment Analysis

The Texas Cancer Center supports the increased use of sphincter-sparing surgery for selected patients with cancer of the rectum. The Texas Cancer Center also supports the position of the NSABP that local recurrence is a maker for distant metastasis, not its cause. Promptly-treated local recurrence does not spread.

CHAPTER 13: SOFT TISSUE SARCOMA

It has now been proven that conservative surgery alone is safe and effective treatment for most patients with soft tissue sarcoma. But, the scientific evidence is often buried by the prevailing prejudice against limited treatment. Many "leading" surgeons in this field still refuse to accept the innocent behavior of promptly-treated local recurrence. They recommend too much surgery and too much radiation therapy.

Since 1995, two major randomized, prospective trials have published their updated results. W. T. Pisters and associates from the Memorial Sloan-Kettering Cancer Center conducted a trial of 164 patients, who were followed for over six years.[67] Local recurrence developed in 18 percent of those given radiation therapy and 29 percent of those who were not treated. The statistical five-year survival rates were statistically similar - 83 percent versus 80 percent, respectively. The authors concluded,"This improvement in local control does not have an impact on rates of distant recurrence or disease-specific survival."

J. C. Yang and colleagues from the National Cancer Institute conducted a randomized trial of 141 patients, who were followed for over 9½ years.[68] Local recurrence rates were lower in patients who received radiation, 1.4 percent for those given radiation therapy versus 23.9 percent for those who were not treated. There was no significant difference in the five-year survival rates. The authors said,"Thus the conclusions regarding adjuvant XRT (radiation) for patients with sarcoma are similar to conclusions reached for . . . primary breast cancer and rectal cancer, where local control was enhanced without significant differences in overall survival."

Surgery without Radiation Therapy

Some institutions have reported favorable experience using surgery alone without radiation therapy. C. P. Karakousis and associates of Roswell Park Cancer Institute in Buffalo New York, treated 116 with wide or radical resection.[69] Nine patients had an amputation. The local recurrence rate among these patients was 10 percent. The authors concluded,"Wide resection, when feasible, provides acceptable local control and may be preferable to local excision plus radiation therapy."

C. P. Gibbs and colleagues of the University of Chicago analyzed 62 patients.[70] Fifty-nine patients (95 percent) went to Chicago for excision alone following limited surgery at a community hospital. Almost five years after treatment, only three patients - those treated with a narrow excision - had developed a local recurrence. The five-year survival rate - free of any cancer - was 85 percent. The authors concluded,"Excellent rates of survival . . . . can be obtained with carefully planned operative treatment alone."

P.L. Fabrizio and associates from the Mayo Clinic in Rochester used surgery alone to treat 24 patients with localized extremity sarcoma.[71] They concluded,"It is appropriate to consider withholding irradiation for selected patients with low-grade tumors resected with a negative margins."

Promptly-treated Local Recurrence Does Not Influence Survival

P.M.F. Choong and associates from the University Hospital in Lund, Sweden, analyzed 134 locally recurrent tumors in patients who did not have metastatic disease.[72] They concluded that the clinical behavior of local recurrence is a better predictor of tumor behavior than the mere presence of local recurrence. Patients with aggressive primary tumors also had aggressive local recurrences and a shortened life expectancy. The local recurrence was an indicator of the poor prognosis - not its cause.

A contrary point of view was expressed by C. S. Trovik and H. C. F. Bauer from the Karolinska Hospital in Stockholm, Sweden.[73] They analyzed their treatment of 379 patients. Among patients with favorable tumors (small size and/or low grade) local recurrence appeared to shorten survival. But, as discussed on page 73 and in the section on breast cancer in this appendix, it is statistically misleading to compare the survival of patients who develop local recurrence to the survival of those who do not.

T. Ueda and colleagues updated their experience at the Osaka University Medical School. In a 1997 study, these investigators concluded,"Multivariate analysis showed that local recurrence after definitive surgery also lost its prognostic significance."[74] S. Singer and associates from Harvard studied 182 patients with extremity sarcomas from 1970 to 1992.[75] They concluded, "Thus, local recurrence does not appear to play a major role in influencing the overall survival."

J. J. Lewis and associates analyzed 911 patients with soft tissue sarcomas of the extremity treated at Memorial Sloan-Kettering Cancer Center from 1982 to 1995.[76] Multivariate analysis demonstrated that local recurrence had no significant effect on survival. They concluded, "Clearly, local recurrence is not a source of metastasis." But, surgeons at Memorial have not embraced this concept and elsewhere their comments are not as clear. N. J. Espat and J. J. Lewis said, ". . . local tumor recurrence is associated with development of distant metastasis. . . . The relationship is an enigma. . . ."[77] Surgeons at Memorial appear to be confused about the relationship between local recurrence and survival. This confusion is further illustrated below.

Perplexing Data from Memorial Sloan-Kettering Cancer Center

M.F. Brennan of Memorial studied two groups of patients: 1) those who were first treated at Memorial Hospital (558 patients) and 2) those who were first treated elsewhere and came to Memorial with a local recurrence (318 patients).[78] All patients had their tumors removed and following surgery the local recurrence rates were similar in both groups. But then Brennan found a surprise. He found that patients who were first treated at a community hospital lived significantly longer than those first treated at Memorial. The five-years survival rates were approximately 80 percent (first treatment elsewhere) versus 55 percent (first treatment at Memorial). Brennan said this information "further obfuscates the problem (of understanding local recurrence)."

Those who are following the theme of this book will find nothing surprising about Brennan's results. Some patients treated at community hospitals died of their disease. (There immune system lost its initial battle against the tumor.) Others who were referred to Memorial may have had a local recurrence, but they were free of apparent distant disease. Their immune system had already prevented the distant spread of tumor cells. They had won their first battle with their cancer and were immunologically strong enough to win the second battle with their local recurrence. In contrast, the group of patients who were first treated at Memorial included some patients with a relatively weak immune system. Their early death decreased the overall survival of this group. Thus, patients who were first treated at a community hospital had an overall survival rate which was greater than that of patients who received their first treatment at Memorial.

Texas Cancer Center Treatment Analysis

The Texas Cancer Center supports the increased use of conservative surgery in the treatment of soft tissue sarcomas. The Texas Cancer Center also supports the position of the NSABP that local recurrence is a marker for distant metastasis, not its cause. Promptly-treated local recurrence does not spread.

CHAPTER 14: CANCER OF THE VAGINA

Radiation therapy continues to play a major role in the treatment of vaginal cancer. There have been no major publications since 1995. For stage I disease brachytherapy alone achieves local control equivalent to that achieved with external beam pelvic radiation.[79] Patients with more advanced disease may benefit from a combination of external radiation and brachytherapy.

Vaginal Melanoma

Patients with vaginal melanoma are usually treated with surgery. D. J. Buchanan and associates from Fullerton, California, reviewed the medical literature and found 66 cases of vaginal melanoma published since 1989.[80] They concluded,"Since no single treatment is clearly preferable, we suggest conservative resection where possible. We find it difficult to support radical surgery as primary treatment for vaginal melanoma. . . ."

An opposing point of view was expressed by K. M. Van Nostrand and associates from the University of Californian, Irvine.[81] They reported on 8

Appendix II

patients from their institution and 119 cases reported since 1949. They compared patients who had been treated with radical surgery to those treated with conservative surgery. They reported a survival advantage following radical surgery. My letter-to-the-editor pointed out that the authors had failed to consider important prognostic factors, such as stages of disease and depth of invasion.[82] I said that the authors had a "bias which favors radical surgery over procedures which preserve bodily form and function." K.M. Van Nostrand replied,"We had no intention . . . to make a statement concerning the need for aggressive cancer surgery in all such instances."[83]

Texas Cancer Center Treatment Analysis

The Texas Cancer Center supports the increased use of conservative surgery and radiation therapy for cancer of the vagina. Vaginal melanoma should be treated like melanoma elsewhere in the body - with narrow margins of excision, as needed for a good cosmetic and functional result.

CHAPTER 15: CANCER OF THE VULVA

Studies of cancer of the vulva fall into two categories: those that look at treatment of the primary lesion, and those that look at treatment of the lymph nodes.

The Primary Lesion

Since 1995, there has been a strong shift toward more conservative surgery. The following publications are representative of that change. There have been no scientific studies which indicate that conservative surgery poses a risk to patient survival.

J. D. Nash and S. Curry of the University of Connecticut said,". . . surgically conservative approaches achieve equivalent outcomes with far less morbidity and cosmetic disfiguration."[84] J. F. Magrina and associates from the Mayo Clinic in Scottsdale, Arizona, reported their experience with 225 patients.[85] Radical surgery was performed on 134 patients and vulvar excision was performed on 91. After 5 years, 14 percent of patients developed local recurrence and 76 percent of patients were alive. There were no significant differences between the two procedures in the development of local recurrence or in overall survival. Surgical complications- both immediate and long term - were greater among patients treated with radical surgery.

N. F. Hacker of the Royal Hospital for Women in New South Wales, Australia, has said,"In recent years, vulvar cancer management has been revolutionized with a more conservative approach being recommended for the primary lesion and a more rational approach to the management of the lymph nodes."[86] T. W. Burke and colleagues at the UT M. D. Anderson Cancer Center treated 76 patients with T1 and T2 vulvar cancers using wide excision and selective inguinal node dissection.[87] Nine women (12 percent) developed local recurrence in the vulva and all were controlled by additional surgery. The statistical 4-year survival rate was 81 percent. The authors concluded that this treatment could be "safely offered" to women with this disease and that patients with local recurrence in the vulva could be salvaged by further therapy. As with other malignancies adjuvant radiation therapy improves local control, but its effect of overall survival is questionable.

The Regional Lymph Nodes

Several investigators have reported favorable experience with lymphatic mapping and sentinel lymph node biopsy.[88,89] The few difficulties that have been reported are related to technical aspects of the procedure and the "learning curve" associated with any new procedure.[90] The increasing use of this technique in patients with breast cancer and malignant melanoma suggests that this procedure will gain acceptance in the treatment of cancer of the vulva.

Texas Cancer Center Treatment Analysis

The Texas Cancer Center supports the increased use of limited surgery for cancer of the vulva.

Preface
1. Evans RA. Host resistance to carcinoma of the breast. *South Med J* 73:1261-1263, 1980.
2. Crile G Jr. *Cancer and Common Sense.* American Book-Stratford Press, Inc.: New York. 1955.
3. Crile G Jr. *The Way It Was: Sex, Surgery, Treasure and Travel.* Kent State University Press: Kent, OH. 1992. p. 316.

Introduction
1. Evans RA. Host resistance to carcinoma of the breast. *South Med J* 73:1261-1263, 1980.

Chapter 1
The History of Cancer Surgery
1. Robinson JO. The history of surgical oncology. In McKenna RJ, Murphy GP (eds): *Fundamentals of Surgical Oncology.* Macmillan Pub. Co.: New York. 1986. p. 60.
2. Halsted WS. The results of operations for the cure of cancer of the breast performed at Johns Hopkins Hospital from June 1889 to January 1894. *Ann Surg* 20:497-555, 1894.
3. Halsted WS. The results of operations for the cure of cancer of the breast performed at Johns Hopkins Hospital from June 1889 to January 1894. *Ann Surg* 20:510, 1894.
4. Paterson JT. *The Dread Disease: Cancer and Modern American Culture.* Harvard University Press: Cambridge, MA. 1987.
5. Haagensen CD. *Diseases of the Breast.* Philadelphia: W. B. Sanders Co. 1986. p. 870.
6. Nuland SB. *Doctors: The Biography of Medicine.* New York: Vintage Books. 1988. p. 406.
7. Crile G Jr. *What Women Should Know about the Breast Cancer Controversy.* Pocket Books: New York. 1974.
8. Paterson JT. *The Dread Disease: Cancer and Modern American Culture.* Harvard University Press: Cambridge, MA. 1987.
9. Paterson JT. *The Dread Disease: Cancer and Modern American Culture.* Harvard University Press: Cambridge, MA. 1987. p. 51.
10. Recht A and Hayes D. Local recurrence. In Harris JR, Henderson IC, Hellman S and Kinne D (eds): *Breast Diseases.* Lippincott: Philadelphia. 1987. pp. 508-524.
11. Carter RL. Significance of local recurrence. In Stoll BA (ed): *Secondary Spread of Breast Cancer.* Year Book Medical Publishers: Chicago. 1977. pp. 31-44.
12. Shimkin MB, Lucia EL, Low-Beer BVA, and Bell HG. Recurrent cancer of the breast. *Cancer* 7:29-46, 1954.
13. Haagensen CD. *Carcinoma of the Breast.* American Cancer Society: New York. 1950.
14. Keynes G. *The Gates of Memory.* Clarendon Press: Oxford. 1981. p. 216.
15. Fitzwilliams DCL. A plea for more local operation in really early breast carcinoma. *BMJ* 2:405-408, 1940.
16. Mustakallio S. Conservative treatment of breast carcinoma—review of 25 years follow up. *Clin Radiol* 23:110-116, 1972.
17. Peters MV. Cutting the "Gordian knot" in early breast cancer. *Ann R Coll Phys Surg Can* 8:186-192, 1975.
18. Adair FE. The role of surgery and irradiation in cancer of the breast. *JAMA* 121:553-559, 1943.
19. Williams IG, Murley RS, and Curwen, MP. Carcinoma of the female breast: conservative and radical surgery. *BMJ* 2:787-796, 1953.
20. Osborne MP, Ormiston N, Harmer CL, and others. Breast conservation in the treatment of early breast cancer. *Cancer* 53:349-355, 1984.
21. Taylor H, Baker R, Fortt RW, and Hermon-Taylor J. Sector mastectomy in selected cases of breast cancer. *Br J Surg* 58:161-163, 1971.
22. Bulman AS, Zeitman A, Phillips RH, and Ellis H. Interim results of treat-

ment of breast cancer with breast conservation for all patients. *Surgery* 101:395-399, 1987.
23. Tagart REB. Partial mastectomy for breast cancer. *BMJ* 2:1286, 1978.
24. Tagart R, Bratherton D, Hartley L, and Sikora K. Partial mastectomy alone in early breast cancer. *BMJ* 290:434, 1985.
25. Williams IG, Murley RS, and Curwen MP. Carcinoma of the female breast; conservative and radical surgery. *BMJ* 2:787-796, 1953.
26. Keynes G. Carcinoma of the breast, the unorthodox view. *Proc Cardiff Med Soc* 40-49, April 1954.
27. Crile G Jr. *Cancer and Common Sense.* American Book-Stratford Press, Inc.: New York, 1955. p. 54.
28. Calle R, Vilcoq JR, Zafrani B, and others. Local control and survival of breast cancer treated by limited surgery followed by irradiation. *Int J Radiat Oncol Bio Phys* 12:873-878, 1986.
29. Sarrazin D, Dewar JA, Arriagada R, and others. Conservative management of breast cancer. *Br J Surg* 73:604-606, 1986.
30. Amalric R, Santamaria F, Robert F, and others. Radiation therapy with or without primary limited surgery for operable breast cancer. *Cancer* 49:30-34, 1982.
31. Spitalier JM, Brandone H, Ayme Y, and others. Traitements curatifs a espérance conservatrice des cancers du sein—généralités-résultats d'ensemble à 5 et 10 ans. [Conservative treatment with the hope of cure for cancers of the breast—general results together at 5 to 10 years.] *Méditer Méd* 170 (Suppl):3-7, 1978.
32. Kurtz JM, Spitalier JM, Amalric R, and others. Mammary recurrences in women younger than forty. *Int J Radiat Oncol Bio Phys* 16:271-276, 1988.
33. Leung S, Otmezguine Y, Calitchi E, and others. Locoregional recurrences following radical external beam irradiation and interstitial implantation for operable breast cancer—a twenty-three year experience. *Radiother Oncol* 5:1-10, 1986.
34. Verhaeghe M, Laurent JC, Clay A, and others. Mastectomie partielle avec curage pour les petits cancers du sein. [Partial mastectomy with scraping for small cancers of the breast.] *Bull Acad Natl Med* 163:836-842, 1979.
35. Kurtz JM, Amalric R, Delouche G, and others. The second ten years: long-term risks of breast conservation in early breast cancer. *Int J Radiat Oncol Bio Phys* 13:1327-1332, 1987.
36. Calle R, Pilleron JP, Schlienger P, and Vilcoq JR. Conservative management of operable breast cancer. *Cancer* 42:2045-2053, 1978.
37. Halsted WS. The results of operations for the cure of cancer of the breast performed at Johns Hopkins Hospital from June 1889 to January 1894. *Ann Surg* 20:497-555, 1894.
38. Editorial: Treatment of early carcinoma of breast. *BMJ* 2:417-418, 1972.
39. Stehlin JS Jr, Evans RA, Gutierrez AA, and others. Treatment of carcinoma of the breast. *Sur Gynecol Obstet* 149:911-922, 1979.
40. Hellman S. Dogma and inquisition in medicine. *Cancer* 71:2430-2433, 1993.
41. Fisher B, Redmond C, Fisher ER, and others. The contribution of recent NSABP clinical trials of primary breast cancer therapy to an understanding of tumor biology—an overview of findings. *Cancer* 46:1009-1025, 1980.
42. Crile G Jr. Possible role of involved regional nodes in preventing metastasis from breast cancer. *Cancer* 24:1283-1285, 1969.
43. Crile G Jr. Simplified treatment of cancer of the breast: early results of a clinical study. *Ann Surg* 153: 745-

761, 1961. (Presented before the Southern Surgical Association, December 6-8, 1960.)
44. Mustakallio S. Conservative treatment of breast carcinoma—review of 25 years follow up. *Clin Radiol* 23:110-116, 1972.
45. Peters MV. Radiation therapy in the management of breast cancer. In *Proceedings of the 6th national cancer conference.* Lippincott: New York. 1970. pp. 163-174.
46. Kurtz JM, Spitalier JM, and Amalric R. Late breast recurrence after lumpectomy and irradiation. *Int J Radiat Oncol Bio Phys* 9:1191-1194, 1983.
47. Fisher B, Anderson S, Fisher ER, and others. Significance of ipsilateral recurrence after lumpectomy. *Lancet* 338:327-331, 1991.
48. Fisher B, Wickerham DL, Deutsch M, Anderson S, Redmond C, and Fisher ER. Breast tumor recurrence following lumpectomy with and without breast irradiation: an overview of recent NSABP findings. *Semin Surg Oncol* 8:153-160, 1992.
49. Brennan MF, Casper ES, Harrison LB, and others. The role of multimodality therapy in soft-tissue sarcoma. *Ann Surg* 214:328-338, 1991.
50. Cascinelli N, van der Esch EP, Breslow A, Morabito A, and Bufalino R. Stage I malignant melanoma of the skin: the problem of resection margins. *Eur J Cancer* 16:1079-1085, 1980.
51. Crile G Jr. *The Way It Was: Sex, Surgery, Treasure, and Travel.* Kent State University Press: Kent, Ohio. 1992. p. 317.

Chapter 2
The Behavior of Cancer
1. Beardsley T. A war not won. *Sci Am* 130-138, January 1994.
2. Liotta LA and Stetler-Stevenson WG. Principles of molecular cell biology of cancer; cancer metastasis. In DeVita VT Jr, Hellman S, and Rosenberg SA (eds.): *Cancer: Principles & Practice of Oncology* (4th edition). J. B. Lippincott Co.: Philadelphia. 1993. p. 134.
3. Kinzler KW and Vogelstein B. Clinical implications of basic research. Cancer therapy meets p53. *N Engl J Med* 331:49-50, 1994.
4. Folkman J. Angiogenesis and breast cancer. *J Clin Oncol* 12:441-443, 1994.
5. Weidner N, Folkman J, Pozza F, Bevilacqua P, Allred EN, Moore DH, and others. Tumor angiogenesis: a new significant and independent prognostic indicator in early-stage breast carcinoma. *J Natl Cancer Inst* 84:1875-1887, 1992.

Chapter 3
The Defense Against Cancer
1. Weiss L. The biology of metastasis. In McKenna RJ and Murphy GP (eds.): *Fundamentals of Surgical Oncology.* Macmillan Pub. Co.: New York. 1986. p. 60.
2. Talmadge JE, Meyers KM, Prieur DJ, and Starkey JR. Role of NK cells in tumour growth and metastasis in *beige* mice. *Nature* 284:622-624, 1980.
3. Hanna N. Role of natural killer cells in control of cancer metastasis. *Cancer Metastasis Rev* 1:45-64, 1982.
4. Trinchieri G and Perussia B. Biology of disease. Human natural killer cells: biologic and pathologic aspects. *Lab Invest* 50:489-512, 1984.
5. Herberman RB and Ortaldo JR. Natural killer cells: Their role in defenses against disease. *Science* 141:24-30, 1981.
6. Fulton A, Heppner G, Roi L, and others. Relationship of natural killer cytotoxicity to clinical and biochemical parameters of primary human breast cancer. *Breast Cancer Res and Treat* 4:109-116, 1984.
7. Mickel RA, Kessler DJ, Taylor JMG, and Lichtenstein A. Natural killer cy-

totoxicity in the peripheral blood, cervical lymph nodes, and tumor of head and neck cancer patients. *Cancer Res* 48:5017-5022, 1988.
8. Schantz SP, Brown BW, Lira E, and others. Evidence for the role of natural immunity in the control of metastatic spread of head and neck cancer. *Cancer Immunol Immunother* 25:141-148, 1987.
9. Mackay IR, Goodyear MDE, Riglar C, and Penschow J. Effect on natural killer cell and antibody-dependent cellular cytotoxicity of adjuvant cytotoxic chemotherapy including melphalan in breast cancer. *Cancer Immunol Immunother* 16:98-100, 1983.
10. Wiltschke C, Tyl E, Speiser P, and others. Increased natural killer cell activity correlates with low or negative expression of the HER-2/neu oncogene in patients with breast cancer. *Cancer* 73:135-139, 1994.
11. Colacchio TA, Yeager MP, and Hildebrandt LW. Perioperative immunomodulation in cancer surgery. *Arch Surg* 176:174-179, 1994.
12. Trinchieri G and Perussia B. Biology of disease. Human natural killer cells: biologic and pathologic aspects. *Lab Invest* 50:489-512, 1984.
13. Ortaldo JR. Regulation of natural killer activity. *Cancer Metastasis Rev* 6:637-651, 1987.
14. Levy JA. Long-term survivors of HIV infection. *Hosp Prac* Oct 15:41-52, 1994.
15. Benacerraf B and McDevitt HO. Histocompatibility-linked immune response genes. *Science* 175:273-279, 1972.
16. Alper CA, Kruskall MS, Marcus-Bagley D, Craven DE, Katz AJ, Brink SJ, and others. Genetic prediction of nonresponse to hepatitis B vaccine. *New Engl J Med* 321:708-712, 1989.
17. Williams RM and Kraus L. Genetic basis of natural killer cell activity in man. *Nat Immun* 11:237, 1993.
18. Pociot F, Briant L, Jongeneel CV, Molvig J, Worsaae H, Abbal M, and others. Association of tumor necrosis factor (TNF) and class II major histocompatibility complex alleles with the secretion of TNF-a and TNF-b by human mononuclear cells: a possible link to insulin-dependent diabetes mellitus. *Eur J Immunol* 23:224-231, 1993.

Chapter 4
The Seed and the Soil
1. Paget S. The distribution of secondary growths in cancer of the breast. *Lancet* 1:571-573, 1889.
2. Evans RA. Host resistance to carcinoma of the breast. *South Med J* 73:1261-1263, 1980.
3. Evans RA. Breast cancer: The dilemma of local recurrence. *Med Hypotheses* 29:151-153, 1989.
4. Evans RA. Preservation surgery for malignant disease: why it works. *South Med J* 82:1534-1537, 1989.
5. Fisher ER, Sass R, Fisher B, Gregorio R, Brown R, and Wickerham L. Pathologic findings from the National Surgical Adjuvant Breast Project (Protocol 6). II. relation of local breast recurrence to multicentricity. *Cancer* 57:1717-1724, 1986. See p. 1723.
6. Fisher B, Anderson S, Fisher ER, and others. Significance of ipsilateral recurrence after lumpectomy. *Lancet* 338:327-331, 1991. See p. 330.
7. Evans RA. Significance of ipsilateral recurrence after lumpectomy. *Lancet* 338:1402, 1991.
8. Papaioannou AN. Hypothesis: increasingly intensive locoregional treatment of breast cancer may promote recurrence. *J Surg Oncol* 30:33-41, 1985.
9. Crile G Jr. How much surgery for breast cancer? *Modern Med* 41:32-38, 1973.
10. Papaioannou AN. Hypothesis: increasingly intensive locoregional treatment of breast cancer may pro-

mote recurrence. *J Surg Oncol* 30:33-41, 1985.
11. Margolese RC. 4. Diagnosis and management of local recurrence after breast-conserving surgery. *Can J Surg* 35:378-381, 1992.
12. Clarke, DH, Le MG, Sarrazin D, and others. Analysis of local regional relapses in patients with early breast cancers treated by excision and radiotherapy: experience of the institut Gustave-Roussy. *Int J Radiat Oncol Bio Phys* 11:137-145, 1985.
13. Cajucom CC, Tsangaris TN, Nemoto T, Driscoll D, Penetrante RB, and Holyoke ED. Results of salvage mastectomy for local recurrence after breast-conserving surgery without radiation therapy. *Cancer* 71:1774-1779, 1993.
14. Kurtz JM, Amalric R, Brandone H, and others. Local recurrence after breast-conserving surgery and radiotherapy: frequency, time course and prognosis. *Cancer* 63:1912-1917, 1989.
15. Barr LC, Brunt AM, Goodman AG, Phillips RH, and Ellis H. Uncontrolled local recurrence after treatment of breast cancer with breast conservation. *Cancer* 64:1203-1207, 1989.
16. Kurtz JM, Jacquemier J, Brandone H, Ayme Y, Hans D, Bressac C, and Spitalier J. Inoperable recurrence after breast-conserving surgical treatment and radiotherapy. *Surg Gynecol Obstet* 172:357-361, 1991.
17. Haffty BG, Fischer D, Beinfield M, and McKhann C. Prognosis following local recurrence in the conservatively treated breast cancer patient. *Int J Radiat Oncol Bio Phys* 21:293-298, 1991.
18. Haffty BG, Goldberg NB, Fischer D, and others. Conservative surgery and radiation therapy in breast carcinoma: local recurrence and prognostic implications. *Int J Radiat Oncol Bio Phys* 17:727-732, 1989.
19. Recht A, Schnitt SJ, Connolly JL, Rose MA, Silver B, Come S, Henderson IC, Slavin S, and Harris JR. Prognosis following local or regional recurrence after conservative surgery and radiotherapy for early stage breast carcinoma. *Int J Radiat Oncol Bio Phys* 16:3-9, 1989.
20. Hayward J and Caleffi M. The significance of local control in the primary treatment of breast cancer. *Arch Surg* 122:1244-1247, 1987.
21. Kolata G. New AIDS findings on why drugs fail. *The New York Times* 1/12/95: A1.

Chapter 5
Principles of Treatment
1. Wong RJ and DeCosse JJ. Cytoreductive surgery. *Surg Gynecol Obstet* 170:276-281, 1990.
2. Welch JS. The postirradiated breast. *Mayo Clin Proc* 61:392-395, 1986.
3. Pizzarello DJ, Roses DF, Newell J, and Barish RJ. The carcinogenicity of radiation therapy. *Surg Gynecol Obstet* 159:189-200, 1984.
4. Mueller CB. The case against the use of adjuvant chemotherapy in breast cancer. *Am Coll Surg Bull* 78(6):25-31, 1993.
5. Bonadonna G and Valagussa P. Dose-response effect of adjuvant chemotherapy in breast cancer. *New Engl J Med* 304:10-15, 1981.
6. Evans RA, Bland KI, McMurtrey MJ, and Ballantyne A. Radionuclide scans not indicated in clinical stage I melanoma. *Surg Gynecol Obstet* 150:532-534, 1980.
7. Schapira DV and Urban N. A minimalist policy for breast cancer surveillance. *JAMA* 265:380-382, 1991.

Chapter 6
Bladder Cancer
1. Thrasher J and Crawford ED. Current management of invasive and metastatic transitional cell carcinoma of the bladder. *J Urol* 149:957-972, 1993.

Notes

Chapter 7
Breast Cancer

1. Early Breast Cancer Trialists' Collaborative Group. Systemic treatment of early breast cancer by hormonal, cytotoxic, immune therapy. *Lancet* 339:1-15 and 71-85, 1992.
2. Mueller CB. The case against the use of adjuvant chemotherapy in breast cancer. *Am Coll Surg Bull* 78(6):25-31, 1993.
3. Greenspan EM. Has the cure of breast cancer with chemotherapy become a reality? *Cancer Invest* 12:98-100, 1994.
4. National Institutes of Health Consensus Development Conference. Treatment of early stage breast cancer. *JAMA* 265:391-395, 1991.
5. Morris J, Farmer A, and Royle G. Recent changes in the surgical management of T1/2 breast cancer in England. *Eur J Cancer* 28A:1709-1712, 1992.
6. Greening WP, Montgomery ACV, Gordon AB, and Gowing NFC. Quadrantic excision and axillary node dissection without radiation therapy: the long-term results of a selective policy in the treatment of stage I breast cancer. *Eur J Surg Oncol* 14:221-225, 1988.
7. The Uppsala-Örebro Breast Cancer Study Group. Sector resection with or without postoperative radiotherapy for stage I breast cancer: a randomized trial. *J Natl Cancer Inst* 82:277-282, 1990.
8. Clark RM, McCulloch PB, Levine MN, Lipa RH, Wilkinson RH, Mahoney LJ, and others. Randomized clinical trial to assess the effectiveness of breast irradiation following lumpectomy and axillary dissection for node-negative breast cancer. *J Natl Cancer Inst* 84:683-689, 1992.
9. Hermann RE, Esselstyn CB, Grundfest-Broniatowski S, and others. Partial mastectomy without radiation is adequate treatment for patients with stages 0 and I carcinoma of the breast. *Surg Gynecol Obstet* 177:247-253, 1993.
10. Nemoto T, Patel LK, Rosner D, Dao TL, Schuh M, and Penetrante R. Factors affecting recurrence in lumpectomy without irradiation for breast cancer. *Cancer* 67:2079-2082, 1991.
11. Moffat FL and Ketcham AS. Breast-conserving surgery and selective adjuvant therapy for stage I and II breast cancer. *Semin Surg Oncol* 8:172-176, 1992.
12. Cady B, Stone MD, and Wayne J. New therapeutic possibilities in primary invasive breast cancer. *Ann Surg* 218:338-349, 1993.
13. Singletary SE, McNeese MD, and Hortobagyi GN. Feasibility of breast-conservation surgery after induction chemotherapy for locally advanced breast carcinoma. *Cancer* 69:2849-2852, 1992.
14. Fisher BF, Costantino J, Redmond C, and others. Lumpectomy compared with lumpectomy and radiation therapy for the treatment of intraductal breast cancer. *N Engl J Med* 328:1581-1586, 1993.

Chapter 8
Cancer of the Cervix

1. Childers JM, Hatch K, and Surwit EA. The role of laparoscopic lymphadenectomy in the management of cervical carcinoma. *Gynecol Oncol* 47:38-43, 1992.
2. Morris M. Early cervical carcinoma: are two treatments better than one? *Gynecol Oncol* 54:1-3, 1994.
3. Nicklin JL, Wright RG, Bell JR, and others. A clinicopathological study of adenocarcinoma *in situ* of the cervix. The influence of cervical HPV infection and other factors, and the role of conservative surgery. *Aust NZ J Obstet Gynaecol* 31:179-183, 1991.

Chapter 9
Malignant Melanoma
1. Koh HK. Cutaneous melanoma. *New Engl J Med* 523:171-182, 1991.
2. Milton GW, Shaw HM, and McCarthy WH. Resection margins for melanoma. *Aust NZ J Surg* 55:225-226, 1985.
3. Heenan PJ, Weeramanthri T, Holman CDJ, and Armstrong BK. Surgical treatment and survival from cutaneous malignant melanoma. *Aust NZ J Surg* 55:229-234, 1985.
4. Olsen G. The malignant melanoma of the skin: new theories based on a study of 500 cases. *Acta Chir Scand* [Suppl.] 365:1-220, 1966.
5. Veronesi U, Adamus J, Bandiera DC, and others. Delayed regional lymph node dissection in stage I melanoma of the skin of the lower extremities. *Cancer* 49:2420-2430, 1982.
6. Sim FH, Taylor WF, Pritchard DJ, and Soule EH. Lymphadenectomy in the management of stage I malignant melanoma: a prospective randomized study. *Mayo Clin Proc* 61:697-705, 1986.
7. Slingluff CL, Stidham KR, Ricci WM, Stanley WE, and Seigler HF. Surgical management of regional lymph nodes in patients with melanoma. *Ann Surg* 219:120-130, 1994.

Chapter 10
Cancer of the Penis
1. Von Eschenbach AC, Johnson DE, Wishnow KI, Babaian RJ, and Tenney D. Results of laser therapy for carcinoma of the penis: organ preservation. *Prog Clin Biol Res* 370:407-412, 1991.
2. Catalona WJ. Modified inguinal lymphadenectomy for carcinoma of the penis with preservation of saphenous veins: technique and preliminary results. *J Urol* 140:306-310, 1988.
3. McDougal WS, Kirchner FK Jr, Edwards RH, and others. Treatment of carcinoma of the penis: The case for primary lymphadenectomy. *J Urol* 136:38, 1986.
4. Fraley EE, Zhang G, Manivel C, and others. The role of ilioinguinal lymphadenectomy and significance of histological differentiation in treatment of carcinoma of the penis. *J Urol* 142:1478, 1989.
5. Lubke WL and Thompson IM. The case for inguinal lymph node dissection in the treatment of T_2-T_4, N_0 penile cancer. *Semin Urol* 11:80-84, 1993.

Chapter 11
Prostate Cancer
1. Garnick MB. Prostate cancer: screening, diagnosis, and management. *Ann Intern Med* 118:804-818, 1993.
2. Stamey TA, Freiha FS, McNeal JE, and others. Localized prostate cancer. *Cancer* 71:933-938, 1993.
3. Schmid HP, McNeal JE, and Stamey TA. Observations on the doubling time of prostate cancer. *Cancer* 71:2031-2040, 1993.
4. Bostwick DG, Graham SD Jr, Napalkov P, and others. Staging of early prostate cancer: a proposed tumor volume-based prognostic index. *Urology* 41:403-411, 1993.
5. Catalona WJ, Hudson MA, Scardino PT, and others. Selection of optimal prostate-specific antigen cutoffs for early detection of prostate cancer: receiver operating characteristic curve. *J Urol* 152:2037-2042, 1994.
6. Catalona WJ, Smith DS, Ratliff TL, and Basler JW. Detection of organ-defined prostate cancer is increased through prostate-specific antigen-based screening. *JAMA* 220:948-954, 1993.
7. Ohori M, Wheeler TM, and Scardino PT. The new American Joint Commission on Cancer and International Union Against Cancer TNM Classification of Prostate Cancer: clinical pathological correlations. *Cancer* 73:104-114, 1994.

Notes

8. Catalona WJ. Management of cancer of the prostate. *N Engl J Med* 331:996-1004, 1994.
9. Morton RA, Steiner MS, and Walsh PC. Cancer control following anatomical radical prostatectomy: an interim report. *J Urol* 145:1197-1200, 1991.
10. Sonda LP. Second-look prostate resection for incidental carcinoma of the prostate. In Altwein JE, Faul P, and Schneider W (eds): *Incidential Carcinoma of the Prostate.* Springer-Verlag: Berlin. 1991. pp. 109-113.
11. Catalona WJ. Managment of cancer of the prostate. *N Engl J Med* 331:996-1004, 1994.
12. Stamey TA, Ferrari MK, and Schmid HP. The value of serial prostate specific antigen determinations 5 years after radiotherapy: steeply increasing values characterize 80% of patients. *J Urol* 150:1856-1859, 1993.
13. Johansson JE, Adami HO, Andersson SO, and others. High 10-year survival rate in patients with early, untreated prostate cancer. *JAMA* 267:2191-2196, 1992.
14. Montorsi F, Guazzoni G, Colombo F, and others. Transrectal microwave hyperthermia for advanced prostate cancer: long-term clinical results. *J Urol* 148:342-345, 1992.
15. Onik GM, Cohen JK, Reyes GD, and others. Transrectal ultrasound-guided percutaneous radical cryosurgical ablation of the prostate. *Cancer* 72:1291-1299, 1993.
16. Von Eschenbach AC, Swanson DA, Babaian RJ, and others. Ultrasound-guided cryoablation of recurrent prostate cancer following radiation therapy. *J Urol* 151:432A, 1994.
17. Thompson IM. Observation alone in the management of localized prostate cancer: the natural history of untreated disease. *Urology* 43:41-46, 1994.
18. Fleming C, Wasson JH, Albertsen PC, and others. A decision analysis of alternative treatment strategies for clinically localized prostate cancer. *JAMA* 269:2650-2668, 1993.
19. Johansson JE, Adami HO, Andersson SO, and others. High 10-year survival rate in patients with early, untreated prostate cancer. *JAMA* 267:2191-2196, 1992.
20. Sonda LP. Second-look prostate resection for incidental carcinoma of the prostate. In Altwein JE, Faul P, and Schneider W (eds): *Incidental Carcinoma of the Prostate.* Springer-Verlag: Berlin. 1991. pp. 109-113.
21. Schmid HP, McNeal JE, and Stamey TA. Observations on the doubling time of prostate cancer. *Cancer* 71:2031-2040, 1993.

Chapter 12
Cancer of the Rectum

1. Winawer SJ, Zauber AG, Ho MN, and others. Prevention of colorectal cancer by colonoscopic polypectomy. *N Engl J Med* 329:1977-1981, 1993.
2. Roswit B, Higgins GA, and Keehn RJ. Preoperative radiation for carcinoma of the rectum and rectosigmoid colon. *Cancer* 35:1597-1602, 1975.
3. Moertel CG, Fleming TR, MacDonald JS, and others. Levamisole and fluorouracil for adjuvant therapy of resected colon carcinoma. *New Engl J Med* 322:352-358, 1990.
4. Cummings BJ. Adjuvant radiation therapy for colorectal cancer. *Cancer* 70:1372-1383, 1992.
5. Bosset JF and Horiot JC. Adjuvant treatment in the curative management of rectal cancer: a critical review of the results of clinical randomized trials. *Eur J Cancer* 29A:770-774, 1993.
6. Wolmark N and Fisher B. An analysis of survival and treatment failure following abdominoperineal and sphincter-saving resection in Dukes' B and C rectal carcinoma. *Ann Surg* 204:480-487, 1986.

7. O'Connell MJ, Martenson JA, Wieand HS, and others. Improving adjuvant therapy for rectal cancer by combining protracted-infusion fluorouracil with radiation therapy after curative surgery. *N Engl J Med* 331:502-507, 1994.
8. Moertel CG, Fleming TR, Macdonald JS, and others. An evaluation of the carcinoembryonic antigen (CEA) test for monitoring patients with resected colon cancer. *JAMA* 270:943-947, 1993.

Chapter 13
Soft Tissue Sarcomas
1. Singh B, Sherry JEH, and Lanza JT. Mohs' micrographic surgery in the management of soft tissue sarcomas of the extremities. *Surgery* 111:718-719, 1992.
2. Geer RJ, Woodruff J, Casper ES, and Brennan MF. Management of small soft-tissue sarcoma of the extremity in adults. *Arch Surg* 127:1285-1289, 1992.
3. Keyhani A and Booher RJ. Pleomorphic rhabdomyosarcoma. *Cancer* 22:956-967, 1968.
4. Ariel IM and Briceno M. Rhabdomyosarcoma of the extremities and trunk: analysis of 150 patients treated by surgical resection. *J Surg Oncol* 7:269-287, 1975.

Chapter 15
Cancer of the Vulva
1. Lin JY, DuBeshter B, Angel C, and Dvoretsky PM. Morbidity and recurrence with modifications of radical vulvectomy and groin dissection. *Gynecol Oncol* 47:80-86, 1992.
2. Podratz KC, Symmonds RE, and Taylor WF. Carcinoma of the vulva: analysis of treatment failures. *Am J Obstet Gynecol* 143:340, 1982.
3. Corney RH, Crowther ME, Everett H, and others. Psychosexual dysfunction in women with gynaecological cancer following radical pelvic surgery. *Brit J Obstet Gynaecol* 100:73-78, 1989.

Chapter 16
Barriers to Change
1. Payer L. *Medicine and Culture*. Henry Holt and Co.: New York. 1988. p. 65.
2. Payer L. *Medicine and Culture*. Henry Holt and Co.: New York. 1988. p. 121.
3. Payer L. *Medicine and Culture*. Henry Holt and Co.: New York. 1988. p. 127.
4. National Institutes of Health Consensus Development Conference. Treatment of early stage breast cancer. *JAMA* 265:391-395, 1991.
5. Morris J, Farmer A, and Royle G. Recent changes in the surgical management of T1/2 breast cancer in England. *Eur J Can* 28A:1709-1712, 1992.
6. Fisher B, Anderson S, Fisher ER, and others. Significance of ipsilateral recurrence after lumpectomy. *Lancet* 338:327-331, 1991.
7. Horrobin DF. The philosophical basis of peer review and the suppression of innovation. *JAMA* 263:1438-1441, 1990.
8. Moss R. *The Cancer Industry*. Paragon House: New York. 1991.
9. Kassirer JF. Incorporating patients' preferences into medical decisions. *N Engl J Med* 330:1895-1896, 1994.
10. Fisher B, Anderson S, Fisher ER, Redmond C, Wickerham DL, Wolmark N, Mamounas EP, Deutsch M, and Margolese R. Significance of ipsilateral recurrence after lumpectomy. *Lancet* 338:327-331, 1991.
11. Cascinelli N, van der Esch EP, Breslow A, Morabito A, and Bufalino R. Stage I malignant melanoma of the skin: the problem of resection margins. *Eur J Can* 16:1079-1085, 1980.
12. Brennan MF, Casper ES, Harrison LB, Shiu MH, Gaynor J, and Hajdu SI. The role of multimodality therapy in soft-tissue sarcoma. *Ann Surg* 214:328-338, 1991.

13. Kuhn TA. *The Structure of Scientific Revolutions*. 2nd ed. University of Chicago Press: Chicago. 1970. p. 6.
14. Planck M. *Philosophy of Physics*. W.W. Norton: New York. 1936.

Appendix

1. Murphy LJT. *The History of Urology*. Charles C. Thomas: Springfield, IL. 1972.
2. Nichols JA and Marshall VF. The treatment of bladder carcinoma by local excision and fulguration. *Cancer* 9:559-565, 1956.
3. Herr HW. Conservative management of muscle-infiltrating bladder cancer: prospective experience. *J Urol* 138:1162-1163, 1987.
4. Herr HW. Transurethral resection in regionally advanced bladder cancer. *Urol Clin Nor Am* 19:695-700, 1992.
5. Sweeney P, Kursh ED, and Resnick MI. Partial cystectomy. *Urol Clin Nor Am* 19:701-711, 1992.
6. Faysal MH and Freiha FS. Evaluation of partial cystectomy for carcinoma of bladder. *Urology* 14:352-356, 1979.
7. Novick AC and Stewart BH. Partial cystectomy in the treatment of primary and secondary carcinoma of the bladder. *J Urol* 116:570-574, 1976.
8. Novick AC and Stewart BH. Partial cystectomy in the treatment of primary and secondary carcinoma of the bladder. *J Urol* 116:570-574, 1976.
9. Kaufman DS, Shipley WU, Griffin PP, and others. Selective bladder preservation by combination treatment of invasive bladder cancer. *N Engl J Med* 329:1377-1382, 1993.
10. Lazovich D, White E, Thomas DB, and Moe RE. Underutilization of breast-conserving surgery and radiation therapy among women with stage I or II breast cancer. *JAMA* 266:3433-3438, 1991.
11. Osteen RT, Steele JD Jr, Menck HR, and Winchester WP. Regional differences in surgical management of breast cancer. *CA-Can J Clin* 42:39-43, 1992.
12. Tate PS, McGee EM, Hopkins SF, Rogers EL, and Page GV. Breast conservation versus mastectomy: patients preferences in a community practice in Kentucky. *J Surg Oncol* 52:213-226, 1993.
13. Fisher B, Redmond C, Poisson R, and others. Eight-year results of a randomized clinical trial comparing total mastectomy and lumpectomy with or without irradiation in the treatment of breast cancer. *N Engl J Med* 320:822-828, 1989.
14. Peters MV. Wedge resection with or without radiation in early breast cancer. *Int J Radiat Oncol Biol Phys* 2:1151-1156, 1977.
15. Crile G Jr, Cooperman A, Esselstyn CB Jr, and Hermann RE. Results of partial mastectomy in 173 patients followed for from five to 10 years. *Surg Gynecol Obstet* 150:563-566, 1980.
16. Crile G Jr and Esselstyn CB Jr. Factors influencing local recurrence of cancer after partial mastectomy. *Cleve Clin J Med* 57:143-146, 1990.
17. Esselstyn CB Jr. A technique for partial mastectomy. *Surg Clinic North Am* 55:1065-1074, 1975.
18. Tagart R, Brather D, Hartley L, and Sikora K. Partial mastectomy alone in early breast cancer. *BMJ* 290:434, 1985.
19. Reed MWR and Morrison JM. Wide local excision as the sole primarily treatment in elderly patients with carcinoma of the breast. *Br J Surg* 76:898-900, 1989.
20. Hermann RE, Grundfest-Broniatowski S, and Esselstyn CB Jr. Breast-conserving surgery: how much is enough? *Semin Surg Oncol* 8:136-139, 1992.
21. Greening WP, Montgomery ACV, Gordon AB, and Gowing NFC. Quadrantic excision and axillary node dissection without radiation

therapy: the long-term results of a selective policy in the treatment of stage I breast cancer. *Eur J Surg Oncol* 14:221-225, 1988.
22. The Uppsala-Örebro Breast Cancer Study Group. Sector resection with or without postoperative radiotherapy for stage I breast cancer: a randomized trial. *J Natl Cancer Inst* 82:277-282, 1990.
23. Hermann RE, Esselstyn CB Jr, Crile G Jr, and others. Results of conservative operations for breast cancer. *Arch Surg* 120:746-751, 1985.
24. Crile G Jr and Esselstyn CB Jr. Factors influencing local recurrence of cancer after partial mastectomy. *Cleve Clin J Med* 57:143-146, 1990.
25. Hermann RE, Esselstyn CB Jr, Grundfest-Broniatowski S, and others. Partial mastectomy without radiation is adequate treatment for patients with stages 0 and I carcinoma of the breast. *Surg Gynecol Obstet* 177:247-253, 1993.
26. Nemoto T, Patel LK, Rosner D, Dao TL, Schuh M, and Penetrante R. Factors affecting recurrence in lumpectomy without irradiation for breast cancer. *Cancer* 67:2079-2082, 1991.
27. Moffat FL and Ketcham AS. Breast-conserving surgery and selective adjuvant therapy for stage I and II breast cancer. *Semin Surg Oncol* 8:172-176, 1992.
28. Fisher B, Wickerham DL, Deutsch M, Anderson S, Redmond C, and Fisher ER. Breast tumor recurrence following lumpectomy with and without breast irradiation: an overview of recent NSABP findings. *Semin Surg Oncol* 8:153-160, 1992.
29. Clark RM, McCulloch PB, Levine MN, Lipa RH, Wilkinson RH, Mahoney LJ, and others. Randomized clinical trial to assess the effectiveness of breast irradiation following lumpectomy and axillary dissection for node-negative breast cancer. *J Natl Cancer Inst* 84:683-689, 1992.

30. Veronesi U, Luini A, Del Vecchio M, and others. Radiotherapy after breast-preserving surgery in women with localized cancer of the breast. *New Engl J Med* 328:1587-1591, 1993.
31. Fisher B, Wickerham DL, Deutsch M, Anderson S, Redmond C, and Fisher ER. Breast tumor recurrence following lumpectomy with and without breast irradiation: an overview of recent NSABP findings. *Semin Surg Oncol* 8:153-160, 1992.
32. Liljegren G, Holmberg L, Adami HO, Westman G, Graffman S, Bergh J, and Uppsala-Örebro Breast Cancer Study Group. Sector resection with or without postoperative radiotherapy for stage I breast cancer: Five-year results of a randomized trial. *J Natl Cancer Inst* 86:717-722, 1994.
33. Burghardt E, Girardi F, Lahousen M, and others. Microinvasive carcinoma of the uterine cervix (International Federation of Gynecology and Obstetrics Stage IA). *Cancer* 67:1037-1045, 1991.
34. Lohe KJ, Burghardt E, Hillemanns HG, and others. Early squamous cell carcinoma of the uterine cervix II. Clinical results of a cooperative study in the management of 419 patients with early stromal invasion and microcarcinoma. *Gynecol Oncol* 6:31-50, 1978.
35. Schink JJC and Lurain JR. Microinvasive cervix cancer. *Int J Gynaec Obstet* 36:5-12, 1991.
36. Kolstad P. Follow-up study of 232 patients with stage Ia1 and 411 patients with stage Ia2 squamous cell carcinoma of the cervix (microinvasive carcinoma). *Gynecol Oncol* 33:265-272, 1989.
37. Ebeling K, Bilek, Johannsmeyer D, and others. Mikroinvasives karzinom der cervix uteri stadium Ia—ergebnisse einer multizentrischen klinikbezogenen analyse. [Microinva-

sive carcinoma of the cervix and uterus stage Ia—results of multicenter hospital-based study.] *Geburtsh u Frauenheilk* [Geburtsh and Frauenheilk] 49:776-781, 1989.
38. Morris M, Mitchell MF, Silva EG, Copeland LJ, and Gershenson DM. Cervical conization as definitive therapy for early invasive squamous carcinoma of the cervix. *Gynecol Oncol* 51:193-196, 1993.
39. Dargent D. Traitement des cancers de l'exocol et du vagin par la chirurgie avec conservation de l'utérus et de ses annexes. [Surgical treatment of exocervical and vaginal carcinoma conserving uterus and ovaries.] *Cah Oncol* 1:21-25, 1992.
40. Greer BE, Figge DC, Tamimi KT, and others. Stage IA$_2$ squamous carcinoma of the cervix: difficult diagnosis and therapeutic dilemma. *Am J Obstet Gynecol* 162:1406-1411, 1990.
41. Rutledge S, Carey MS, Prichard H, Allen HH, Kocha W, and Kirk ME. Conservative surgery for recurrent or persistent carcinoma of the cervix following irradiation: Is exenteration always necessary? *Gynecol Oncol* 52:353-359, 1994.
42. Sivanesaratnam V, Jayalakshmi P, and Loo C. Surgical management of early invasive cancer of the cervix associated with pregnancy. *Gynecol Oncol* 48:68-75, 1993.
43. Monk BJ and Montz FJ. Invasive cervical cancer complicating intrauterine pregnancy: treatment with radical hysterectomy. *Obstet Gynecol* 80:199-203, 1992.
44. Duggan B, Muderspach LI, Roman LD, and others. Cervical cancer in pregnancy: reporting on planned delay in therapy. *Obstet Gynecol* 82:598-602, 1993.
45. Handley WS. The pathology of melanotic growths in relation to their operative treatment. Lecture II. *Lancet* 1:996-1003, 1907.
46. McNeer G and Cantin J. Local failure in the treatment of melanoma. *Am J Roentgenol* 99:791-808, 1967.
47. Petersen NC, Bodenham DC, and Lloyd OC. Malignant melanoma of the skin. *Br J Plast Surg* 15:49-116, 1962.
48. Wong CK. A study of melanocytes in the normal skin surrounding malignant melanomata [melanoma]. *Dermatologica* 141:215-225, 1970.
49. Cochran AJ. Histology and prognosis in malignant melanoma. *J Pathol* 97:459-468, 1969.
50. Olsen G. The malignant melanoma of the skin: new theories based on a study of 500 cases. *Acta Chir Scand* [Suppl.] 365:1-220, 1966.
51. Morton DL. Current management of malignant melanoma. *Ann Surg* 212:123-124, 1990.
52. Cascinelli N, van der Esch EP, Breslow A, Morabito A, and Bufalino R. Stage I malignant melanoma of the skin: the problem of resection margins. *Eur J Cancer* 16:1079-1085, 1980.
53. Schmoeckel C, Bockelbrink A, Bockelbrink H, and Braun-Falco O. Low- and high-risk malignant melanoma. III. Prognostic significance of the resection margin. *Eur J Clin Oncol* 19:245-249, 1983.
54. Heenan PJ, Weeramanthri T, Holman CDJ, and Armstrong BK. Surgical treatment and survival from cutaneous malignant melanoma. *Aust NZ J Surg* 55:229-234, 1985.
55. Heenan PJ, English DR, Holman CDJ, and others. The effects of surgical treatment on survival and local recurrence of cutaneous malignant melanoma. *Cancer* 69:421-426, 1992.
56. Pitt TTE. Aspects of surgical treatment for malignant melanoma: The place of biopsy and wide excision. *Aust NZ J Surg* 47:757-766, 1977.
57. Ackerman AB and Scheiner AM. How wide and deep is wide and deep enough? *Human Pathol* 14:743-744, 1983.

58. Elder DE, Guerry D, Heiberger R, LaRossa D, and others. Optimal resection margin for cutaneous malignant melanoma. *Plast Reconst Surg* 71:66-72, 1983.
59. Aitken DR, Clausen K, Klein JP, and James AG. The extent of primary melanoma excision. A re-evaluation—how wide is wide? *Ann Surg* 198:634-641, 1983.
60. Aitken DR, James AG, and Carey LC. Local cutaneous recurrence after conservative excision of malignant melanoma. *Arch Surg* 119:643-646, 1984.
61. Lehman JA, Cross FS, and Richey DG. Clinical study of forty-nine patients with malignant melanoma. *Cancer* 19:611-619, 1966.
62. O'Rourke MGE and Altmann CR. Melanoma recurrence after excision; is a wide margin justified? *Ann Surg* 217:2-5, 1993.
63. Seigler HF. Clinicopathologic factors relating to surgical margins for cutaneous melanoma. *Ann Surg* 217:1, 1992.
64. Brown M and Goldsmith LA. Excision margins for melanoma in awkward places like the eyelid. *JAMA* 269:588-589, 1993.
65. Balch CM, Milton GW, Cascinelli N, and Sim FH. Elective lymph node dissection: pros and cons. In Balch CM, Houghton AN, Milton GW, and Sober AJ (eds): *Cutaneous Melanoma*. J. B. Lippincott: Philadelphia. 1992.
66. McCarthy WH, Shaw HM, Cascinelli N, Santinami N, and Belli F. Elective lymph node dissection for melanoma: two perspectives. *World J Surg* 16:203-213, 1992.
67. Sutherland CM and Mather FJ. Prophylactic lymph node dissection for malignant melanoma: What to do while we wait. *J Surg Oncol* 51:1-4, 1992.
68. Balch CM, Soong SJ, Milton GW, and others. A comparison of prognostic factors and surgical results in 1,786 patients with localized (stage I) melanoma treated in Alabama, USA and New South Wales, Australia. *Ann Surg* 196:677-684, 1982.
69. Veronesi U, Adamus J, Bandiera DC, and others. Delayed regional lymph node dissection in stage I melanoma of the skin of the lower extremities. *Cancer* 49:2420-2430, 1982.
70. Sim FH, Taylor WF, Pritchard DJ, and Soule EH. Lymphadenectomy in the management of stage I malignant melanoma: a prospective randomized study. *Mayo Clin Proc* 61:697-705, 1986.
71. Balch CM, Murad TM, Soong SJ, and others. A multifactorial analysis of melanoma: Prognostic histopathological features comparing Clark's and Breslow's methods. *Ann Surg* 188:732-742, 1978.
72. Balch CM, Soong SJ, Shaw HM, Urist MM, and McCarthy WH. Analysis of prognostic factors in 8500 patients with cutaneous melanoma. In Balch CM, Houghton AN, Milton GW, and Sober AJ (eds): *Cutaneous Melanoma*. J. B. Lippincott: Philadelphia. 1992.
73. McCarthy WH, Shaw HM, Thompson JF, and Milton GW. Time and frequency of recurrence of cutaneous stage I malignant melanoma with guidelines for follow-up study. *Surg Gynecol Obstet* 166:497-502, 1988.
74. Veronesi U, Adamus J, Bandiera DC, and others. Delayed regional lymph node dissection in stage I melanoma of the skin of the lower extremities. *Cancer* 49:2420-2430, 1982.
75. Mohs FE, Snow SN, and Larson PO. Mohs micrographic surgery for penile tumors. *Urol Clin Nor Am* 19:291-304, 1992.
76. Brown MD, Zachery CB, Grekin RE, and others. Penile tumors: their management with Mohs micro-

graphic surgery. *J Dermatol Surg Oncol* 13:1163-1167, 1987.
77. Mikhail GR. Cancers of the genitalia and the perineum. In Mikhail GR (ed): *Mohs Micrographic Surgery*. W. B. Saunders: Philadelphia. 1991. pp. 160-237.
78. Malek RS. Laser treatment of premalignant and malignant squamous cell lesions of the penis. *Lasers Surg Med* 12:246-253, 1992.
79. Horenblas S, Tinteren HV, Delemarre JFM, Boon TA, Moonen LMF, and Lustig V. Squamous cell carcinoma of the penis. II. Treatment of the primary tumor. *J Urol* 147:1533-1538, 1992.
80. Schellhammer PF, Jordan GH, and Schlossberg SM. Tumors of the penis. In Walsh PC, Retik AB, Stamey TA, and Vaughan ED Jr (eds): *Campbell's Urology*, Vol. II, 6th ed. W. B. Saunders Co.: Philadelphia. 1992.
81. McDougal WS, Kirchner FK, Edwards RH, and Killion LT. Treatment of carcinoma of the penis: The case for primary lymphadenectomy. *J Urol* 136:38-41, 1986.
82. Narayana AS, Olney LE, Loening SA, Weimar GW, and Culp DA. Carcinoma of the penis. Analysis of 219 cases. *Cancer* 49:2185-2192, 1982.
83. Jensen MS. Cancer of the penis in Denmark 1942 to 1962 (511 cases). *Dan Med Bull* 24:66-72, 1977.
84. Cabanas RM. Anatomy and biopsy of sentinel lymph nodes. *Urol Clin Nor Am* 19:267-276, 1992.
85. Kamat MR, Kulkarni JN, and Tongaonkar HB. Carcinoma of the penis: the Indian experience. *J Surg Oncol* 52:50-55, 1993.
86. Ravi R. Prophylactic lymphadenectomy vs. observation in node-negative patients with invasive carcinoma of the penis. *Jpn J Clin Oncol* 23:53-58, 1993.
87. McDougal WS, Kirchner FK Jr, Edwards RH, and others. Treatment of carcinoma of the penis: The case for primary lymphadenectomy. *J Urol* 136:38, 1986.
88. Fraley EE, Zhang G, Manivel C, and others. The role of ilioinguinal lymphadenectomy and significance of histological differentiation in treatment of carcinoma of the penis. *J Urol* 142:1478, 1989.
89. Lubke WL and Thompson IM. The case for inguinal lymph node dissection in the treatment of T_2-T_4, N_0 penile cancer. *Semin Urol* 11:80-84, 1993.
90. Catalona WJ, Smith DS, Ratliff TL, and Basler JW. Detection of organ-defined prostate cancer is increased through prostate-specific antigen-based screening. *JAMA* 220:948-954, 1993.
91. Catalona WJ, Richie JP, Ahmann FR, and others. Comparison of digital rectal examination and serum prostate specific antigen in the early detection of prostate cancer: results of a multicenter clinical trial of 6,630 men. *J Urol* 151:1283-1290, 1994.
92. Lu-Yao G, McLerran D, Wasson J, and others. An assessment of radical prostatectomy. *JAMA* 269:2633-2636, 1993.
93. Paulson DF. Randomized series of treatment with surgery versus radiation for prostate adenocarcinoma. *NCI Monographs* 7:127-131, 1988.
94. Matzkin H, Patel JP, Altwein JE, and Soloway MS. Stage $T1_a$ carcinoma of prostate. *Urology* 43:11-21, 1994.
95. Brendler CB and Walsh PC. The role of radical prostatectomy in the treatment of prostate cancer. *CA-Can J Clin* 42:212-222, 1992.
96. Blute ML, Zincke H, and Farrow GM. Long-term followup of young patients with stage A adenocarcinoma of the prostate. *J Urol* 136:840-843, 1986.
97. Ziegler M, Becht E, Zwergel T, and others. Incidental carcinoma of the prostate: diagnostic second transurethral resection and therapeutic con-

sequences. In Altwein JE, Faul P, and Schneider W (eds): *Incidental Carcinoma of the Prostate.* Springer-Verlag: Berlin. 1991. pp. 128–132.
98. Marberger M. Incidental discovery of prostatic carcinoma with transurethral resection and the possible consequences. In Altwein JE, Faul P, and Schneider W (eds): *Incidental Carcinoma of the Prostate.* Springer-Verlag: Berlin. 1991. pp. 114–118.
99. Fleming C, Wasson JH, Albertsen PC, and others. A decision analysis of alternative treatment strategies for clinically localized prostate cancer. *JAMA* 269:2650–2668, 1993.
100. Wasson JH, Cushman CC, Bruskewitz RC, and others. A structured literature review of treatment for localized prostate cancer. *Arch Fam Med* 2:487–493, 1993.
101. Catalona WJ. Management of cancer of the prostate. *N Engl J Med* 331:996–1004, 1994.
102. Walsh PC. Prostate cancer kills: strategy to reduce deaths. *Urology* 44:463–466, 1994.
103. Adolfsson J, Steineck G, and Whitmore WF Jr. Recent results of management of palpable clinically localized prostate cancer. *Cancer* 72:310–322, 1993.
104. Whitmore WF Jr, Warner JA, and Thompson IM. Expectant management of localized prostatic cancer. *Cancer* 67:1091–1096, 1991.
105. Jewett HJ. Radical perineal prostatectomy for palpable, clinically localized, non-obstructive cancer: experience at the Johns Hopkins Hospital, 1909–1963. *J Urol* 124:492–494, 1980.
106. Partin AW, Lee BR, Carmichael M, Walsh P, and Epstein P. Radical prostatectomy for high grade disease: a reevaluation 1994. *J Urol* 151:1583–1586, 1994.
107. Chodak GW, Thisted RA, Gerber GS, and others. Results of conservative management of clinically localized prostate cancer. *N Engl J Med* 330:242–248, 1994.
108. Sonda LP. Second-look prostate resection for incidental carcinoma of the prostate. In Altwein JE, Faul P, and Schneider W (eds): *Incidental Carcinoma of the Prostate.* Springer-Verlag: Berlin. 1991. pp. 109–113.
109. Zelefsky MJ, Whitmore WF Jr, Leibel SA, Wallner KE, and Fuks Z. Impact of transurethral resection on the long-term outcome of patients with prostate carcinoma. *J Urol* 150:1860–1864, 1993.
110. Stamey TA and McNeal JE. Adenocarcinoma of the prostate. In Walsh PC, Retik AB, Stamey TA, and Vaughan ED Jr. (eds): *Campbell's Urology,* Vol. II, 6th ed. W. B. Saunders Co.: Philadelphia. 1992.
111. Neerhut GJ, Wheeler TM, Dunn JK, and Scardino PT. Residual tumor after transurethral resection of the prostate: features of incidentally found prostate cancer in transurethral and radical prostatectomy specimens. In Altwein JE, Faul P, and Schneider W (eds): *Incidental Carcinoma of the Prostate.* Springer-Verlag: Berlin. 1991. pp. 119–121.
112. Rogers E, Ohori M, Kassabian VS, and others. Salvage radical prostatectomy: outcome measured by serum prostate specific antigen levels. *J Urol* 153:104–110, 1995.
113. Thompson IM. Observation alone in the management of localized prostate cancer: the natural history of untreated disease. *Urology* 43:41–46, 1994.
114. Glass RE, Ritchie JK, Thompson HR, and Mann CV. and The results of surgical treatment of cancer of the rectum by radical resection and extended abdomino-iliac lymphadenectomy. *Br J Surg* 72:599–601, 1985.
115. Welch JP and Welch CE. Cancer of the rectum. Where are we? Where are we going? *Arch Surg* 128:687–702, 1993.

116. Stearns MW. The choice among anterior resection, the pull-through and abdominoperineal resection of the rectum. *Cancer* 34:969, 1974.
117. Marks G, Mohiuddin M, Masoni L, and Montori A. High-dose preoperative radiation therapy as the key to extending sphincter-preservation surgery for cancer of the distal rectum. *Surg Oncol Clin North Am* 1:71-86, 1992.
118. Enker WE, Paty PB, Minsky BD, and Cohen AM. Restorative or preservative operations in the treatment of rectal cancer. *Surg Oncol Clin North Am* 1:57-69, 1992.
119. O'Connell MJ, Martenson JA, Wieand HS, and others. Improving adjuvant therapy for rectal cancer by combining protracted-infusion fluorouracil with radiation therapy after curative surgery. *N Engl J Med* 1:502-507, 1994.
120. Fuhrman GM, Talamonti MS, and Curley SA. Sphincter-preserving extended resection for locally advanced rectosigmoid carcinoma involving the urinary bladder. *J Surg Oncol* 50:77-80, 1992.
121. Culp CE and Jackson RJ. Reappraisal of conservative management of certain selected cancer of the rectum. In Najarian JS and Delaney JP (eds): *Surgery of the Gastrointestinal Tract.* Stratton: New York. 1974. pp. 511-519.
122. DeCosse JJ, Wong RJ, Quan SHQ, and others. Conservative treatment of distal rectal cancer by local excision. *Cancer* 63:219-223, 1989.
123. Graham RA, Garney L, and Jessup JM. Local excision of rectal carcinoma. *Am J Surg* 160:306-311, 1990.
124. Papillon J. Intracavitary irradiation of early rectal cancer for cure. *Cancer* 36:696-701, 1975.
125. Beart RW Jr and Biggers O. Local excision of rectal cancer. *Prob Gen Surg* 2:240-243, 1985.
126. Minsky BD. Clinical experience with local excision and postoperative radiation therapy for rectal cancer. *Dis Colon Rectum* 36:405-409, 1993.
127. Minsky BD, Cohen AM, Enker WE, and Mies C. Sphicter preservation in rectal cancer by local excision and postoperative therapy. *Cancer* 67:908-914, 1991.
128. Adloff M, Arnaud JP, Schloegel M, and others. Factor influencing local recurrence after abdominoperineal resection for cancer of the rectum. *Dis Colon Rectum* 28:413-415, 1985.
129. Meijer S, de Rooij PD, Derksen EJ, Boutkan H, and Cuesta MA. Cryosurgery for locally recurrent rectal cancer. *Eur J Surg Oncol* 18:255-257, 1992.
130. Cuthbertson AM and Simpson RL. Curative local excision of rectal adenocarcinoma. *Aust NZ J Surg* 56:229-231, 1986.
131. Stulc JP, Davidson B, Herrera L, and Petrelli NJ. The prognostic significance of anastomotic recurrence from colorectal adenocarcinoma. Read before the Forty-third Annual Meeting of the Society of Surgical Oncology, Washington, DC. May 21, 1990.
132. Stahl TJ, Murray JJ, Coller JA, and others. Sphincter-saving alternatives in the management of adenocarcinoma involving the distal rectum. *Arch Surg* 128:545-550, 1993.
133. Wolmark N and Fisher B. An analysis of survival and treatment failure following abdominoperineal and sphincter-saving resection in Dukes' B and C rectal carcinoma. *Ann Surg* 204:480-487, 1986.
134. Paty PB, Enker WE, Cohen AM, and Lauwers GY. Treatment of rectal cancer by low anterior resection with coloanal anastomosis. *Ann Surg* 219:365-373, 1994.
135. Warren S and Sommer GNJ. Fibrosarcoma of the soft parts with special reference to recurrence and metastasis. *Arch Surg* 33:425-450, 1936.

136. Stout AP. Fibrosarcoma: the malignant tumor of fibroblasts. *Cancer* 3:30-63, 1948.
137. Lieberman Z and Ackerman LV. Principles in management of soft tissue sarcomas. A clinical and pathological review of one hundred cases. *Surgery* 35:350-365, 1954.
138. Emrich LJ, Ruka W, Driscoll DL, and Karakousis CP. The effect of local recurrence on survival time in adult high-grade soft tissue sarcoma. *J Clin Epidemiol* 42:105-110, 1989.
139. Cantin J, McNeer GP, Chu FC, and Booher RJ. The problem of local recurrence after treatment of soft tissue sarcoma. *Ann Surg* 168:47-53, 1968.
140. Giuliano AE, Eilber FR, and Morton DL. The management of locally recurrent soft-tissue sarcoma. *Ann Surg* 196:87-91, 1982.
141. Atkinson L, Garvan JM, and Newton NC. Behavior and management of soft connective tissue sarcomas. *Cancer* 16:1552-1562, 1963.
142. Lindberg RD, Martin RG, Romsdahl MM, and Barkley HT. Conservative surgery and postoperative radiotherapy in 300 adults with soft-tissue sarcomas. *Cancer* 47:2391-2397, 1981.
143. Suit HD, Mankin HJ, Wood WC, and Proppe KH. Preoperative, intraoperative, and postoperative radiation in the treatment of primary soft tissue sarcoma. *Cancer* 55:2659-2667, 1985.
144. Suit HD, Mankin HJ, Wood WC, and Gebhardt MC. Treatment of the patient with stage M0 soft tissue sarcomas. *J Clin Oncol* 6:854-862, 1988.
145. Leibel SA, Tranbaugh RF, Wara WM, Beckstead JH, Bovill EG, and Phillips TL. Soft-tissue sarcomas of the extremities. Survival and patterns of failure with conservative surgery and postoperative irradiation compared to surgery alone. *Cancer* 50:1076-1083, 1982.

146. Lawrence W, Donegan WL, Natarajan N, and others. Adult soft tissue sarcomas: a pattern of care survey of the American College of Surgeons. *Ann Surg* 205:349-359, 1987.
147. Potter DA, Kinsella T, Glatstein E, and others. High-grade soft tissue sarcomas of the extremities. *Cancer* 58:190-205, 1986.
148. Rööser B. Prognosis in soft tissue sarcoma. *Acta Orthop Scand* [supp. 225] 58:1-52, 1987.
149. Gustafson P, Rööser B, and Rydholm A. Is local recurrence of minor importance for metastases in soft tissue sarcoma? *Cancer* 67:2083-2086, 1991.
150. Ueda T, Aozasa K, Tsujimoto M, Hamada H, Hayashi H, Ono K, and Matsumoto K. Multivariant analysis for clinical prognostic factors in 163 patients with soft tissue sarcoma. *Cancer* 62:1444-1450, 1988.
151. Brennan MF, Shiu MH, Collin C, and others. Extremity soft tissue sarcomas. *Cancer Treat Symp* 3:71-81, 1985.
152. Brennan MF. Management of extremity soft-tissue sarcoma. *Am J Surg* 158:71-78, 1989.
153. Brennan MF, Casper ES, Harrison LB, and others. The role of multimodality therapy in soft-tissue sarcoma. *Ann Surg* 214:328-338, 1991.
154. Collin C, Godbold J, Hajdu S, and Brennan M. Localized extremity soft tissue sarcoma: An analysis of factors affecting survival. *J Clin Oncol* 5:601-612, 1987.
155. Markhede G, Angervall L, and Stener B. A multivariate analysis of the prognosis after surgical treatment of soft-tissue tumors. *Cancer* 49:1721-1733, 1982.
156. Stotter AT, A'Hern RP, Fisher C, and others. The influence of local recurrence of extremity soft tissue sarcoma on metastasis and survival. *Cancer* 65:1119-1129, 1990.

157. Margolese RG. 4. Diagnosis and management of local recurrence after breast-conservation surgery. *Can J Surg* 35:378-381, 1992.
158. Fisher B, Anderson S, Fisher ER, and others. Significance of ipsilateral recurrence after lumpectomy. *Lancet* 338:327-331, 1991.
159. Senekjian EK, Frey KW, Anderson D, and Herbst AL. Local therapy in stage I clear cell adenocarcinoma of the vagina. *Cancer* 60:1319-1324, 1987.
160. Hoffman MS, DeCesare SL, Roberts WS, and others. Upper vaginectomy for in situ and occult, superficially invasive carcinoma of the vagina. *Am J Obstet Gynecol* 166:30-33, 1992.
161. Hacker NF, Van der Velden J. Conservative management of early vulvar cancer. *Cancer* 71:1673-1677, 1993.
162. Heaps JM, Fu YS, Montz FJ, and others. Surgical-pathologic variables predictive of local recurrence in squamous cell carcinoma of the vulva. *Gynecol Oncol* 38:309-314, 1990.
163. Dipasquale C, Pellizzari P, and Cataldi A. Conservative surgery in vulvar-vaginal neoplasias and fertility. *European J of Gynaecol Oncol* 12:415-417, 1991.
164. Burke TW, Stringer CA, Gershenson DM, and others. Radical wide excision and selective inguinal node dissection for squamous cell carcinoma of the vulva. *Gynecol Oncol* 38:328-332, 1990.
165. Heaps JM, Fu YS, Montz FJ, and others. Surgical-pathologic variable predictive of local recurrence in squamous cell carcinoma of the vulva. *Gynecol Oncol* 38:309-314, 1990.
166. Hopkins MP, Reid GC, and Morley GW. The surgical management of recurrent squamous cell carcinoma of the vulva. *Obstet Gynecol* 75:1001, 1990.
167. Dipasquale C, Pellizzari P, and Cataldi A. Conservative surgery in vulvar-vaginal neoplasias and fertility. *Eur J Gynaecol Oncol* 12:415-417, 1991.
168. DiSaia PJ and Creasman WT. *Clinical Gynecologic Oncology*. Mosby Year Book: St. Louis. 1992. p. 260.
169. Podratz KC, Symmonds RE, and Taylor WF. Carcinoma of the vulva: analysis of treatment failures. *Am J Obstet Gynecol* 143:340-351, 1982.
170. Piura B, Masotina A, Murdoch J, and others. Recurrent squamous cell carcinoma of the vulva: a study of 73 cases. *Gynecol Oncol* 48:189-195, 1993.
171. Hopkins MP, Reid GC, and Morley GW. Radical vulvectomy: The decision for the incision. *Cancer* 72:799-803, 1993.
172. Rogo KO, Andersson R, Edbom G, and Stendahl U. Conservative surgery for vulvovaginal melanoma. *Eur J Gynaecol Oncol* 12:113-119, 1991.
173. Davidson T, Kissin M, and Westbury G. Vulvo-vaginal melanoma—should radical surgery be abandoned? *Brit J Obstet Gynaecol* 94:473-476, 1987.
174. Lin JY, DuBeshter B, Angel C, and Dvoretsky PM. Morbidity and recurrence with modifications of radical vulvectomy and groin dissection. *Gynecol Oncol* 47:80-86, 1992.
175. DiSaia PJ, Creasman WT, and Rich WM. An alternate approach to early cancer of the vulva. *Am J Obstet Gynecol* 133:825-832, 1979.
176. Homesley HD, Bundy BN, Sedlis A, and Adcock L. Radiation therapy versus pelvic lymph node resection for carcinoma of the vulva with positive groin nodes. *Obstet Gynecol* 68:733-740, 1986.

Notes II

These are the notes to the revised edition. The references listed under Appendix II include medical articles published since 1994.

Preface to the Revised Edition
1. Henderson IC. Paradigmatic shifts in the management of breast cancer. N Engl J Med 332:951-952, 1995.
2. Evans RA. Adjuvant chemotherapy in breast cancer. N Engl J Med 333;596-597, 1995. (letter)
3. Hellman S. Stopping metastases at their source. N Engl J Med 337:996-997, 1997.
4. Evans RA. Radiation therapy and chemotherapy in high-risk beast cancer. N Engl J Med 338:331, 1998. (letter)
5. Evans RA. Host resistance to carcinoma of the breast. South Med J 73:1261-1263, 1980.
6. Balch CM, Soong S-J, Bartolucci AA, and others. Efficacy of an elective regional lymph node dissection of 1 to 4 mm thick melanomas for patients 60 years of age and younger. Ann Surg 224:255-266, 1996.
7. Evans RA. Elective lymph node dissection for clinical stage I malignant melanoma. J Surg Oncol 57:31-2, 1994. (letter)
8. Evans RA. Review and current perspectives of cutaneous malignant melanoma. J Am Coll Surg 179:764-767, 1994. (letter)
9. Evans RA. Elective lymph node dissection for malignant melanoma: the tumor burden of nodal disease. Anticancer Res 15:575-80, 1995.
10. Evans RA. Elective lymph node dissection (ELND) for malignant melanoma. Ann Surg 221:435-6, 1995. (letter)
11. Evans RA. Malignant melanoma: primary surgical management (excision and node dissection) based upon pathology and staging. Cancer 76:2384-5, 1995.(letter)
12. Evans RA. Melanoma recurrence surveillance: Patient or physician based? Ann Surg 223:445-6, 1996. (letter)
13. Evans RA. Recent advances in the care of the patient with malignant melanoma. Ann Surg 227:607-8, 1998. (letter)

Appendix II
1. Laufer M. Transurethral resection and partial cystectomy for invasive bladder cancer. Semin Urol Oncol 18:296-299, 2000.
2. Herr HW. Transurethral resection of muscle-invasive bladder cancer: 10-year outcome. J Clin Oncol 19:89-93, 2001.
3. Kim HL, Steinberg GD. The current status of bladder preservation in the treatment of muscle invasive bladder cancer. J Urol 164:627-632, 2000.
4. Sternberg CN, Pansadoro V, Calabro F, Marini L, van Rijn A, Carli PD, and others. Neo-adjuvant chemotherapy and bladder preservation in locally advanced transitional cell carcinoma of the bladder. Ann Oncol 10:1301-5, 1999.
5. Herr HW, Bajorin DF, Scher HI. Neoadjuvant chemotherapy and bladder-sparing surgery for invasive bladder cancer: ten-year outcome. J Clin Oncol 16:1298-301, 1998.
6. Montie JE. Against bladder sparing surgery. J Urol 162:452-7, 1999.

7. Tester W, Caplan R, Heaney J, and others. Neoadjuvant combined modality program with selective organ preservation for invasive bladder cancer: Results of Radiation Therapy Oncology Group Phase II Trail 8892. J Clin Oncol 14:119-126, 1996.
8. Early Breast Cancer Trialists' Collaborative Group. Favourable and unfavourable effects on long-term survival of radiotherapy for early breast cancer: an overview of the randomized trials. Lancet 355:1757-1770, 2000.
9. Atkins CD. Breast cancer survival advantage with radiotherapy. Lancet 356:1269, 2000.
10. De Csepel J, Tartter PI, Gajdos C. When not to give radiation therapy after breast conservation for breast cancer. J Surg Oncol 74:273-277, 2000.
11. Gruenberger T, Gorlitzer M, Soliman T, Rudas M, Mittlboeck M, Gnant M, and others. It is possible to omit postoperative irradiation in a highly selected group of elderly breast cancer patients. Breast Cancer Res Treat 50:37-46, 1998.
12. Sader C, Ingram D, Hastrich D. Management of breast cancer in the elderly by complete local excision and tamoxifen alone. Aust N Z J Surg 69:790-793, 1999.
13. Fisher B, Costantino J, Redmond C, and others. Lumpectomy and radiation therapy for the treatment of intraductal breast cancer: findings from the National Surgical Adjuvant Breast and Bowel Project B-17. J Clin Oncol 16:441-452, 1998.
14. Fisher B, Dignam J, Wolmark N, and others. Tamoxifen in treatment of intraductal breast cancer: National Surgical Adjuvant Breast and Bowel Project B-24 randomized controlled trial. Lancet 353:1993-2000, 1999.
15. Silverstein MJ, Lagios MS, Groshen S, Waisman JR, Lewinsky BS, Martino S, and others. The influence of margin width on local control of ductal carcinoma in situ of the breast. N Engl J Med 340:1455-1461, 1999.
16. Schwartz GF, Solin LJ, Olivotto IA, Ernster VL, Pressman PI. Consensus Conference on the Treatment of In Situ Ductal Carcinoma of the Breast, April 22-25, 1999. Cancer 88:946-954, 2000.
17. Haffty BG, Reiss M, Beinfield M, Fischer D, Ward B, and McKhann C. Ipsilateral breast tumor recurrence as a predictor of distant disease: Implication for systemic therapy at the time of local relapse. J Clin Oncol 14:52-57, 1996.
18. Fortin A, Larochelle M, Laverdiere J, Lavertu S, Tremblay D. Local failure is responsible for the decrease in survival for patients with breast cancer treated with conservative surgery and postoperative radiotherapy. J Clin Oncol 17:101-109, 1999.
19. Evans RA. Host resistance to carcinoma of the breast. South Med J 73:1261-1263, 1980.
20. Dargent D, Martin X, Sacchetoni A, Mathevet P. Laparoscopic vaginal radical trachelectomy: A treatment to preserve the fertility of cervical carcinoma patients. Cancer 88:1877-1882, 2000.
21. Roy M, Plante M. Pregnancies after radical vaginal trachelectomy for early-stage cervical cancer. Am J Obstet Gynecol 179:1491-1496, 1998.

22. Roy M, Plante M. Radical vaginal trachelectomy for invasive cervical cancer. [French] J Gynecol Obstet Biol Reprod (Paris) 29:279-281, 2000.
23. Covens A, Shaw P, Murphy J, DePetrillo D, Lickrish G, Laframboise S, Rosen B. Is radical trachelectomy a safe alternative to radical hysterectomy for patients with stage IA-B carcinoma of the cervix? Cancer 86:2272-2279, 1999.
24. Yaegashi N, Sato S, InoueY, Noda K, Yajima A. Conservative surgical treatment in cervical cancer with 3 to 5 mm stromal invasion in the absence of confluent invasion and lymph-vascular space involvement. Gynecol Oncol 54:333-337, 1994.
25. Zitelli JA, Brown C, Hanussa BH. Mohs micrographic surgery for the treatment of primary cutaneous melanoma. J Am Acad Dermatol 37:236-45, 1997.
26. Snow SN, Mohs FE, Oriba HA, Dudley CM, Leverson CM, Hetzer M. Cutaneous malignant melanoma treated by Mohs surgery. Review of the treatment of 179 cases from the Mohs Melanoma Registry. Dermatol Surg 23:1055-60, 1997.
27. Heaton KM, Sussman JJ, Gershenwald JE, Lee JF, Reintgen DS, Mansfield PF, Ross MI. Surgical marg and prognostic factors in patients with thick (> 4 mm) primary melanoma. Ann Surg Oncol 5:322-8, 1998.
28. Hudson DA, Krige JE, Grobbelaar AO, Morgan B, Grover R. Melanoma of the face: the safety of narrow excision margins. Scand J Plast Reconstr Surg Hand Surg 32:97-104, 1998.
29. Dong XD, Tyler D, Johnson JL, DeMatos P, Seigler HF. Analysis of prognosis and disease progression after local recurrence of melanoma. Cancer 88:1063-1071, 2000.
30. Balch CM, Soong S-J, Bartolucci AA, and others. Efficacy of an elective regional lymph node dissection of 1 to 4 mm thick melanomas for patients 60 years of age and younger. Ann Surg 224:255-266, 1996.
31. Evans RA. Elective lymph node dissection for clinical stage I malignant melanoma. J Surg Oncol 57:31-2, 1994. (letter)
32. Evans RA. Review and current perspectives of cutaneous malignant melanoma. J Am Coll Surg 179:764-767, 1994. (letter)
33. Evans RA. Elective lymph node dissection for malignant melanoma: the tumor burden of nodal disease. Anticancer Res 15:575-80, 1995.
34. Evans RA. Elective lymph node dissection (ELND) for malignant melanoma. Ann Surg 221:435-6, 1995. (letter)
35. Evans RA. Malignant melanoma: primary surgical management (excision and node dissection) based upon pathology and staging. Cancer 76:2384-5, 1995.(letter)
36. Evans RA. Melanoma recurrence surveillance: Patient or physician based? Ann Surg 223:445-6, 1996. (letter)
37. Evans RA. Recent advances in the care of the patient with malignant melanoma. Ann Surg 227:607-8, 1998. (letter)
38. Soria JC, Fizazi K, Piron D, Kramer A, Gerbaulet A, Haie-Meder C and others. Squamous cell

carcinoma of the penis: multivariate analysis of prognostic factors and natural history in monocentric study with a conservative policy. Ann Oncol 8:1089-1098, 1997.
39. Chaudhary AJ, Ghosh S, Bhalavat RL, Kulkarni JN and Sequeira BV. Interstitial brachytherapy in carcinoma of the penis. Strahlenther Onkol 175: 17-20, 1999.
40. Sarin R, Norman AR, Steel GG, and Horwich A. Treatment results and prognostic factors in 101 men treated for squamous carcinoma of the penis. Int J Radiat Oncol Biol Phys 38:713-722, 1997.
41. Tietjen DN, Malek RS. Laser therapy of squamous cell dysplasia and carcinoma of the penis. Urology 52:559-565, 1998.
42. Windahl T and Hellsten S. Laser treatment of localized squamous cell carcinoma of the penis. J Urol 154:1020-1023, 1995.
43. Gotsadze D, Matveev B, Zak B, Mamaladze V. Is conservative organ-sparing treatment of penile carcinoma justified? Eur Urol 38:306-312, 2000.
44. Theodorescu D, Russo P, Zhang ZF, Morash C, Fair WR. Outcomes of initial surveillance of invasive squamous cell carcinoma of the penis and negative nodes. J Urol 155:1626-1631, 1996.
45. Pettaway CA, Pisters LL, Dinney CP, and others. Sentinel lymph nodes dissection for penile carcinoma: the M. D. Anderson Cancer Center experience. J Urol 154:1999-2003, 1995.
46. Fowler FJ Jr, McNaughton Collins M, Albertsen PC, Zietman A, Elliott DB, Barry MJ Comparison of recommendations by urologists and radiation oncologists for treatment of clinically localized prostate cancer. JAMA. 283:3217-3222, 2000.
47. Labrie F, Candas B, Dupont A, and others. Screening decreases prostate cancer death: First analysis of the 1988 Quebec prospective randomized controlled trial. Prostate 38:83-91, 1999.
48. Ragde H, Korb L. Brachytherapy for clinically localized prostate cancer. Semin Surg Oncol 18:45-51, 2000.
49. Sharkey J, Chovnick S, Behar R, Otheguy J, Rabinowitz R. Re: radical prostatectomy for localized prostate cancer provides durable cancer control with excellent quality of life: a structured debate. J Urol 165:192-193, 2000.
50. Walsh PC. Editorial comment: Taking on prostate cancer. J Urol 156:1518-1548, 1996.
51. Evans RA. RE: Editorial comment: Taking on prostate cancer. J Urol 156:1528-1529, 1996.
52. Lundgren R, Nordle O, Josefsson K. Immediate estrogen or estramustine phosphate therapy versus deferred endocrine treatment in nonmetastatic prostate cancer: a randomized multicenter study with 15 years of followup. The South Sweden Prostate Cancer Study Group. J Urol 153:15480-1586, 1995.
53. The Medical Research Council Prostate Cancer Working Party Investigators Group. Immediate versus delayed treatment for advanced prostate cancer: initial results of the Medical Research Council Trial. Br J Urol 79:235-246, 1997.

54. Strum SB, Scholtz MS, McDermed JE. Intermittent androgen deprivation in prostate cancer patients: factors predictive of prolonged time off therapy. The Oncologist 5:45-52, 2000.
55. Stone NN, Stock RG. Neoadjuvant hormonal therapy improves the outcomes of patients undergoing radioactive seed implantation for localized prostate cancer. Mol Urol 3:239-244, 1999.
56. Adolfsson J. The natural history of early prostate cancer and the impact of endocrine treatment. Eur Urol 36:3-8, 1999.
57. D'Amico A, Scholtz D, Loffredo M, Dugal R, Hurwitz M, Kaplan I, and others. Biochemical outcome following external beam radiation therapy with or without androgen suppression for clinically localized prostate cancer. JAMA 284:1280-1283, 2000.
58. Cohen JK, Miller RJ, Benoit R, Rooker GM, Merlotti L. Five year outcome of PSA and biopsy following cryosurgery as primary treatment for localized prostate cancer. J Urol 159 (suppl):252, 1998.
59. Labrie F. Screening and early treatment of prostate cancer are accumulating strong evidence and support. Prostate 43:215-222, 2000.
60. Ng AK, Recht A, Busse PM. Sphincter preservation therapy for distal rectal carcinoma. Cancer 79:671-683, 1997.
61. Valentini V, Coco C, Cellini N, Picciocchi A, Genovesi D, Mantini G, Barbaro B, et al. Preoperative chemoradiation for extraperitoneal T3 rectal cancer: Acute toxicity, tumor response and sphincter preservation. Int J Radiation Oncology Biol Phys 40:1067-1075. 1998.
62. Graham RA, Hackford AW, Wazer DE. Local excision of rectal carcinoma: a safe alternative for more advanced tumors? J Surg Oncol 70:235-238, 1999.
63. Mohiuddin M, Regine WF, Marks GJ, Marks JW. High-dose preoperative radiation and the challenge of sphincter-preservation surgery for cancer of the distal 2 cm of the rectum. Int J Radiat Oncol Biol Phys 40:569-574, 1998.
64. Janjan NA, Crane CN, Feig BW and others. Prospective trial of preoperative concomitant boost radiotherapy with continuous infusion 5-fluorouracil for locally advanced rectal cancer. Int J Radiat Oncol Biol Phys 47:713-718, 2000.
65. Shibata D, Guillem JG, Lanouette N and others. Functional and quality-of-life outcomes in patients with rectal cancer after combined modality therapy, intraoperative radiation therapy, and sphincter preservation. Dis Colon Rectum. 43:752-758, 2000.
66. Garcia-Aguilar J, Mellgren A, Sirivongs P, Buie D, Madoff RD, Rothenberger DA. Local excision of rectal cancer without adjuvant therapy: a word of caution. Ann Surg 231:345-351, 2000.
67. Pisters PWT, Harrison LB, Leung DHY, Woodruff JM, Casper ES, Brennan MF. Long-term results of a prospective randomized trial of adjuvant brachytherapy in soft tissue sarcoma. J Clin Oncol 14:859-868, 1996.
68. Yang JC, Chang AE, Baker R, Sindelar WF, Danforth DN, and others. Randomized prospective

study of the benefit of adjuvant radiation therapy in the treatment of soft tissue sarcoma of the extremity. J Clin Oncol 16:197-203, 1998.
69. Karakousis CP, Proimakis C, Walsh DL. Primary soft tissue sarcoma of the extremities in adults. Br J Surg 82:1208-1212, 1995.
70. Gibbs CP, Peabody TD, Mundt AJ and others. Oncological outcomes of operative treatment of subcutaneous soft-tissue sarcomas of the extremities. J Bone Joint Surg Ann 79:888-897, 1997.
71. Fabrizio PL, Stafford SL, Pritchard DJ. Extremity soft-tissue sarcomas selectively treated with surgery alone. Int J Radiat Oncol Biol Phys 48:227-232, 2000.
72. Choong PFM, Gustafson P, Rydholm A. Size and timing of local recurrence predicts metastasis in soft tissue sarcoma. Acta Orthop Scand 66:147-152, 1995.
73. Trovik CS and Bauer HCF Bauer. Local recurrence of soft tissue sarcoma a risk factor for late metastases. Acta Orthop Scand 65:553-558, 1994
74. Ueda T, Toshikawa H, Mori S, Myoui A, Kuratsu S, Uchida A. Influence of local recurrence of the prognosis of soft-tissue sarcoma. J Bone Joint Surg (Br) 79:B:553-557, 1997.
75. Singer S, Corson JM, Gonin R, Labow B, Eberlein TJ. Prognostic factors predictive of survival and local recurrence for extremity soft tissue sarcoma. Ann Surg 219:165-173, 1994.
76. Lewis JJ, Leung D, Heslin M, Woodruff JM, Brennan MF. Association of local recurrence with subsequent survival in extremity soft tissue sarcoma. J Clin Oncol 15:646-52, 1997.
77. Espat NJ and Lewis JJ. The biological significance of failure at the primary site on ultimate survival in soft tissue sarcoma. Semin Radiat Oncol 9:369-377, 1999.
78. Brennan MF. The enigma of local recurrence. Ann Surg Oncol 4:1-12, 1997.
79. Perez CA, Grigsby PW, Garipagaoglu M, Mutch DG, Lockett MA. Factors affecting long-term outcome of irradiation in carcinoma of the vagina. Int J Radiation Oncol Biol Phys 44:37-45, 1999.
80. Buchanan DJ, Schlaerth J, Kurosaki T. Primary vaginal melanoma: Thirteen-year disease-free survival after wide local excision and review of recent literature. Am J Obstet Gynecol 178:1177-1184, 1998.
81. Van Nostrand KM, Lucci JA 3rd, Schell M. Berman ML, Manetta A, DiSaia PJ. Primary vaginal melanoma: improved survival with radical pelvic surgery. Gynecol Oncol 55:234-237, 1994.
82. Evans RA. Primary vaginal melanoma: improved survival with radical pelvic surgery. Gynecol Oncol 59:164-165, 1995. (letter)
83. Van Nostrand KM. Primary vaginal melanoma: improved survival with radical pelvic surgery. Gynecol Oncol 59:165. (letter)
84. Nash JD and Curry S. Vulvar cancer. Surg Oncol Clin N Am 7:335-346, 1998.
85. Magrina JF, Gonzales-Bosquet J, Weaver AL, and others. Primary squamous cell cancer of the vulva: radical versus modified radical vulvar surgery. Gynecol Oncol

71:116-121, 1998.

86. Hacker NF. Current management of early vulvar cancer. Ann Acad Med Singapore 27:688-692, 1998.

87. Burke TW, Levenback C, Coleman RL, Morris M, Silva EG, and Gershenson DM. Surgical therapy of T1 and T2 vulvar carcinoma: further experience with radical wide excision and selective inguinal lymphadenectomy. Gynecol Oncol 57:215-220, 1995.

88. Grendys EC Jr, Salud C, Durfee JK, Fiorica JV. Lymphatic mapping in gynecologic malignancies. Surg Oncol Clin N Am 8:541-553, 1999.

89. Bowles J, Terada KY, Coel MN, Wong JH. Preoperative lymphoscintigraphy in the evaluation of squamous cell cancer of the vulva. Clin Nucl Med 24:235-238, 1999.

90. de Hullu JA, Doting E, Piers DA and others. Sentinel lymph node identification with technetium-99m-labeled nanocolloid in squamous cell cancer of the vulva. J Nucl Med 39:1381-1385, 1998.

Glossary

Italicized words are defined elsewhere in the Glossary.

Abdominoperineal resection (APR). The removal of the entire rectum and lymph nodes. Surgeons operate within the abdomen and also around the anus. The patient is left with a permanent *colostomy*.

Adenocarcinoma. Cancer that arises from glandular or fluid-producing tissue.

Adhesion molecule. A molecule that allows a cancer cell to move through normal tissue.

Adjuvant therapy. *Radiation therapy* or *chemotherapy* administered after the visible cancer has been removed. It is therapy used "in addition to" surgery.

AJCC system. One of several *staging systems* devised by the American Joint Committee on Cancer, some of them in cooperation with the Union Internationale Contra Cancer (AJCC-UICC systems). Some of these systems are based on the *TNM system*. There are AJCC (or AJCC-UICC) systems for *malignant melanoma*, *soft tissue sarcoma*, and cancers of the bladder, prostate, and rectum.

Alkaloid. A class of *chemotherapy* drugs that interfere with cell division.

Alkylating agent. A class of *chemotherapy* drugs that either break *DNA* strands or interfere with their division.

Anal canal. The last inch of the rectum.

Anal verge. The ridge formed by the *external sphincter* at the bottom of the *anal canal*.

Androgen. A male sex hormone that can stimulate the growth of some prostate cancers. *Testosterone* is the most prominent type of androgen.

Aneuploid cell. A cancer cell with an abnormal number of *chromosomes* (something other than twenty-three pairs). Such cells divide rapidly, leading to a worse prognosis.

Antiandrogen. A class of *hormonal therapy* agents that prevent androgens from helping prostate cancers to grow.

Antibiotic. A class of *chemotherapy* drugs that damage *DNA* or prevent DNA from making *RNA*.

Antibody. A substance produced by *lymphocytes* in reponse to an *antigen*. Antibodies are most effective against threats from outside the cell, such as bacteria.

Antiestrogen. A class of *hormonal therapy* agents that prevent *estrogen* from helping breast cancers to grow.

Antigen. A substance that can provoke an immune response in an animal or a human being.

Antimetabolite. A class of *chemotherapy* drugs that interfere with chemical reactions necessary for *DNA synthesis*.

Anus. The opening at the bottom of the *anal canal*.

Aorta. The body's main artery. It leads away from the heart's main pumping chamber.

Apoptosis. A form of programmed cell death. A *lymphokine* can cause a cancer cell to destroy itself in this way.

Atypical intraductal hyperplasia. See *intraductal hyperplasia*.

AUA system. A *staging system* for prostate cancer devised by the American Urological Association.

Axillary dissection. The removal of lymph nodes in the armpit.

Axillary lymph nodes. The nodes in the armpit.

B cell. A *lymphocyte* that produces antibodies in reaction to *antigens*.

Bacillus Calmette-Guerin (BCG). A bacterium that stimulates the immune response. It is used in *biological therapy*.

Barium enema. An X-ray of the large intestine after the introduction of barium, which can outline abnormalities.

Base. A substance that forms the "rungs" in the ladder-like *DNA* molecule. The sequence of bases (there are only four) determine the genetic code, which in turn determines such inherited traits as eye color and blood type.

Basement membrane. The thin membrane between the *epithelial cells* and the underlying connective tissue that supports the production of these cells.

Basic science. The study of cancer in the laboratory, at the chemical level.

Glossary

Benign prostatic hypertrophy (BPH). A benign enlargement of the prostate. It often occurs as a man ages.

Biological response modifier (BRM). A substance that increases the body's immune response to cancer.

Biological therapy. The use of *biological response modifiers* to treat cancer. It is also called immunotherapy.

Biopsy. The removal of a tissue sample to determine whether it is malignant or not. This tissue can be treated as either a *frozen section* or a *permanent section*.

Bone marrow transplantation. A therapy in which a patient's own bone marrow is removed so that high-dose *chemotherapy* can be given. The patient's ability to make white blood cells, which are formed in the marrow, is restored by giving the bone marrow cells back to the patient after the chemotherapy treatments are over.

Brachytherapy. Another term for *interstitial radiation*, in which radioactive seeds are introduced directly into a tumor. This term is used because this type of therapy can be done in a short (*brachy-*) period of time.

Breslow's thickness. A system that measures how far (in millimeters) a *malignant melanoma* has penetrated into the skin.

Carcinoembryonic antigen (CEA). A substance in the blood stream that may be elevated in some patients with rectal cancer and some other malignancies. If the level of CEA in the blood falls after surgery, and then rises, it may signal a recurrence.

Carcinogen. A substance that stimulates cancer development.

Carcinoma. Cancer that arises from the *epithelial cells* that line the body surfaces inside and out.

Cell-mediated immunity. The aspect of the immune response that is controlled by *killer T cells*. It is most effective against threats from inside the cell, such as viruses or *DNA* abnormalities.

Cellular matrix. The "glue" that holds normal cells together.

Centrifugal spread theory. A theory, developed in the nineteenth century, which stated that cancer spreads by direct extension, for example, breast cancer spreading to the liver by growing through the layers of tissue that separate the breast and the liver. It was disproved once doctors discovered that cancer spreads through the circulation of cancer cells in the blood stream.

Cervical intraepithelial neoplasia (CIN). A premalignant change in the cervix that can lead to cancer *in situ*.

Chemotherapy. The use of drugs to treat cancer.

Chromosome. The part of the cell that controls both cell function and cell division. A human cell contains twenty-three pairs of chromosomes. Each chromosome is made up of *genes*, which in turn are made up of *DNA*.

Clark's levels. A system that measures how many layers of skin a *malignant melanoma* has penetrated.

Clinical science. The study of cancer in human beings.

Clinical staging. The observations on how far a cancer has spread made by a doctor on physical examination without the benefit of a pathologist's examination of the regional lymph nodes or other tissue.

Coley's toxin. A vaccine developed by William Coley in the 1890s and used by him to treat cancer. It was an early form of *biological therapy*.

Coloanal anastomosis. A procedure in which, after the tumor is removed, the lower colon is pulled into and sewn to the anus.

Colony-stimulating factors (CSF). Naturally-occurring substances that stimulate the growth of white blood cells. They are used in *biological therapy*.

Colostomy. A procedure in which the large intestine is attached to the abdominal wall. The patient defecates into an external bag.

Colposcopy. The examination of the cervix through a scope placed into the vagina.

Cone biopsy. See *conization*.

Conization. The removal of a cone-shaped piece of cervical tissue. It is used both to diagnose and to treat early cancer.

Cryosurgery. Surgery performed with a probe that freezes tissue.

Cystectomy. See *partial cystectomy* and *radical cystectomy*.

Cystoscope. A lighted tube used to examine the bladder, prostate, and *urethra*.

Cystoscopy. An examination of the bladder through a *cystoscope*.

Cytokine. A chemical that regulates and stimulates white blood cells. When used in treatment, cytokines are called *biological response modifiers*.

Cytoplasm. The part of the cell that contains the machinery needed to perform that cell's particular function, such as the production of hormones or other proteins. Activity in the cytoplasm is directed by the cell's *nucleus*.

Debulking surgery. Surgery performed to reduce the mass of a tumor. Often, it is done before *chemotherapy* or *radiation therapy*.

Glossary

Depth of invasion. The number of layers of tissue that a cancer has penetrated.

Diethylstilbestrol (DES). A synthetic *estrogen* used to treat metastatic prostate cancer. It has also been found to be a cancer-causing agent in women whose mothers took DES to prevent miscarriage in the 1950s and 1960s.

Differentiated (low grade). A cancer that is slow-growing. The cells are distinctive, that is, they resemble the cells from which they arose. Such tumors are less likely to spread.

Digital rectal examination (DRE). A check for prostate enlargement and rectal polyps. It is done by a physician inserting a gloved finger into the rectum.

Diploid cell. A cancer cell with the normal number of *chromosomes* (twenty-three pairs). These cells do not divide so rapidly, leading to a better prognosis.

Disease-free survival. The amount of time a patient lives after treatment without any evidence of cancer.

DNA (deoxyribonucleic acid). The basic "stuff" of which *genes* and *chromosomes* are made. Its structure resembles a twisted ladder or spiral staircase. By "unzipping" the ladder down the middle, it can either reproduce itself (as part of cell division) or form another molecule called *RNA* (as part of cell function).

DNA ploidy. The number of *chromosomes* within the cell; a normal cell has twenty-three pairs. Measured by *flow cytometry*.

DNA synthesis (S phase). The process by which the *DNA* molecule reproduces itself prior to cell division.

Doubling time. The time it takes a cell to go through a complete cell-division cycle. Since cancers are groups of endlessly dividing cells, they are also said to have doubling times.

Dukes system. A *staging system* for rectal cancer. It is named after the doctor who devised it.

Elective lymph node dissection (ELND). The removal of lymph nodes before they become enlarged. At this point, the nodes may or may not contain cancer.

Electrocautery. The use of an electric current to either cut tissue or to control bleeding.

Endocavitary radiation. See *intracavitary radiation*.

Endocervical canal. The opening through the cervix into the uterus.

Endothelial cell. A cell that lines a blood vessel.

Epidermis. The topmost layer of skin.

Epithelial cell. A cell that lines the body's surfaces inside and out. Those that produce mucous are called mucosal epithelial cells (*mucous epithelium*).

Estrogen. A female sex hormone that slows the growth of some prostate cancers.

Excisional biopsy. A *biopsy* in which the entire tumor or lesion is removed.

Extensive intraductal component (EIC). The presence of *intraductal carcinoma* throughout the breast. Patients with EIC are at a greater risk of developing local recurrence.

External sphincter. The muscle that surrounds the *anus*. It is under voluntary control.

External-beam radiation. Radiation from outside of the body.

Fibrocystic changes. Tender breast lumps. They are commonplace, and differ from breast cancer in that the latter usually forms a nontender lump.

Fibrosarcoma. A common *soft tissue sarcoma* arising from connective tissue.

FIGO system. A *staging system* devised by the International Federation of Gynecology and Obstetrics. There are FIGO systems for cancers of the cervix, vagina, and vulva.

Fistula. An abnormal opening or channel through which fluid can pass.

Flow cytometry. A test that measures the percentage of cells in a tissue sample that have the normal number of *chromosomes* (twenty-three pairs). It can also measure the number of cells that are in the *DNA synthesis* phase of cell division.

Fractionating. The division of *radiation therapy* over several days. This is done to reduce side effects.

Frozen section. *Biopsied* tissue that is frozen, cut, stained, and examined. It is used when curative surgery, if needed, is to immediately follow the biopsy.

Fulguration. The burning away of tissue.

Gene. A packet of *DNA* in a specific location on a *chromosome*. Genes contain the information that determines inherited traits, such as eye color and blood type.

Genome. All the information contained in a complete set (twenty-three pairs) of human *chromosomes*.

Gleason grade. A system for measuring *tumor grade* in prostate cancer. Grades range from 2 to 10.

Grading system. A system, generally low, intermediate, and high or 1, 2, and 3, that measures *tumor grade*, or how aggressive a tumor looks when examined under the microscope.

Gray (Gy). The current unit of radiation. It replaces the rad; 100 rads equal one gray.

High grade. A term used to describe a fast-growing cancer. Such a cancer is likely to spread.

Hormonal therapy. The administration of either sex hormones or proteins that regulate hormones in order to affect the growth of cancer cells.

Hormone receptor. The part of the cell membrane that recognizes a specific hormone; the receptor and the hormone fit together like a key in a lock. Cancer cells that contain such receptors (receptor positive) are more like normal cells, and therefore less aggressive. Cancer cells that don't contain such receptors (receptor negative) are less like normal cells, and therefore more aggressive.

Human papillomavirus (HPV). A virus that is associated with cervical, vaginal, and vulvar cancer.

Hyperthermia. The use of microwaves or other heat sources to heat, and thus destroy, cancer cells.

Hysterectomy. See *modified radical hysterectomy, radical hysterectomy,* and *total hysterectomy*.

Ileal conduit. A piece of small intestine that is attached to the ureters (the tubes leading away from the kidney) and to the abdominal wall, so that the patient urinates into a plastic bag outside of the body.

Imaging procedure. A procedure, such as an MRI, X-ray, or scan, that can detect abnormalities, such as cancer, within the body.

Immune surveillance theory. A theory, proposed by biologist Lewis Thomas, which states that the immune system is constantly on guard against cancer. Cancer cells form frequently and are usually disposed of before they can form tumors. The theory has been neither proved nor disproved.

In situ. A cancer that only involves the topmost layer of cells (*in situ* means "in place").

Incisional biopsy. A *biopsy* in which a wedge of tissue is cut out of the tumor.

Incomplete prostatectomy. An operation that removes part of the prostate gland. It is usually used to treat *benign prostatic hypertrophy*.

Perineal, retropubic, and *suprapubic prostatectomies,* along with *transurethral resection of the prostate,* are all incomplete prostatectomies.

Inflammatory breast cancer. An aggressive form of breast cancer, once fatal in most cases within a year. *Multidrug therapy* has been shown to improve survival rates.

Informed-consent laws. Laws that require physicians to offer breast-sparing treatment options to breast cancer patients.

Inhibitor of steroid hormone production. A class of *hormonal therapy* agents that block the production of various steroid-type hormones.

Interferon. A group of proteins produced by the immune system that slow the growth of tumor cells and regulate white blood cells. They are used in *biological therapy.*

Interleukin. A group of hormones that stimulate the immune system by causing *B* and *T cells* to multiply rapidly. They are used in *biological therapy.*

Internal sphincter. The muscle that lies within the rectal wall. It is under automatic (nonvoluntary) control.

Interstitial radiation. *Radiation therapy* delivered directly into the tumor through the use of radioactive seeds or needles.

Intracavitary radiation. *Radiation therapy* delivered into the female reproductive tract through the use of hollow applicators into which radioactive material is placed. When used in the rectum, it is called **endocavitary radiation.**

Intraductal carcinoma. Cancer that arises from the cells lining the ducts that carry milk within the breast.

Intraductal hyperplasia. Buildup of extra cells in the breast ducts, similar to callus formation. If these cells begin to look abnormal, the condition is called **atypical intraductal hyperplasia**. It may lead to the development of breast cancer.

In-transit metastases. *Metastases* that develop when *malignant melanoma* cells lodge within the skin between the primary tumor and the regional lymph nodes.

Intravenous pyelogram. An X-ray of the kidneys after a dye has been introduced through a vein to produce contrast.

Invasive cancer. Cancer that has penetrated beyond the topmost cell layer in an organ.

Ionizing radiation. The type of radiation used to treat cancer. It disrupts atoms by knocking electrons out of place, which disrupts chemical bonds, which in turn causes the cell to die.

Glossary

Jackson system. A *staging system* for penile cancer. It is named after the doctor who devised it.

Jewett-Strong-Marshall system. A *staging system* for bladder cancer. It is named after the doctors who devised it.

Killer T cell. A *lymphocyte* that attaches to a cancer cell and kills it with toxic chemicals after becoming sensitized to the cancer cell's *antigen*.

Lamina propria. The layer under a *mucous epithelium*, such as the *transitional epithelium* in the bladder. Cancers are considered invasive after they penetrate the lamina propria.

Laparoscopic surgery. Surgery performed by the introduction of tubes into the abdomen, through which the surgeon can manipulate cutters while watching the operation on a monitor.

Laser surgery. Surgery performed with a laser beam, which boils the water inside of cells and causes them to explode.

Leukemia. Cancer that arises from the white blood cells when it occurs among cells that are circulating in the blood stream.

Levator ani muscles. A sling of voluntary muscles from which the rectum is suspended.

Liposarcoma. A common *soft tissue sarcoma* that arises from fat tissue.

Lobular carcinoma. Cancer that arises from the milk-producing lobules within the breast.

Local excision. The removal of a tumor, usually with a narrow *margin* of healthy tissue around it.

Local recurrence. Cancer that reappears at the site of a removed tumor.

Local treatment. Treatment that eliminates cancer cells in a specific part of the body.

Loop electrosurgical excision procedure (LEEP). A form of *electrocautery* that uses a wire loop instead of a metal tip.

Low anterior resection (LAR). The removal of an intestinal segment that contains a rectal cancer in which the remaining colon is attached to the remaining rectum, often with surgical staples.

Low grade. A term used to describe a slow-growing cancer. Such a cancer is less likely to spread.

Lumpectomy. The removal of a breast tumor with a narrow *margin* of healthy tissue around it.

Luteinizing hormone. A hormone sent from the *pituitary gland* to the gonads. In men, it increases *testosterone* production. In women, it causes the ovaries to release eggs.

Luteinizing hormone-releasing hormone (LHRH). A hormone sent by the hypothalamus, a part of the brain, to the *pituitary gland*, directing it to send *luteinizing hormone* to the testicles or ovaries.

Lymphangiogram. An X-ray of the lymph vessels after a dye is introduced to produce contrast.

Lymphatic vessel. A vessel that carries lymph, the clear fluid that bathes all the body's cells, to the lymph nodes and on to the blood stream.

Lymphocyte. A type of white blood cell that participates in the immune response against cancer.

Lymphokine. A chemical produced by a *lymphocyte* that stimulates and regulates the functioning of other cells.

Lymphoma. Cancer that arises from the white blood cells in organs that contain many of these cells, such as the spleen or the lymph nodes.

Macrophages. White blood cells that ingest and process foreign matter, including cancer cells. They pass the processed *antigens* they encounter to *lymphocytes*.

Major histocompatibility complex (MHC). The set of genes that controls white blood cell type. There are only four red blood cell types, but many, many white blood cell types.

Malignant melanoma. A life-threatening skin cancer that arises from melanocytes, the cells that produce pigment. Most skin cancers are not malignant melanomas, and are not life-threatening.

Mammogram. An X-ray of the breast. It uses less radiation than other X-rays.

Margin (surgical margin). The border of healthy tissue (usually, at least 2 cm if possible) that is removed along with a tumor.

Mastectomy. See *modified radical mastectomy, partial mastectomy, quadrentectomy,* and *radical mastectomy.*

Melanocyte. A cell that produces melanin, which determines skin color. *Malignant melanoma* usually arises from this cell.

Metastasis. The spread of cancer through the blood stream. The distant colonies of cancer cells thus formed are called **metastases**.

Microinvasive carcinoma. An early stage of cancer of the vulva or cervix. It is defined by various specialists from 1 mm of invasion to 5 mm.

Glossary

Microwave thermal therapy. A form of *hyperthermia* that uses heat generated by microwaves to treat prostate cancer.

Mitosis. The process of cell division in which each daughter cell has a complete set of chromosomes.

Modified radical hysterectomy. The removal of the uterus, the cervix, and the upper third of the vagina. Some of the supporting ligaments normally removed in a standard *radical hysterectomy* are left. This reduces bladder dysfunction.

Modified radical mastectomy. The removal of the breast and the lymph nodes under the arm. The pectoral muscle under the breast, normally removed in a standard *radical mastectomy*, is left. This eliminates the "washboard" effect that results from the skin lying directly on top of the ribs.

Modified radical vulvectomy. The removal of only the side of the vulva affected by the cancer, along with the lymph nodes on that side. Instead of being removed in one large piece, as in a *radical vulvectomy*, the vulva and the nodes are removed with separate, smaller incisions. This reduces postoperative complications.

Mohs micrographic surgery. A technique used for cancers on the body's surface, especially skin cancer. The surgeon removes the lesion and cuts fragments from it. These are checked by a pathologist for tumor cells. The surgeon continues to remove tissue, fragment by fragment, until the *margins* are free of tumor cells.

Monoclonal antibody. An *antibody* that recognizes a specific tumor *antigen*. These antibodies can be linked to drugs or radioactive chemicals that can then be delivered directly to the tumor. This experimental technology is used in *biological therapy* and to make tumors show up on scans.

Mucous epithelium. An internal body surface composed of cells that secrete mucus, such as that which coats the inside of the mouth.

Multicentricity. The observation that sometimes if a tumor is present, there are small areas throughout the organ (such as the breast) that resemble early cancer. However, it has been found that these changes do not always lead to the development of cancer.

Multidisciplinary treatment. The idea that the surgeon, radiation therapist, and *oncologist* should work together as a team to plan an integrated course of treatment, as opposed to having the patient go to each separately.

Multidrug therapy. *Chemotherapy* in which a number of drugs are given at once.

Multivariate analysis. A statistical method that considers the effect of many factors on an outcome such as survival, and weighs the importance of each factor.

Muscularis. The muscular layer of the bowel.

National Surgical Adjuvant Breast Project (NSABP). A research effort organized in 1957 to study various aspects of breast cancer treatment. The trials performed by this group disproved many of the standard medical beliefs regarding breast cancer.

Natural killer (NK) cell. A large *lymphocyte* that contains chemicals toxic to tumor cells. The killing ability of these cells is called NK cytotoxicity.

Needle biopsy. A *biopsy* in which a needle is used to remove a tissue sample for study by a pathologist.

Needle localization. The use of X-rays to place needles into a suspicious lesion in the breast.

Negative. The state of lymph nodes or *margins* when they do not contain cancer.

Neoadjuvant therapy. *Radiation therapy* or *chemotherapy* administered before surgery.

Nucleus. The "headquarters" of the cell, where the *chromosomes* are and from which all cell activities, including cell division, are directed. The cell is divided into two parts, the nucleus and the *cytoplasm*.

Oncogene. A *gene* that has been transformed into a cancer-causing gene. This can occur because of genetic abnormalities, toxins, or viruses.

Oncologist. A doctor who specializes in the treatment and study of cancer.

Orchiectomy. The removal of the testicles.

Paclitaxel. A *chemotherapy* drug that interferes with cell division and other cell functions.

Palliative surgery. Surgery performed to relieve symptoms in cases of incurable cancer.

Papanicolaou (Pap) smear. A sample of cells taken from the cervix during a standard gynecological examination to check for premalignant or malignant changes. It is named for the doctor who devised it.

Papillary dermis. The layer of skin beneath the *epidermis*. It contains small, nipple-like formations of connective tissue or collagen.

Papilloma. An outgrowth of tissue into a body cavity, such as the bladder. Papillomas can be either benign or malignant.

Parametrium. The tissue surrounding the uterus and cervix.

Glossary

Partial cystectomy. The removal of a bladder tumor along with a *margin* of healthy tissue.

Partial mastectomy. The removal of a breast tumor plus a 2-cm *margin* of healthy tissue.

Pathological staging. The observations on how far a cancer has spread after a pathologist has examined the regional lymph nodes and other tissue.

Penectomy. The removal of the penis.

Perfusion, isolated regional. A form of *hyperthermia* used to treat *malignant melanoma*, in which an extremity is placed on a heart-lung machine while being perfused with heated blood containing a high dosage of chemotheraputic drugs.

Perineal prostatectomy. The removal of a portion of the prostate gland through an incision between the scrotum and the anus. It is an *incomplete prostatectomy*.

Perineum. The area between the anus and either the scrotum in men or the vulva in women.

Permanent section. *Biopsied* tissue that is placed in paraffin, cut into thin slices, stained, and examined. It is then kept on file.

Photodynamic therapy. An experimental treatment that uses laser light shining on chemically altered cells to create toxins within the cells.

Pituitary gland. A gland at the base of the brain that regulates the production of hormones.

Polyp. A growth arising from a mucous membrane.

Positive. The state of lymph nodes or *margins* when they contain cancer.

Practice parameters. A range of therapies that are considered by the medical establishment to be acceptable in the treatment of a specific disease.

Primary tumor. The tumor that forms when cancer first arises. It can spread to lymph nodes in the immediate area and *metastasize* to distant organs.

Progestin. A class of *hormonal therapy* agents that are used to treat breast and prostate cancer.

Prolapse. A condition that occurs when the vagina or the uterus falls out of position.

Prospective study. See *randomized prospective trial*.

Prostatectomy. See *incomplete prostatectomy* and *radical prostatectomy*.

Prostate-specific antigen (PSA). A substance produced by all prostate cells, both normal and malignant. Malignant cells leak about ten times more PSA into the blood stream than normal ones.

Protease. An enzyme that can disrupt proteins, including the *basement membrane* of a particular type of tissue.

Pull-through procedure. A procedure in which, after the tumor is removed, the colon is pulled down through the rectum and the mucosal lining of the rectum is stripped away so that the colon and rectum will stick together.

Quadrentectomy. The removal of a full quarter of the breast surrounding a tumor.

Radiation therapy. The use of radiation to treat cancer.

Radical cystectomy. The removal of the bladder, the surrounding tissue, the pelvic lymph nodes, and parts of the interior reproductive organs.

Radical hysterectomy. The removal of the uterus (including the cervix and upper third of the vagina), the *parametrial* tissues and ligaments, and the pelvic lymph nodes.

Radical mastectomy. The removal of the breast, the underlying chest muscles, and the lymph nodes in the armpit.

Radical pelvic exenteration. The removal of most of the important pelvic structures, including the uterus, cervix, vagina, bladder, and rectum.

Radical prostatectomy. The removal of the prostate gland, the *seminal vesicles*, and the pelvic lymph nodes.

Radical vulvectomy. The removal of the vulva along with the lymph nodes in both groin areas, all in one piece.

Randomized prospective trial. A study in which patients (with their consent) are assigned randomly to one form of treatment or another. These studies follow strict rules and can take years to complete.

Reconstructive surgery. Surgery performed to reconstruct a part of the body (such as the breast) after removal of a tumor.

Releasing factor antagonist. A class of *hormonal therapy* agents that prevent the *pituitary gland* from stimulating the gonads into producing sex hormones by sending a false signal to the pituitary.

Resection. Surgical removal or excision of tissue.

Response rate. The response of a tumor to *chemotherapy*. A complete response (remission) refers to a cancer that has disappeared according to the most precise imaging technique available (and even the most

Glossary

precise cannot detect individual cancer cells). A partial response refers to a cancer that has shrunk to less than half its original size.

Reticular dermis. The layer of skin beneath the *papillary dermis*. It contains hair follicles.

Retroperitoneum. The area beneath and behind the abdominal cavity.

Retropubic prostatectomy. The removal of a portion of the prostate gland through a low abdominal incision. The surgeon goes behind the pubic bone in front of the bladder. It is an *incomplete prostatectomy*.

Retrospective study. A study that looks at the experience of a particular doctor or a particular hospital by examining patient charts.

Ribosome. A structure in the *cytoplasm* that creates proteins, based on instructions from the *RNA*.

RNA (ribonucleic acid). A substance that is very similar to *DNA*, being composed of a different sugar and containing one *base* that is different from those in DNA. DNA forms RNA, which in turn directs protein formation.

S phase. See *DNA synthesis*.

Salvage. The removal of an organ (such as the breast) when a tumor reappears (*local recurrence*) after conservative surgery.

Sarcoma. Cancer that arises from a body tissue, such as muscle or fat, as opposed to that which arises from specific organs. Hard tissue sarcomas arise from bone and cartilage, soft tissue sarcomas from other tissues.

Screening. The testing of apparently healthy individuals for a disease. Screening has been proven useful in detecting some kinds of cancer, but controversial in detecting others.

Self breast examination. An examination of the breasts conducted by the woman herself, preferably on a monthly basis.

Seminal vesicles. Structures near the prostate gland that secrete and store a component of semen.

Serosa. The outer covering of the bowel.

Sigmoid colon. The last 18 inches of the colon. It is so called because it is shaped like an S (*sigma* in Greek).

Sigmoidscope. A scope that allows the doctor to view the *sigmoid colon* and rectum.

Sign. An abnormality found by a doctor.

Skinny needle biopsy. A *biopsy* in which a very thin needle is passed through the tumor several times. Only individual cells (as opposed to tissue structures) can be examined.

Soft tissue sarcoma. A *sarcoma* of the soft tissues.

Squamous cell. A type of body lining cell that is flat and scaly.

Staging procedure. Surgery in which tissue is removed to see how far cancer has spread, for example, removal of lymph nodes that are not swollen to see if they contain microscopic cancer.

Staging system. A system used to determine the stage, or extent, of a cancer. Cancers in different parts of the body have their own staging systems.

Stereotaxic breast biopsy. A *biopsy* that precisely locates a suspicious area within the breast. It requires special equipment.

Subcutaneous tissue. The tissue underneath the skin. It is made up mostly of fat.

Suprapubic prostatectomy. The removal of a portion of the prostate gland through a low abdominal incision. The surgeon approaches the prostate from above the bladder. It is an *incomplete prostatectomy*.

Surgical margin See *margin*.

Symptom. An abnormality found by a patient.

Systemic treatment. Treatment that kills cancer cells throughout the body.

T cell. See *killer T cell* and *T helper cell*.

T helper cell. A *lymphocyte* that can guide the immune response towards either *cell-mediated immunity* (a T$_H$1 cell) or *antibody* production (a T$_H$2 cell).

Tandem and ovoids. Containers of radioactive material placed in the upper vagina and uterus to deliver *radiation therapy* directly to a cervical tumor.

Telomerase. An enzyme produced by most cancer cells that stops the loss of *telomeres* during cell division. This prevents cell death, and thus allows the cancer cell to keep dividing.

Telomere. A chain of *DNA* that is attached to the end of the *chromosomal* DNA. Each time a cell divides, telomeres are lost. Loss of all telomeres leads to cell death.

Testosterone. A male sex hormone that can stimulate the growth of some prostate cancers.

Theraputic lymph node dissection. The removal of enlarged lymph nodes that contain cancer.

TNM system. A general *staging system* based on tumor size (T), lymph

Glossary

node involvement (N), and presence of distant metastases (M). It has been adapted to cancers of various organs, but its complexity makes it more useful for research than for clinical practice.

Total hysterectomy. The removal of the uterus and cervix.

Trachelectomy. The removal of the cervix.

Traditional system. A *staging system* for breast cancer.

Transcription. The process by which *DNA* uses the genetic code to create *RNA*, which in turn *translates* this information into protein formation.

Transition zone. The area within the *endocervical canal* where the tissue that lines the cervix meets the tissue that lines the uterus.

Transitional epithelium. The cells that line the inside of the bladder.

Translation. The process by which *RNA*, having received instructions from *DNA* in the cell *nucleus*, orders the production of proteins in the *cytoplasm* by the *ribosomes*.

Transrectal ultrasound (TRUS). *Ultrasound* of the prostate or other tissues surrounding the rectum, taken through the rectum.

Transurethral resection (TUR). The removal of bladder tumors through a *cystoscope*.

Transurethral resection of the prostate (TURP). The removal of small pieces of prostate tissue through a scope placed in the urethra. It is an *incomplete prostatectomy*.

Trigone. The area at the bottom of the bladder through which the *ureters* and *urethra* pass.

Tumor angiogenesis factor. A hormone produced by normal growing tissue and some cancer cells that stimulates the growth of small blood vessels into the tissue or tumor.

Tumor grade. The term used to describe how a tumor cell looks under the microscope and how rapidly it is dividing. See *high grade* and *low grade*.

Tumor necrosis factor. A protein produced by some white blood cells that can kill some tumor cells. It is used in *biological therapy*.

Tumor-associated antigens. *Antigens* on cancer cells that identify them as malignant.

Tumor-patient conflict. The battle that goes on between the cancer and the patient's immune system. I believe the body can fight against the spread of cancer even after a tumor develops—it has not been "defeated" just because a tumor has established itself locally.

Tumor-suppressor gene. A gene that hinders tumor formation by slowing down *DNA* duplication.

Type I recurrence. A form of *local recurrence* that only happens after conservative surgery. It is the regrowth of cancer from malignant cells left behind after the operation.

Type II recurrence. A form of *local recurrence* that can happen after either conservative surgery or radical surgery. It is the regrowth of cancer from malignant cells that travel back to the surgical site from a distant *metastasis*.

Ultrasound. The use of high-frequency sound waves to create a picture of internal organs.

Undifferentiated (high grade). A cancer that is fast-growing. The cells are not distinctive, that is, they do not resemble the cells from which they arose. Such tumors are likely to spread.

Ureters. The tubes that carry urine from the kidneys to the bladder.

Urethra. The tube that carries urine from the bladder to outside the body.

Urine cytology. The examination of cells found in the urine, using a microscope.

Vaginal intraepithelial neoplasia (VAIN). Noninvasive cancer of the vagina.

Vaginectomy. The removal of the vagina.

Vascularization. The formation of blood vessels.

Vulvar intraepithelial neoplasia (VIN). Noninvasive cancer of the vulva.

Vulvectomy. See *modified radical vulvectomy* and *radical vulvectomy*.

Watchful waiting. An approach towards the management of prostate cancer, primarily in older patients, in which the cancer is carefully monitored. This spares the patient the side effects of aggressive treatment at a time of life when the prostate cancer is not likely to cause his death. But the cancer may be treated if it grows rapidly.

Wide excision. The removal of the tumor with a *margin* of healthy tissue around it, usually 2 cm or more.

Index

Abdominoperineal resection (APR), 193
Ablation, 195
Adair, Frank, 21
Adenine, 43, 44, 45
Adenocarcinoma, 84, 140, 169, 188, 219
Adhesion molecules, 56
Adjuvant therapy
   chemotherapy, 100–101
   radiation therapy, 97
Adriamycin, 98, 119, 207
Aflatoxin, 45
Age, mammograms and, 126–127
AJCC staging system
   for malignant melanoma, 155, 156
   for soft tissue sarcoma, 205, 206
Alkaloids, 98
Alkylating agents, 99
AMA. See American Medical Association.
American Cancer Society, 18
American Joint Committee on Cancer (AJCC), 88, 205
American Medical Association (AMA), xvi
American Society for the Control of Cancer, 18
Amino acid, 45
Aminoglutethimide, 107
Anal canal, 188
Anal verge, 188
Androgens, 105, 179
Anesthesia
   complications with, 94
   surgery and, 14

Aneuploid cells, 49, 170
Angiosarcoma, 203
Aniline dyes, bladder cancer and, 112
Antiandrogen, 107, 180
Antibiotics, 98
Antibodies, 63
Antiestrogen, 107
Antigens, 60
Antimetabolites, 99
Anus, 188
Apoplexy, 18
Apoptosis, 64
APR. See Abdominoperineal resection.
Areola, 124
AUA staging system, 173–174
Auchincloss, Hugh, 25
Autocrines, 51
Axillary dissection, 131
Axillary lymph nodes, xiv

B cells, 63–64
Bacillus Calmette-Guerin (BCG), 109, 119
Baclesse, F., 24
Barium enema, 190, 213
Basement membrane, 52, 53
BCG. See Bacillus Calmette-Guerin.
Benign prostatic hypertrophy (BPH), 173, 176
Biological response modifiers (BRMs), 66, 107–108
Biological therapy, 107–108
   for bladder cancer, 119
   for malignant melanoma, 156–157
   types of, 108–109

355

Biopsy
　for breast cancer, 127-128
　for cervical cancer, 141
　diagnosis and, 86-87
　for malignant melanoma, 155
　for penile cancer, 162
　for prostate cancer, 171, 172, 173
　for rectal cancer, 190
　for soft tissue sarcoma, 204-205
　types of, 90-91
　for vaginal cancer, 213
　for vulvar cancer, 220
Bladder, physiology of, 113
Bladder cancer
　analysis of, 119-121
　biological therapy for, 119
　causes of, 112
　chemotherapy for, 119
　diagnosis of, 114-115
　follow-up for, 122
　grades of, 113-114
　incidence of, 112
　radiation therapy for, 118-119
　recurrence of, 112, 117, 120
　screening for, 114
　signs and symptoms of, 114
　spread of, 114
　stages of, 115, 116, 117
　surgery for, 115-118
　treatment according to stage, 121-122
　treatments for, 115-119
　types of, 113
Bladder dysfunction
　hysterectomy and, 144
　radical prostatectomy and, 176
Bladder infections, chronic, bladder cancer and, 112
Bleeding, surgery and, 94
Bleomycin, 98, 146
Blood, in stool, test for, 189
Blood clots, surgery and, 94-95
Blood tests, 85-86
Bonadonna, Gianni, 101
Bone marrow transplantation, 99
Bowel. *See* Rectum.
BPH. *See* Benign prostatic hypertrophy.

Brachytherapy, 96
Breast, physiology of, 123-124
Breast cancer
　analysis of, 133-135
　causes of, 45-46, 47
　chemotherapy for, 131-133
　diagnosis of, 127-128
　follow-up for, 138
　grades of, 124-125
　hormonal therapy for, 132, 133
　incidence of, 123
　mammograms for, 126-127
　radiation therapy for, 131
　recurrence rates of, 134-135
　risk factors for, 126
　screening for, 125-126
　signs and symptoms of, 127
　spread of, 38, 85, 125
　special considerations for treatment, 137-138
　stages of, 128, 129, 130
　surgery for, 129-131
　treatment according to stage, 135-138
　treatments for, 129-133
　types of, 124
Breast-removing surgery, 129-130
Breast-sparing surgery, xiii, 24-27, 30-31, 130-131
　radiation with, 133-134
Breathing difficulties, surgery and, 94
Brennan, Murray, 32
Breslow, Alexander, 153
Breslow's grading system (Breslow's thickness), 153, 154
British Medical Journal, 26
BRMs. *See* Biological response modifiers.

Caffeine, bladder cancer and, 112
Cancer
　body's reaction to, 58-61
　causes of, 45-48
　chemotherapy for, 98-105
　chromosome number and, 49
　definition of, 2
　diagnosis of, 86-87

Index

grades of, 48-49, 84-85
growth of, 48-52
hormonal therapy for, 105-107
hormone production and, 51-52
hormone receptors and, 49-51
radiation therapy for, 95-98
recurrence and, 73-75
screening for, 85-86
signs of, 86
spread of, 35-38, 52-56, 85
stages of, 87-89
surgery for, 89-95
symptoms of, 86
TNM staging and, 88
treatment of, 89-110
types of, 83-84
See also Bladder cancer; Breast cancer; Cervical cancer; Malignant melanoma; Penile cancer; Prostate cancer; Rectal cancer; Soft tissue sarcoma; Vaginal cancer; Vulvar cancer.

Cancer and Common Sense (Crile), xvi, 22
Carcinoembryonic antigen (CEA), 60, 190, 200-201
Carcinoid, 188
Carcinomas, epithelial cells and, 52, 84
CEA. *See* Carcinoembryonic antigen.
Cell
  division, mistakes in, 46-47
  function, 43-45
  production, 42-43
  sampling, 85
Cell-mediated immunity, 64
Centrifugal spread, 15
Cervical cancer
  analysis of, 147-148
  bladder cancer and, 112
  causes of, 139
  chemotherapy for, 146-147
  diagnosis of, 141
  follow-up for, 150
  grades of, 140
  incidence of, 139
  pregnancy and, 149-150

radiation therapy for, 146
recurrence of, 147
screening for, 141
signs and symptoms of, 141
spread of, 140-141
stages of, 141-142, 143
surgery for, 142-146
treatment according to stage, 148-150
treatments for, 142-147
types of, 140
Cervical intraepithelial neoplasia (CIN), 140
Cervix, physiology of, 139-140
Chemotherapy, 24, 98
  adjuvant, 100-101
  for bladder cancer, 119
  bone marrow transplantation, 99
  for breast cancer, 131-133
  cancer death rates and, 102
  for cervical cancer, 146-147
  for malignant melanoma, 156
  for penile cancer, 164
  for prostate cancer, 179
  for rectal cancer, 196, 200
  resistance to, 99-100
  side effects of, 102, 105
  for soft tissue sarcoma, 207
  types of, 9899
Chest X-ray
  soft tissue sarcoma and, 204
  vaginal cancer and, 213
Chromosome number, cancer growth and. *See* DNA ploidy.
Chromosomes, 42-43
Cigarette smoking, bladder cancer and, 112
CIN. *See* Cervical intraepithelial neoplasia.
Cisplatin, 99, 119, 146
Clark's grading system (Clark's levels), 153, 154
Cleveland Clinic, 2
Cobalt-60, 95
Coley, William, 58-59
Coley's toxin, 59, 109
Colon, physiology of, 187
Colon cancer. *See* Rectal cancer.

Coloanal anastomosis, 194
Colony-stimulating factors (CSF), 66, 109
Colostomy, 193, 194
Colposcopic examination, 141
Commando operation, 18
Cone biopsy, 141
Conization, 142, 147
Connective tissue, 52, 53
Conservative surgery, 1, 3, 72-73.
    Also see Breast-sparing surgery.
Cope, Oliver, 25
Cortisone, function of, 105-106
Crawford, E. D., 121
Crile, George Jr., xiii-xiv, xvi-xvii, 22, 25, 29, 33, 74
Crile, George Sr., 18
Cryosurgery, 91-92
    for cervical cancer, 145
    for prostate cancer, 181
    for rectal cancer, 195
CSF. *See* Colony-stimulating factors.
Curie, Marie, 20, 95
Curie, Pierre, 20, 95
Cushing, Harvey, 17
Cyclophosphamide, 99
Cystectomy, 115-118
Cytokines, 66
Cytoplasm, 42
Cytoscopic examination, 114, 213
Cytosine, 43, 44, 45
Cytotoxic cells, 64

Dargent, D., 149
Death rates, cancer
    female, 103
    male, 104
Debulking surgery, 93
Deoxyribonucleic acid (DNA), 42-43
    cell division and, 44
    protein formation and, 44-45
    structure of, 43-44
    synthesis, 44
Dermis, 152
DES. *See* Diethylstilbestrol.
DiLuzio, Nicholas, xi

Diarrhea
    chemotherapy and, 105
    radiation therapy and, 97, 118
Diethylstilbestrol (DES), 106
    for prostate cancer, 179
    vaginal cancer and, 211
Differentiation of cells, 44
Digital rectal examination (DRE), 171, 189
Diploid cells, 49, 170
Disease-free survival, 100-101
Distant metastases, 77-79
    local recurrence and, 73-74
DNA. *See* Deoxyribonucleic acid.
DNA ploidy
    breast cancer and, 125
    cancer growth and, 49
    penile cancer and, 162
    prostate cancer and, 170
Doctors: The Biography of Medicine (Nuland), 17
Double helix, 43
Doubling time, 44
Doxorubicin, 98
DRE. *See* Digital rectal examination.
DTIC, for malignant melanoma, 156
Dukes, C. E., 190
Dukes staging system, 190, 191

Efudex, 164
EIC. *See* Extensive intraductal component.
Elective lymph node dissection (ELND), 158-159, 163, 165
Electrocautery, 91
ELND. *See* Elective lymph node dissection.
Endocavitary radiation, 97, 195
Endocervical canal, 140
Endothelial cells, 52, 53
Enucleation, 183
Epidermis, 152
Epithelial cells, 52, 53, 84, 188, 211
Estramustine, 107, 179
Estrogen, 106
    breast cancer and, 105, 125
    for prostate cancer, 105, 179

Index

Estrogen-receptor positive cells, breast cancer and, 125
Etoposide, 98
Ewing, James, 19, 59
Excisional biopsy, 90, 205
Experimental local treatment, prostate cancer and, 180
Extensive intraductal component (EIC), 137
External sphincter, 188
External-beam radiation, 96
    for bladder cancer, 118
    for cervical cancer, 146
    for penile cancer, 163–164
    for prostate cancer, 178
    for vaginal cancer, 215
    for vulvar cancer, 222

Fast-growing cancer, 49
Fatigue, radiation therapy and, 97
Fear, dealing with, 4–5
Fertility, cervical cancer and, 142–145, 147–148
Fibrocystic changes, 127
Fibrosarcoma, 203
Fibrous histiocytoma, malignant, 203
Fidler, Isaiah, 56
FIGO staging system
    for cervical cancer, 141, 143
    for vaginal cancer, 213, 214
    for vulvar cancer, 220, 221
Fisher, Bernard F., 28, 138
Fistulas, 144, 164, 215
Fitzwilliams, Duncan, 20
5-fluorouracil, 99, 146, 196, 215
Flow cytometry, 49
Flutamide, 107, 180
Fractionating, 96
Frozen section, 87, 193
Fulguration
    for bladder cancer, 118
    for penile cancer, 164
    for rectal cancer, 195
Fulton, Amy, 65

Gates of Memory, The (Keynes), 20
Genes, 43

Genetic testing, 85–86
Genome, human, 43
Gleason scoring system, 170
Glutamine, radiation therapy and, 146
Goserelin acetate, 180
Grading
    of bladder cancer, 113–114
    of breast cancer, 124–125
    of cervical cancer, 140
    of malignant melanoma, 152–153
    of penile cancer, 162
    of prostate cancer, 170
    of rectal cancer, 188
    of soft tissue sarcoma, 203–204
    of tumors, 48–49, 84–85
    of vaginal cancer, 212
    of vulvar cancer, 219
Grant, Ulysses S., 16
Gray, as a unit of measure, 96
Growth factors, 51
Guanine, 43, 44, 45

Haagensen, Cushman, 19
Hair loss
    chemotherapy and, 105
    radiation therapy and, 97
Halsted, William S., 14–17, 18, 20, 26, 28, 129
Halsted radical mastectomy. *See* Radical mastectomy.
Handley, Sampson, 18
Harvey, Samuel, 17
Hellman, Samuel, 26
Hematoporphyrin, 118
Hemicorpectomy, 18
Henderson, Lawrence, 18
High grade cancer, 49
Hodgkin's disease, 84
Hormonal therapy, 105
    for breast cancer, 132, 133
    for prostate cancer, 179–180
    types of, 106–107
Hormone production, 105–106
    cancer growth and, 51–52
Hormone receptors, cancer growth and, 49–51
Horrobin, David, 231

Hospice movement, 228-229
Hot flashes, progestins and, 107
HPV. *See* Human papillomavirus.
Hull, F. M., 228
Human papillomavirus (HPV), 139, 140, 211, 218
  antigens and, 61
Hydroxyurea, 147
Hyperthermia treatment, 109-110
Hypothalamus, function of, 105
Hysterectomy, 143-144

Ileal conduit, 116
Imaging procedures, 85-86
Immune system
  cancer and, 61-67, 69-70, 75-77
  MHC cells and, 67-69
Impotence
  progestins and, 107
  radical cystectomy and, 116
  radical prostatectomy and, 176
In situ cancer
  of bladder, 113
  of breast, 124, 138
In-transit metastases, 153
Incisional biopsy, 90, 205
Incomplete prostatectomy, 176-177
Infections, surgery and, 95
Inflammatory breast cancer, 133
Inhibitor of steroid hormone production, 107
Interferon, 66, 108, 119
Interleukin, 66, 108
Internal sphincter, 188
International Union Against Cancer, 88
Interstitial radiation, 96
  cervical cancer and, 146
  penile cancer and, 164
  prostate cancer and, 178
  rectal cancer and, 195
  vaginal cancer and, 214-215
Intra-abdominal abscesses, 95
Intracavitary radiation, 96-97
  for cervical cancer, 146
  for vaginal cancer, 214
Intraductal carcinoma, 124
Intraduct hyperplasia, 124

Intravenous pyelogram, 213
Ionizing radiation, 95-96
Iridium-192 implants, 119
Isolated regional perfusion, 109-110, 157

Jackson, S. M., 163
Jackson staging system, 163, 164
Jernigan, Dan, xvi
Jewett-Strong-Marshall staging system, 115, 117

Karkinoma, 15
Kassirer, Jerome, 232
Ketoconazole, 107
Keynes, Geoffrey, 20, 21, 22
Keynes, John Maynard, 20
Killer T cells, 64, 68
Kuhn, Thomas S., xvi, 235

Labia majora, 218
Labia minora, 218
LAK cells, 108
Lamina propria, 113
Lancet, 131-132
Laparoscope, 118, 145
Laparoscopic surgery, 92, 118, 145, 178, 214, 222
LAR. *See* Low anterior resection.
Large recurrence, 75
Laser surgery, 92
  for prostate cancer, 180
Laser therapy, for bladder cancer, 118
Latent cancer, prostate, 169-170
LEEP. *See* Loop electrosurgical excision procedure.
Leiomyosarcoma, 203
Leucovorin, 99, 196
Leukemia, 84
  radiation therapy and, 240
Leuprolide, 107, 180
Leupron, 180
Leutenizing hormone, 106
Leutenizing hormone-releasing hormone (LHRH), 106
Levamisole, 196
Levator ani muscles, 188

Index

LHRH. *See* Leutenizing hormone-releasing hormone.
Limb-sparing surgery, 206, 207
Lindskog, Gustaf, 17
Liotta, Lance, 36
Liposarcoma, 203
Lister, Joseph, 14
Lobular carcinoma, 124
Lobules, breast, 123
Local excision, 20–21
   for malignant melanoma, 155–156
   for rectal cancer, 194
   for vulvar cancer, 222
Local recurrence. *See* Recurrence.
Loop electrosurgical excision procedure (LEEP), 144–145
Low anterior resection (LAR), 193–194
Low grade cancer, 48
Lumpectomy, 8, 30, 130
Lymph node sampling, 177–178
Lymph nodes, spread of cancer and, 85
Lymphangiogram, 213
Lymphangiosarcoma, 203
Lymphatic vessels, cancer spread and, 53
Lymphocytes, 63–65
Lymphokine-activated killer (LAK) cells, 108
Lymphokines, 64
Lymphoma, 84, 188

Macrophages, 63, 66, 108
McWhirter, Robert, 21
Major histocompatibility complex (MHC), 67–69
Malignant melanoma
   analysis of, 157–159
   biological therapy for, 156–157
   causes of, 151
   chemotherapy for, 156
   diagnosis of, 155
   follow-up for, 160
   grades of, 152–153, 154
   hyperthermia for, 109, 157
   incidence of, 151
   penile cancer and, 161–162
   rectal cancer and, 188
   recurrence of, 152, 157–159
   screening for, 153
   signs and symptoms of, 153
   spread of, 151–152, 153
   stages of, 155, 156
   surgery for, 155–156
   treatment according to stage, 159–160
   treatments for, 155–157
   types of, 152
   vulvar cancer and, 219
Mammograms, 85–86, 126–127
Margolese, Richard, 74
Mastectomy, 15–16, 22–24, 27, 129–131
   salvage, 25
Matas, Rudolf, 20
Measurement terms, 3–4
Medicine and Culture (Payer), 228
Megestrol, 106
Melanocytes, 152
Melanoma, malignant. *See* Malignant melanoma.
Metastases, development of, 54
Metastatic prostate cancer, diethylstilbestrol for, 106
Methotrexate, 99, 119
Methyl cholanthrene, antigens and, 61
Metric terms, 3–4
MHC. *See* Major histocompatibility complex.
Microwave thermal therapy, 110, 180–181
Miles, Ernest, 18
Mitomycin, 119, 146
Mitosis, 44
Modified radical hysterectomy, 144
Modified radical mastectomy, 129–130
Modified radical vulvectomy, 220–221
Mohs micrographic surgery, 92
   for penile cancer, 163
   for soft tissue sarcoma, 206
Monoclonal antibodies, 109

Montague, Eleanor, xiii
Mouth
 dryness, radiation therapy and, 97
 sores, chemotherapy and, 105
Mucosa, 188, 211, 218
Mucosal epithelial cells, 52
Mucous epithelium, 188
Muscularis, rectal cancer and, 189
Multicentricity, 30, 124
Multidrug therapy, 100, 133
Murley, Reginald, 21, 22
Mustakallio, Sakari, 20, 30
Myc gene, 45

NASA, 34
National Cancer Institute, 21, 36
National Surgical Adjuvant Breast Project (NSABP), xiii, 8, 9, 28-29, 38, 41
Natural killer (NK) cells, 64-65
Nausea
 chemotherapy and, 105
 radiation therapy and, 97
Needle biopsy, 90
 for breast cancer, 127
 for prostate cancer, 173
 for soft tissue sarcoma, 205
Needle localization, 127
Neurofibrosarcoma, 203
Nitrogen mustard, 98
Nixon, Richard, 34
NK cells. *See* Natural killer cells.
NSABP. *See* National Surgical Adjuvant Breast Project.
Nucleus, 42
Nuland, Sherwin, 17

Oncogene, 45
Oncologist, 49
Orchiectomy, 179
Ortaldo, John, 65
Ovoids, 146

Paclitaxel, 99
Paget, Stephen, 71, 77
Palliative surgery, 93

Pap smear, 85, 86, 139, 141, 212, 219
Papillary dermis, 152
Papilloma, 113
Papillon, Jean, 195
Paracrines, 51
Parametrium, cervical cancer and, 141
Partial cystectomy, 116-118
Partial mastectomy, 131
Pathologist, role of, in diagnosis, 86-87
Payer, Lynn, 228, 229
Penectomy, 163
Penile cancer
 analysis of, 164-165
 causes of, 161
 chemotherapy for, 164
 diagnosis of, 162
 follow-up for, 167
 grades of, 162
 incidence of, 161
 radiation therapy for, 163-164
 recurrence of, 165
 screening for, 162
 signs and symptoms of, 162
 spread of, 162
 stages of, 163, 164
 surgery for, 163
 treatment according to stage, 165-167
 treatments for, 163-164
 types of, 161
Penis, physiology of, 161
Perineal prostatectomy, 177
Perineum, 173, 218
Permanent section, 87
Peters, Vera, 20, 30
Phenacetin, bladder cancer and, 112
Photodynamic therapy, 118
Pituitary gland, function of, 105
Planck, Max, 235
Polyps, rectal cancer and, 189-190
Pregnancy, cervical cancer and, 149-150
Primary tumor, 83

Index

Progesterone, breast cancer and, 105, 125
Progestins, 106–107
Prostate cancer
   analysis of, 181–184
   chemotherapy for, 179
   cryosurgery for, 181
   diagnosis of, 173
   follow-up for, 186
   grades of, 170
   hormonal therapy for, 179–180
   incidence of, 168
   laser surgery for, 180
   microwave thermal therapy for, 110, 180–181
   radiation therapy for, 178
   screening for, 171–173
   signs and symptoms of, 173
   spread of, 170–171
   stages of, 173, 174, 175
   surgery for, 175–178
   treatment according to stage, 184–186
   treatments for, 174–181
   types of, 169–170
   watchful waiting for, 181, 182–184
Prostate gland, physiology of, 169
Prostate-specific antigen (PSA), 61, 86, 93, 168, 171–172, 182–184
Prostatectomy, 176–177
Proteases, 53
PSA. See Prostate-specific antigen.
Pull-through procedure, 194

Quadrantectomy, 27, 131

Rad, 96
Radiation therapy, 95–96
   bladder cancer and, 112
   for bladder cancer, 118–119
   for breast cancer, 131
   for cervical cancer, 146
   introduction of, 20
   for penile cancer, 163–164
   for prostate cancer, 178
   for rectal cancer, 195–196
   side effects of, 97–98
   for soft tissue sarcoma, 207
   types of, 96–97
   for vaginal cancer, 214–215
   for vulvar cancer, 222
Radical cystectomy, 115–116
Radical hysterectomy, 143–144
Radical mastectomy, 15–16, 22–24, 129
Radical pelvic exenteration, 144
Radical prostatectomy, 176
Radical surgery, xii
   development of, 18–19, 22–24
   theory behind, 15–16
Radical vaginectomy, 213
Radical vulvectomy, 220–222
Ras gene, 53
Receptors, cell, 45
Reconstructive surgery, 94
Rectal cancer
   analysis of, 196–197
   causes of, 187
   chemotherapy for, 196, 200
   diagnosis of, 190
   incidence of, 187
   malignant melanoma and, 188
   radiation therapy for, 195–196, 200
   recurrence rates of, 197
   screening for, 189–190
   signs and symptoms of, 190
   spread of, 189
   stages of, 190, 191, 192
   surgery for, 193–195
   treatment according to stage, 197–200
   treatments for, 193–196
   types of, 188
Rectum, physiology of, 187–188, 192
Recurrence, 73–75
   bladder cancer and, 112, 117, 120
   breast cancer and, 134–135
   cervical cancer and, 147
   danger from, 73–75
   local, nature of, 5–6, 7–8, 19, 29, 30–31, 32, 73–75
   malignant melanoma and, 157–158
   penile cancer and, 165

rectal cancer and, 197
  soft tissue sarcoma and, 208, 209-210
  types of, 74-75
  vaginal cancer and, 215
  vulvar cancer and, 223
Releasing factor antagonist, 107, 180
Removal of metastases, 93-94
Resection for cure, 91-92
Response rates, 101
Reticular dermis, 152
Retroperitoneum, liposarcoma and, 203
Retropubic prostatectomy, 176
Retrospective studies, 40-41
Rhabdomyosarcoma, 203
Ribonucleic acid (RNA)
  formation of, 44
  translation of, 44-45
RNA. *See* Ribonucleic acid.

Salvage mastectomy, 25
Sarcoma. *See* Soft tissue sarcoma.
Saunders, Cicely, 228-229
Schapira, David, 111
Screening, 85-86
  for bladder cancer, 114
  for breast cancer, 125-126
  for cervical cancer, 141
  for malignant melanoma, 153
  for penile cancer, 162
  for prostate cancer, 171-173
  for rectal cancer, 189-190
  for soft tissue sarcoma, 204
  for vaginal cancer, 212
  for vulvar cancer, 219
Second-look surgery, 93
Serosa, rectal cancer and, 189
Sigmoid colon, 187
Sigmoidoscopic examination, 189-190, 213
Simpson, Sir James, 14
Skin, physiology of, 152
Skin cancer. *See* Malignant melanoma.
Skin irritation, radiation therapy and, 97

Skinny needle biopsy, 90
  for breast cancer, 127
Slow-growing cancers, 48
Smoking, bladder cancer and, 112
Society of Gynecologic Oncology, 142
Soft tissue sarcoma, 32, 84
  analysis of, 207-208
  chemotherapy for, 207
  causes of, 202
  diagnosis of, 204-205
  follow-up for, 210
  grades of, 203-204
  incidence of, 202
  penile cancer and, 162
  radiation therapy for, 207
  recurrence of, 208, 209-210
  screening for, 204
  signs and symptoms of, 204
  spread of, 204
  stages of, 205, 206
  surgery for, 205-206
  treatment according to stage, 208-210
  treatments for, 205-207
  types of, 203
Solid tumor, definition of, 3
Southern Medical Journal, xiv
Spitalier, J. M., 30
Squamous cells, 113, 140, 161
Stages of disease, 87-88, 89
  of bladder cancer, 115, 116, 117
  of breast cancer, 128, 129, 130
  of cervical cancer, 141-142, 143
  of malignant melanoma, 155, 156
  of penile cancer, 163, 164
  of prostate cancer, 173, 174, 175
  of rectal cancer, 190, 191, 192
  of soft tissue sarcoma, 205, 206
  of vaginal cancer, 213, 214
  of vulvar cancer, 220, 221
Staging procedures, 92
  for cervical cancer, 142, 145-146
Stamey, T. A., 171, 178, 183
"Standards for Breast Conservation Treatment," 230
Stereotaxic breast biopsy, 128
Steroid hormones, function of, 106

Stehlin, John Jr., xiii, 26
Structure of Scientific Revolutions, The (Kuhn), 235
Subcutaneous tissue, 152
Submucosa, rectal cancer and, 189
Sucralfate, radiation therapy and, 146
Suprapubic prostatectomy, 176
Suramin, 179
Surgery
    for bladder cancer, 115–118
    for breast cancer, 129–131
    breast-sparing, xiii, 24–27, 30–31, 130–131
    for cervical cancer, 142–146
    complications of, 94–95
    conservative, 1, 3, 72–73
    limb-sparing, 206, 207
    for malignant melanoma, 155–156
    for penile cancer, 163
    for prostate cancer, 174–181
    radical, vii, 15–16, 18–19, 22–24
    for rectal cancer, 193–195
    for soft tissue sarcoma, 205–206
    types of, 89–95
    for vaginal cancer, 213–214
    for vulvar cancer, 220–222
Synovial sarcoma, 203

T helper cells, 64
Tamoxifen, 107, 125, 132, 133
Tandem, 146
Taxol, 99
Telomerase, 47
Telomeres, 47
Testing, for cancer. *See* Screening.
Testosterone, 105, 106, 179–180
The Way It Was (Crile), 33
Therapeutic lymph node dissection, 163
Thomas, Lewis, 57–58
Thrasher, J., 121
Thymine, 43, 44, 45
Thyroid hormone, function of, 105–106
TNM staging system, 88, 89
    for bladder cancer, 115, 116
    for breast cancer, 128, 129
    for prostate cancer, 173, 175
    for rectal cancer, 190, 191
Total hysterectomy, 144
Trachelectomy, 144
Traditional staging system, 128–129, 130
Transcription, ribonucleic acid and, 44
Transition zone, 145
Transitional epithelial cells, 113
Transrectal ultrasound (TRUS), 171
Transurethral resection (TUR), 118, 120
Transurethral resection of the prostate (TURP), 173, 177
Treatment
    biological therapy, 107–109
    chemotherapy, 98–105
    considerations for, 238
    hormonal therapy, 105–107
    local, 89
    radiation therapy, 95–98
    questions about, 238–242
    surgical, 89–95
    systemic, 89
    See also individual types of cancer.
Treatment, according to stage
    for bladder cancer, 121–122
    for breast cancer, 135–138
    for cervical cancer, 148–150
    for malignant melanoma, 159–160
    for penile cancer, 165–167
    for prostate cancer, 184–186
    for rectal cancer, 197–200
    for soft tissue sarcoma, 208–210
    for vaginal cancer, 215–216
    for vulvar cancer, 224–226
Trigone, 113
Trinchieri, Giorgio, 65
TRUS. *See* Transrectal ultrasound.
Tryptophan, 45
Tumor
    definition of, 2–3
    excision, 130
    See also Cancer.
Tumor angiogenesis factor, 51
Tumor necrosis factor, 66, 109

Tumor-associated antigens, 60–61
Tumor-patient conflict, xv–xvi, 8–10, 75–76, 78–79
TUR. *See* Transurethral resection.
TURP. *See* Transurethral resection of the prostate.

Ulcerative colitis, rectal cancer and, 190
Ultrasound examination, 190
Uracil, 44, 45
Urban, Jerome, 23
Urban, Nicole, 111
Ureters, 113
Urethra, 113
Urinary frequency, radiation therapy and, 97

Vagina, physiology of, 211
Vaginal cancer
  analysis of, 215
  causes of, 211
  diagnosis of, 213
  follow-up for, 216–217
  grades of, 212
  incidence of, 211
  radiation therapy for, 214–215
  recurrence of, 215
  screening for, 212
  signs and symptoms of, 212
  spread of, 212
  stages of, 213, 214
  surgery for, 213–214
  treatment according to stage, 215–216
  treatments for, 213–215
  types of, 212
Vaginal intraepithelial neoplasia (VAIN), 212
Vaginectomy, 213
VAIN. *See* Vaginal intraepithelial neoplasia.
Veronesi, Umberto, 27
VIN. *See* Vulvar intraepithelial neoplasm.
Vinblastine, 119, 179
Vincristine, 98
Virchow, Rudolf, 14–15, 55

Viruses, antigen production and, 61
Vomiting
  chemotherapy and, 105
  radiation therapy and, 97
Vulva, physiology of, 218
Vulvar cancer
  analysis of, 223–224
  causes of, 218
  diagnosis of, 220
  follow-up for, 226
  grades of, 219
  hyperthermia for, 222
  incidence of, 218
  radiation therapy for, 222
  recurrence of, 223
  screening for, 219
  signs and symptoms of, 220
  spread of, 219
  stages of, 220, 221
  surgery for, 220–222
  treatment according to stage, 224–226
  treatments for, 220–223
  types of, 219
Vulvar intraepithelial neoplasm (VIN), 219
Vulvectomy, 220–222

Watchful waiting, 181
  age and, 182
  follow-up during, 183–184
  tumor reduction before, 182–183
Weight gain, progestins and, 107
Wertheim, Ernst, 18
White blood cells, cancer and, 62–63
Wide excision, 91, 130–131
Williams, I. G., 21

X-ray
  cancer detection and, 85–86
  soft tissue sarcoma and, 204
  vaginal cancer and, 213

Young, Hugh, 18, 177

Zoladex, 180

The Last Word

DR. PETER DE IPOLYI INTRODUCES DR. JOHN STEHLIN

For the past twenty-seven years, my great teacher, Dr. John Stehlin has been my partner in the practice of Oncology Surgery. It is a pleasure to introduce this remarkable man and to put this book into perspective.

In 1957, Dr. Stehlin began practicing at a large cancer hospital, in charge of the Melanoma and Sarcoma Service. At that time, the main thrust of cancer treatment was surgery, because the other forms of therapy, such as chemotherapy or radiation therapy were more primitive. In addition, American cancer treatment was still heavily influenced by Dr. William Halsted, the first Surgery Department Chairman at Johns Hopkins Medical School in Baltimore. Dr. Halsted is now considered the Father of American Surgery. His overwhelming influence is discussed by Dr. Evans in this book.

Early in his career, Dr. Stehlin recognized the serious shortcomings of the standard approaches of cancer treatment. It was clear to him that larger and more mutilating operations were not producing more cures. He became convinced that the only road to better results would lead to the combination of surgery with chemotherapy and radiation. This began the approach now called the multidisciplinary treatment of cancer. This led to the concept of formulating treatment plans among different specialists, combining everyone's opinion from the very start.

The other serious deficit Dr. Stehlin observed was the tendency to focus only on the disease, not on the person who has the disease. During his entire career, Dr. Stehlin has studied the psychological effects of cancer, and has promoted the concept of treating those effects, bringing the psychotherapists and religious counselors into the patient care team.

Another important concept which Dr. Stehlin formulated is what we call our tri-partnership. We believe the best results for the patient will come from the three of us, the patient, the clinical doctor, and the research scientist working hand in hand to produce better opportunities for cure. To accomplish this, he established a research laboratory dedicated to projects directly involved in patient treatment.

In 1970, Dr. Stehlin made a bold and severely criticized step by recommending breast-sparing surgery as the preferred operation for breast cancer. Loud, vitriolic criticism followed for someone who dared to challenge the most sacred tenet of American surgeons. To the benefit of many thousands of women, he held fast, and breast-sparing surgery is today the standard operation for the most prevalent life-threatening cancer in women in this country. We have worked to expand the role of less radical surgery in other areas such as melanoma, sarcoma, rectal cancer and others. I know of no other source which presents this information as clearly as does Dr. Evans in this book.

There has been great change in the treatment of cancer in the past fifty years. Much of the credit belongs to Dr. Stehlin. He pioneered a movement to save patients from the devastating effects of unnecessarily aggressive surgery. He operated on individuals, not cases. He counseled families, not just patients. He addressed the psychological, as well as the physical pain of every illness. Dr. Stehlin has affected the lives of thousands of men and women with cancer, and in the process has left an indelible mark on the art and science of cancer surgery.

Peter de Ipolyi, M.D.
Houston, Texas
March, 2001

DR. STEHLIN HAS THE LAST WORD

In 1957, I began the practice of cancer surgery at a large cancer hospital. My dream was to see every person in the hospital working to heal and support the patient. I wanted to include physicians of all specialties as equal partners in our treatment. This was a paradigm shift in the treatment of cancer patients, and it proved to be very difficult to harness the activities of so many people in a large, bureaucratic institution. Running beneath the surface were the currents of excess ego and professional jealousy. For this reason I entered the private practice of Surgical Oncology, where I could draw together individuals who wanted to unite forces in a concerted attack on our mutual adversary – cancer.

I helped to foster a second paradigm shift that has also been very rewarding. I call it the tri-partnership of cancer treatment. Tripartnership means that the patient, the treating physician, and the research scientist make up a triangle of mutual endeavor to overcome the disease. I believe this has given us the best progress.

In order for this concept to work, it requires one to embrace one of my core beliefs, an acceptance of the inherent sacredness of the human being. One must embrace as I have, our responsibility to be truthful, to always provide hope, and to respect the autonomy of the patient. This means that we must accept the patient as a partner, not an object in treatment.

This brings me to the question of this book. It is heartening to know that I have taught those who follow me in this most challenging of surgical specialities. One of my former pupils, Dr. Richard Evans, has taken up my challenge to do more for others. He has expanded on my belief in conservative surgery for breast cancer. He has demonstrated its validity for other cancers, as well. He has also suggested a rational explanation for the success of conservative surgery - a explanation that is based upon one of our most important weapons - the immune system. Dick shared his ideas with me over 20 years ago. I believed in them then, and I believe in them today.

Dick believes as I do that knowledge is power. He has written a book which I believe will empower patients by giving them knowledge. He believes as I do that any doctor worth his salt welcomes the informed patient, because it is always easier to treat people with life threatening diseases together, not as some godly being manipulating mere mortals. As I said, it is gratifying to see a book such as this which has as its primary purpose better, and less mutilating cancer surgery.

John S. Stehlin, Jr.
Houston, Texas
March, 2001

You'll Want Your Friends and Loved Ones to be Prepared
The Gift That May Change a Life

Visit your local bookstore or order here

❑ YES, please send me ____ copies of *The Cancer Breakthrough You've Never Heard of* at $16.95 each, plus $4 shipping and handling per book. Foreign orders must be accompanied by a postal money order in U.S. dollars. Please allow time for delivery. Domestic - 2 weeks, North America - 4 weeks, Overseas - 6 weeks.

A check or money order to the Texas Cancer Center for $ _____ is enclosed.

Please charge my   ❑ Visa   ❑ Master Card   ❑ AmEx

Name_____
Organization_____
Street Address_____
City/State/Zip_____
Phone_____ E-mail _____
Credit Card # _____ Exp. Date _____
Signature _____

Please mail your check to:

Texas Cancer Center
1011 Augusta Dr., Suite 210
Houston, Texas 77057

Or you may contact us with your credit card order:
713-975-6270
FAX: 713-977-2716
raevans@iapc.net   www.texascancercenter.com

Consultation Services Are Also Available

About the Author

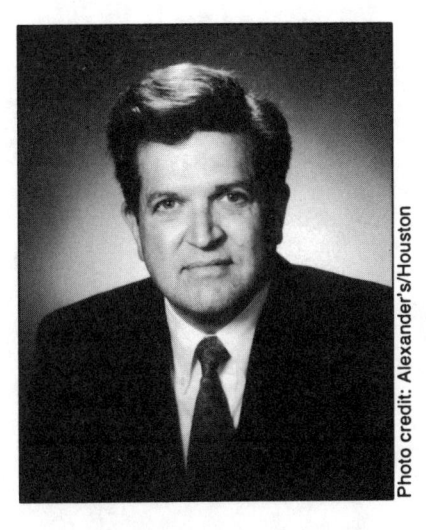

Richard Evans, MD, received his Bachelor of Arts degree from Rice University in Houston, and his Doctor of Medicine and Master of Science degrees from Tulane Medical School in New Orleans. He pursued postgraduate studies at the University of California—San Francisco and the Stanford University School of Medicine. Dr. Evans then returned to Houston for training in general surgery at St. Joseph's Hospital, where he also received a fellowship in surgical oncology working under conservative cancer surgery pioneer Dr. John Stehlin, and at M.D. Anderson Hospital. His articles and letters supporting the use of conservative cancer surgery have been published in numerous medical and surgical journals. Certified by the American Board of Surgery, Dr. Evans has practiced medicine in Houston since 1978.

Suggested Readings

Many excellent laymen's books are available on the subject of cancer treatment. I suggest you study one or two of them. I have tried not to rewrite and repeat information that is already easily available. I focus on information that supports a change toward more conservative treatment, information not always included in the books listed here.

Dr. Susan Love's Breast Book by Susan M. Love, M.D. and Karen Lindsey in one of the most comprehensive books about the breast for the lay reader. *Everyone's Guide to Cancer Therapy* by Malin Dollinger, M.D., Ernest H. Rosenbaum, M.D., and Greg Cable is also lengthy, with a well-illustrated treatment section. *Choices, Realistic Alternatives in Cancer Treatment* by Marion Mora and Eve Potts is in a question-and-answer format. It has over 900 pages of easy to understand charts, illustrations, and text. From these books you can learn in detail about different types of cancer, routes of tumor spread, risk factors, screening methods, sign and symptoms, diagnostic techniques, staging, and what to expect at each phase of treatment. They also provide reliable information about the diagnosis of cancer, the importance of good nutrition, how to care for yourself before and after surgery, and the emotional impact of cancer. But these books all tend to recommend more traditional forms of treatment.